Step-by-Step Massage Therapy Protocols for Common Conditions

Charlotte Michael Versagi, LMT, NCTMB

Author, Consultant, Instructor
Sun City West, Arizona

With contributions from:
Rita D. Woods, BS, LMT, NCTMB
Darien Lourde, Inc.
Dahlonega, Georgia

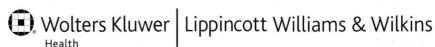
Wolters Kluwer | Lippincott Williams & Wilkins
Health

Philadelphia • Baltimore • New York • London
Buenos Aires • Hong Kong • Sydney • Tokyo

Acquisitions Editor: Kelley Squazzo
Product Manager: Linda G. Francis
Development Editor: Betsy Dilernia
Marketing Manager: Shauna Kelley
Design Coordinator: Teresa Mallon
Production Service: Absolute Service, Inc./Maryland Composition

Printed in China

Library of Congress Cataloging-in-Publication Data

Versagi, Charlotte Michael.
  Step-by-step massage therapy protocols for common conditions / Charlotte Michael Versagi ; with contributions from Rita D. Woods.
      p. ; cm.
  Includes bibliographical references and index.
  ISBN 978-0-7817-8715-4
  1. Massage therapy. 2. Chronic pain—Alternative treatment. I. Woods, Rita D. II. Title.
  [DNLM: 1. Massage—methods. WB 537]
  RM722.V37 2012
  615.8'22—dc23
                                                                                2011013473

Care has been taken to confirm the accuracy of the information presented and to describe generally accepted practices. However, the authors, editors, and publisher are not responsible for errors or omissions or for any consequences from application of the information in this book and make no warranty, expressed or implied, with respect to the currency, completeness, or accuracy of the contents of the publication. Application of the information in a particular situation remains the professional responsibility of the practitioner.

The authors, editors, and publisher have exerted every effort to ensure that drug selection and dosage set forth in this text are in accordance with current recommendations and practice at the time of publication. However, in view of ongoing research, changes in government regulations, and the constant flow of information relating to drug therapy and drug reactions, the reader is urged to check the package insert for each drug for any change in indications and dosage and for added warnings and precautions. This is particularly important when the recommended agent is a new or infrequently employed drug.

Some drugs and medical devices presented in the publication have Food and Drug Administration (FDA) clearance for limited use in restricted research settings. It is the responsibility of the health care provider to ascertain the FDA status of each drug or device planned for use in their clinical practice.

To purchase additional copies of this book, call our customer service department at (800) 638-3030 or fax orders to (301) 223-2320. International customers should call (301) 223-2300.

Visit Lippincott Williams & Wilkins on the Internet: at LWW.com. Lippincott Williams & Wilkins customer service representatives are available from 8:30 am to 6 pm, EST.

10 9 8 7 6 5 4 3 2 1

CCS0711

Charlotte Michael Versagi began her career in massage therapy in 1998. Before that, she attended nursing school, pretended to be a theater major, and worked for the Vatican Library in Rome. Since focusing on massage therapy, she has specialized in manual lymphatic drainage and complete decongestive physiotherapy as well as the clinical aspects of massage. In that journey, she has become the educational director of a 100-hour oncology massage program at Beaumont Hospitals in Royal Oak, Michigan, and a research associate at the same institution. She has also been on the faculty of a 1,000-hour clinical massage therapy program serving as massage, anatomy, and pathophysiology instructor. Having moved from hospitals to the massage franchise arena, she is currently the general manager at a Massage Envy franchise in Arizona, serves as the education coordinator for continuing education courses for all Massage Envy Arizona therapists, and recently won the Therapist of the Year Award for the Surprise, Arizona franchise. She has served as the past president, membership chair, and therapist of the year for American Massage Therapy Association (AMTA) in Michigan. She now dedicates most of her time to traveling and teaching oncology, lymphatic, and medical massage across the country.

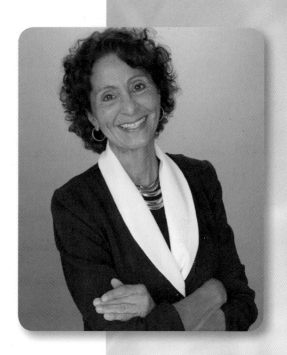

Whether they are advanced students or seasoned practitioners, many massage therapists feel uncertain when faced with a medical condition they have never encountered before. *Step-by-Step Massage Therapy Protocols for Common Conditions* is intended to give massage therapists the knowledge and the confidence to think critically, assess wisely, and treat clients with the techniques already practiced in massage school, while steering them away from doing harm. Courses using this book as a text will be helping prepare their students to play a key role as part of a health care team in relieving pain and helping clients deal effectively with medical conditions.

Massage therapists, by definition, are compassionate. We also enter the professional world with varying levels of education. Unfortunately, sometimes we are told that the basic skills we learn in massage school combined with our limited years of education are not enough to "make a difference" in the realm of pain. The intent of this book is to convince you that nothing is further from the truth.

THE CONDITIONS

This book will teach how to treat approximately 40 of the most common conditions massage therapists see in their practices. The conditions were chosen from two sources: I looked at my client files after a decade of running a private practice and a massage therapy clinic and combined those files with my work in hospitals as a clinical massage therapist, noting the frequency with which people sought out massage therapy for these conditions. Then, a panel of experts and colleagues reviewed the list and agreed that these are the conditions most massage therapists are likely to encounter in a well-rounded practice. Notably absent is any discussion of cancer. This is because cancer does not fit in any "step-by-step" format, because its manifestations in the body vary so widely, as do treatments and responses to them.

The conditions covered in this book are not exotic or especially complicated, and neither are the techniques used to treat them. The basic techniques learned in massage therapy school will serve the reader well in using this book. Armed with basic skills and the step-by-step protocols offered in this book, the massage therapist will be able to confidently and intelligently begin working on clients with these conditions almost immediately.

FOUNDATIONAL CHAPTERS

Chapters 1 through 5 contain foundational knowledge that is essential for the intelligent application of the treatment protocols found in the second half of the book. Chapter 1 defines the differences between relaxation, clinical, and medical massage while distinguishing the use of the words "client" versus "patient." This chapter also explains how to work as a member of a health care team, use a treatment protocol, and work with client charts.

Chapter 2 takes an in-depth look at how the body responds to the common massage modalities learned in massage school. This chapter contains clear illustrations as well as the physiologic effects of effleurage, petrissage, kneading, tapotement, stroking, jostling/vibration, rocking, deep and resisted breathing, cross-fiber friction, use of heat and cold, muscle stripping, compression, and passive/active range of motion (ROM).

Chapter 3 explains what happens, physiologically, when the body is in pain. The essential pain-spasm-pain cycle is explained; once this is investigated and paralleled with a client's condition, this information can be helpful in breaking most pain cycles. This chapter also includes a review of trigger points, the gate control theory of pain, and the universal 0–10 pain scale; additionally, one way to "sneak up" on pain in the body is described. The all-important psychological and social issues surrounding pain are also discussed.

Chapter 4 is dedicated to medications. Most clients will be taking medications and intelligent massage therapy work that includes knowledge of the effects of those medications, with some red flags that must be considered occasionally. This chapter is not a *Physician's Desk Reference*, nor is it intended to rival any of the fine texts already published on medications and massage.

Whether or not the massage therapist and the client reach their agreed-upon goals is as dependent upon what the client does at home as what the therapist does during treatment. Chapter 5 helps the massage therapist determine client self-care that is easy and aimed at a high rate of compliance. The basic "homework" techniques of stretching, strengthening, ROM exercises, water intake, and use of Epsom salts will be explained. This chapter will also explain how and when to refer a client to other health care professionals.

PROTOCOL CHAPTERS

Part II offers the student or practitioner very specific, step-by-step protocols for relieving pain in clients with such conditions as ankylosing spondylosis, multiple sclerosis, cerebral palsy, constipation, fibromyalgia, Bell's palsy, carpal tunnel syndrome, and many more conditions commonly encountered in a massage practice. In addition to giving you background information on the condition and the kinds of treatment a client may already be undergoing, the protocols provide a beginning, middle, and ending point for massage therapy. They suggest exact timeframes to spend on each technique and specific client homework assignments.

Each chapter will feature the following information and instructions for the clinical massage treatment of that specific pathophysiology/condition:

- General Information
- Pathophysiology
- Overall Signs and Symptoms
- Signs and Symptoms Massage Therapy Can Address
- Treatment Options
- Massage Therapist Assessment
- Thinking It Through
- Therapeutic Goals
- Massage Session Frequency
- Massage Protocol
- Contraindications and Cautions
- Massage Therapist Tips
- Homework
- Review
- Bibliography

ADDITIONAL RESOURCES

Step-by-Step Massage Therapy Protocols for Common Conditions includes additional resources for instructors, students, and practitioners. These are available at the book's companion website at http://thePoint.lww.com/Versagi and include the following:

- Access to the searchable eBook for this text
- Sample SOAP notes and Homework sheet
- A dermatome map

A NOTE ABOUT THE PROTOCOLS

This book is not intended to mire the massage therapist, whether a student who is just starting out or a practitioner with years of experience, in a formulaic trap of "This is how you must treat this condition and everything else is incorrect." One of the blessings of being a massage therapist is bringing one's own various modalities, special knowledge, and unique spirit to the treatment table.

However, if you really wanted to make a soufflé and had only a basic idea of how to use eggs, the oven, and your pan, you'd need some very specific instructions the first time you made your creation. Just so, this text teaches students and practitioners exactly what needs to be done to care for the client with Bell's palsy, for example. Just as you start creating your own recipes after you've made your first couple of soufflés, so you'll be able to adjust the massage protocols in the text for each unique massage situation, or design protocols of your own after you've worked with the ones in this text. Teachers of massage can use the protocols as a framework for helping students develop critical thinking skills for working with clients in a variety of clinical situations.

If I accomplish anything in this book, it's to free massage therapists from the worry and panic we all feel when caring for human beings in pain. Freed from the worry of "not knowing exactly what to do," I hope the content of this text allows you to bring the best of your education and your great spirit to the table so you can be joyful on this journey of helping to heal lives.

Feedback is always welcome, and your constructive comments will be considered for future editions of this text.

Charlotte Michael Versagi, LMT, NCTMB
Sun City West, Arizona

- Rita Diane Woods, who walked across a campus and into my life and has now helped me bring this project to fruition
- Anne Marie Drew for caring about words (albeit Shakespearean) as much as I do
- Frank Paul Versagi, Debbie Martin, and Muriel Versagi for being there
- Jane Brown and Linda Ingraham of Carnegie Institute for allowing me to teach
- Gail Elliott Evo and Karen Armstrong of the Integrative Medicine Department at Beaumont Hospitals in Michigan for supporting and continuing a great oncology massage program
- Tammy Evans of Massage Envy in Surprise, Arizona for introducing me to a whole different way of managing human beings
- Steve Cook and especially Carol Thomas of Massage Envy Arizona for allowing me to create a wonderful educational opportunity for therapists in Arizona
- Jill and Eddie Lopez, awesome Massage Envy owners, for granting me the honor of working with them
- Gayle MacDonald, Tracy Walton, and Ruth Werner for serving as ongoing inspiration
- Allan May for being my best friend and constant support
- From LWW: former acquisition editors Pete Darcy and John Goucher for seeing the value in this project; acquisition editor Kelley Squazzo for carrying it forward; product manager Linda Francis for her inestimable help from beginning to end, and her unending patience and humor with unerring guidance; Betsy Dilernia for her tireless attention to the big-picture plan and the details that make it happen; and Shauna Kelley for spreading the word now that the book is completed
- All the patients and clients who allowed me into the room to work on their precious bodies to learn everything I had to learn to create this book
- And, finally, Michael, Rafael, and Cara Mia

DEDICATION

To my father, Frank James Versagi, who taught the four of us the power of words and the importance of logical thinking—and that the two should really somehow be related.

Reviewers

- Patricia Berak, MBA, BHSA, NCBTMB
  Baker College of Clinton Township
  Center Line, MI

- Julie Finn, NCTMB
  JB Therapeutic & Sports Massage
  Walled Lake, MI

- Tiffany Hemrick, LMBT
  Davidson County Community College
  Lexington, NC

- Jeffrey Lutz, CMTPT
  The Pain Treatment & Wellness Center
  Greensburg, PA

- Celina McKenzie, NCTMB
  Minnesota School of Business
  Elk River, MN

PART I GROUNDWORK: FUNDAMENTAL KNOWLEDGE FOR INTELLIGENT HANDS 1

Chapter 1	Defining and Practicing Clinical Massage	2
Chapter 2	Physiologic Effects of Basic Massage Strokes and Techniques	10
Chapter 3	The Physiology of Muscular Activity and Pain	22
Chapter 4	Medications for Common Medical Conditions	31
Chapter 5	Beyond the Table: Client Homework and Referring Out	45

PART II STEP-BY-STEP MASSAGE THERAPY PROTOCOLS 55

Chapter 6	Ankylosing Spondylosis	56
Chapter 7	Bell's Palsy	63
Chapter 8	Bursitis	71
Chapter 9	Carpal Tunnel Syndrome	78
Chapter 10	Cerebral Palsy	85
Chapter 11	Chronic Fatigue Syndrome	94
Chapter 12	Constipation	101
Chapter 13	Degenerative Disc Disease	110
Chapter 14	Delayed Onset Muscle Soreness	118
Chapter 15	Fibromyalgia	124
Chapter 16	Frozen Shoulder	131
Chapter 17	Headache—Migraine	137
Chapter 18	Headache—Tension	143
Chapter 19	Human Immunodeficiency Virus and Acquired Immunodeficiency Syndrome	150
Chapter 20	Hyperkyphosis	158
Chapter 21	Iliotibial Band Syndrome	167
Chapter 22	Insomnia	176
Chapter 23	Multiple Sclerosis	182

Contents

Chapter 24	Muscle Spasm	190
Chapter 25	Neuropathy: Diabetic Peripheral Neuropathy and Chemotherapy-Induced Peripheral Neuropathy	196
Chapter 26	Osteoarthritis	203
Chapter 27	Parkinson's Disease	210
Chapter 28	Piriformis Syndrome	218
Chapter 29	Plantar Fasciitis	226
Chapter 30	Post-Polio Syndrome	235
Chapter 31	Post-traumatic Stress Disorder	241
Chapter 32	Raynaud's Phenomenon	247
Chapter 33	Rheumatoid Arthritis	252
Chapter 34	Scars	259
Chapter 35	Sciatica	266
Chapter 36	Scoliosis	273
Chapter 37	Sprain and Strain	281
Chapter 38	Stress	288
Chapter 39	Stroke	294
Chapter 40	Temporomandibular Joint Dysfunction	303
Chapter 41	Tendinosis	311
Chapter 42	Thoracic Outlet Syndrome	316
Chapter 43	Trigger Points	324
Chapter 44	Whiplash	332

INDEX 338

Part I

Groundwork: Fundamental Knowledge for Intelligent Hands

Defining and Practicing Clinical Massage

RELAXATION VERSUS CLINICAL MASSAGE

The massage industry is fairly comfortable with the distinction between "relaxation" and "clinical" or "therapeutic" massage. *Relaxation massage* is the term generally used for clients who do not have major or even minor medical conditions; the whole-body session is usually performed in a non-medical environment, and the ultimate goal is relaxation.

Clinical or therapeutic massage attempts to address chronic pain, injury, and immobility. The focused—and sometimes very localized—work performed for such medical conditions as arthritis, plantar fasciitis, and Bell's palsy, for example, is more appropriately termed *clinical* rather than relaxation massage.

It is not a black-and-white issue. If the clinical therapist is skilled, careful, and even graceful, there is good reason for the therapeutic massage client to reach a state of profound relaxation, even though relaxation was not the primary focus of the session. In addition, often during a relaxation massage, the therapist will take a detour to address a condition she discovered in midstream.

This text is a reference for massage therapists working in any environment. One therapist may work in a spa applying mud packs and turning over clients every 65 minutes when a client asks her to address bilateral knee arthritis. Another may be in a hospital setting working with oncology patients when she is asked, "Can you just help me fall asleep?" The line between clinical and relaxation massage is becoming blurred and can no longer be defined by practice location alone. With the growth of "medical spas," and now even "hospital-based spas," combined with the preponderance of massage therapists working out of their homes, as well as others teaming up with physicians as part of a health care team, the physical setting has become secondary to the type of work performed by the trained therapist.

What about "medical massage"? Massage school owners, state massage regulators, national massage associations, and national authors have weighed in on trying to define this term. National experts in our field have written extensively on the struggle to define medical massage. This book will not address that argument. It focuses on treating chronic and medical conditions with the assumption that the work is being performed by well-trained massage therapists interested in stopping the cycle of pain.

MASSAGE THERAPY TRAINING

Massage school training is an important consideration in treating client conditions. In some locations, it is appropriate to train in a 100-hour massage therapy course, to then be called a "practitioner" and to perform relaxation massage in a spare room. This is not, however, the background assumed for the readers of this book.

In the U.S., the minimum educational standard set by most massage therapy schools is 500 hours of supervised educational work that is focused on anatomy, physiology, pathophysiology, ethics, basic massage techniques, and some advanced modalities. A solid argument could be made that 500 hours of supervised educational work only scratches the surface, and clinical work should not be attempted without ample training following this basic education. In fact, Canada requires a minimum of 1000–2000 hours for graduation from a massage therapy program.

If a student has been earnest in her training, has mastered the basic skills that will be reviewed in Chapter 2, and carefully studies the pathophysiology of a condition before attempting to treat, there is ample reason, supported by evidence-based practice, to believe that treatment will be effective and pain will diminish.

Scope of Practice

Every medical and allied health profession is regulated closely to ensure the safe care of patients and clients. Dentists are not allowed to perform appendectomies because the procedure is outside of their training and scope of practice. Massage therapists join these regulated ranks by performing carefully within the mind-set of a scope of professional limitations. Yet because state regulation and licensing vary so widely, as does the level of massage education, clearly defining the massage therapist's scope of practice can be challenging. Add to the quandary that many massage therapists are now practicing as part of a health care team in either a hospital or clinic, and the issue becomes muddied further. Another consideration is the addition of continuing education skills gained after massage school graduation; these skills often clearly place one therapist at a considerably different level of practice than another. And finally, many nurses are now moving over into massage therapy, as are physical therapists, psychotherapists, and even some physicians.

Taking all of these into consideration, the following can remind readers of their ethical and professional boundaries as they practice massage therapy. The massage therapist:

- Does not diagnose
- Assesses the client's soft tissue
- Determines appropriate modalities based on her level of massage therapy skills
- Does not combine professional skill sets (e.g., nurse and therapist, psychotherapist and massage therapist)
- Does not prescribe or suggest oral or topical medications or supplements
- Practices with a clear understanding of indications, cautions, and contraindications when treating conditions
- Refers to another health care professional or massage therapist when the client's needs exceed her competence or confidence level

Perhaps one final example can help the therapist determine her scope of practice. The use of rest, ice, compression, and elevation (RICE) immediately after a joint injury or blunt trauma permeates every basic first aid and parent-preparedness class. Most households have ice packs (or bags of peas) stashed in the freezer and compression bandages in the home first aid kit. However, seen from a massage therapists' standpoint, if a client were on the table with swelling from a recent ankle injury, the therapist:

- Can suggest rest
- Can apply an ice pack if she's been trained to do so in her massage therapy curriculum
- Cannot apply compression
- Would use caution in elevating an extremity and would consider the client's overall medical condition and history

The phrase *scope of practice* should not be perceived as an obstacle to safe, effective, and comforting care. It is simply a reasonable control for this growing profession as it carves its niche within the health care model.

CLIENT OR PATIENT?

Are those who receive massage therapy appropriately called "clients" or "patients"? The assumptions made in this text are as follows:

- *Client:* The massage therapist alone is treating a person who found the therapist through word of mouth, advertising, or any other non-medical referral. In this case, the therapist is not treating a condition or necessarily documenting progress but is providing mostly relaxation massage.
- *Patient:* The therapist is functioning as part of a health care team, or is treating a specific condition and documenting progress in a solo practice or health care setting. For example, the patient sees the massage therapist as a result of a verbal referral from an orthopedic surgeon and is simultaneously being seen by a physical therapist. In this case, the massage therapist, physical therapist, and physician are all communicating about the patient's care. Further, if any physician writes a prescription for massage therapy, or if the therapist is working in a hospital or chiropractic setting, the person receiving the care is a patient.

Within this text, the terms will be used interchangeably because some readers may be addressing the conditions in a solo practice and others may have an active physician–therapist relationship.

TREATMENT PROTOCOLS: DETERMINING THE RECIPE FOR CARE

The word "protocol" is used here as it is in medicine and science: a plan of care or formula for how to get from point A to point B. In the case of massage therapy, the protocol consists of the steps taken in a therapeutic massage session to treat the client. It requires therapeutic knowledge of three basic ingredients:

1. The pathophysiology of the condition to be treated
2. The appropriate choice of strokes and modalities, as well as duration and amount of pressure, for example
3. The physiologic effects of the massage therapy strokes and modalities to be used

Along with the step-by-step protocols found in Part II of this book, knowledge in these three areas will equip practicing therapists to confidently treat clients who have the most common medical conditions.

KNOWING THE STROKE AND HOW TO APPLY IT

Using effleurage on an agitated newborn is different from using effleurage on a pre-event marathon runner. Pressure, rhythm, and duration are important factors in the application of every massage technique. Yet, determining the appropriate pressure to use has been a consideration for every massage therapist since she began training. One person's idea of "deep work" varies from another's. But depth, as well as the perception of depth, matters greatly in the effectiveness of the therapeutic session.

Tracy Walton, LMT, MS; Langdon Roberts, MA, CMT; and the Touch Research Institute are responsible for much of our current knowledge about the efficacies of various pressures used in massage therapy. Walton developed a formal five-point pressure scale for her hospital research studies to ensure consistency among massage therapists and for the purpose of safe application of her patient protocols.

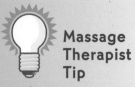

Massage Therapist Tip

"Recipes" as Starting Points

Providing a treatment plan "recipe" may seem simplistic, but it is a good way to start. You may have recently graduated from massage therapy school, or perhaps you graduated years ago and need to refresh your clinical massage thinking skills. In either case, massage therapy is a science *and* an art. You, as an individual therapist, bring unique skills to the table. The protocols included in this book are intended to outline a safe, effective, and clinically justifiable way to immediately start treating clients. But it is expected that you will add your own special skills, techniques, and intentions to these suggestions.

Langdon Roberts created NeuroMassage, a unique therapeutic system that combines biofeedback and bodywork to improve health by making intentional changes in the relationships among the brain, the nerves, the organs, and the muscles. At the 2004 American Massage Therapy Association (AMTA) National Convention, Roberts' poster presentation detailed the effects of massage pressure with the following abbreviated conclusions:

- Using deep pressure massage (without warming tissues first) *produces an increase in muscle tension.*
- Applying light and moderate pressure prior to deep pressure *prevents an increase in muscle tension.*
- When muscle tension was increased because of deep pressure, *light pressure produced muscle relaxation.*
- Using as much force as a client will accept without experiencing pain, *without adequate warm-up, is likely to produce a substantial increase in muscle tension* during and immediately following massage. Starting light may allow more access to deep muscle layers with less work for the therapist, as well as decreased risk and less discomfort for the client.

The Touch Research Institute's work on pressure indicates a profound difference between the effects of moderate pressure and the effects of light pressure. The distinction is made because of the stimulating effects of light pressure, as opposed to the positive physiologic changes from the application of moderate pressure. Suggested indicators for the amount of pressure to use for each condition are found in the step-by-step protocols.

WHEN MASSAGE THERAPY IS CONTRAINDICATED

Even with the best intention and the highest skills, massage therapists may, at times, treat inappropriately. A contraindication for massage therapy exists when massage is inappropriate or unsafe to perform because the therapist could cause harm to the client. Various terms are used, describing "local" or "regional" and "absolute," "total," or "systemic" contraindications. For example, a rash of unknown origin on the anterior forearm would be a local or regional contraindication, whereas a fever of unknown origin not being treated with antibiotics would be an absolute, total, or systemic contraindication.

It is worth noting, however, the difference between *modifying a massage session* while using an appropriate caution and a contraindication for the total massage. A client who is 9 months pregnant will be placed on her side, her proximal or medial thighs will not be massaged, and any tortuous varicosities will be avoided. This is modifying or taking certain precautions with the massage given the client's condition, but third-trimester (uncomplicated) pregnancy is not a contraindication for massage.

It's important for therapists to keep appropriate and responsible cautions in mind. However, it is not possible for even the most seasoned therapist to know every contraindication. In addition, a massage contraindication often depends on these factors:

- The condition
- The patient
- The treatment setting
- The skill level of the massage therapist

Although working on a client with a high fever in the midst of a bout of bacterial pneumonia would be absolutely contraindicated for a beginning massage therapist, if the client (1) had completed a 3-day course of antibiotics, (2) was being treated by a lymphatic massage specialist, and (3) was told what to expect as a result of the work, then the treatment would be appropriate and safe.

Absolute Contraindications for Massage Therapy

Given the shades of gray that exist in most client care, and the fact that the greater the therapist's knowledge, the more skills he may bring to the table, the following are commonly accepted absolute contraindications:

- Thrombus (stationary blood clot) located anywhere in the body
- Medical conditions requiring immediate medical attention
- Unstable vascular damage
- Gangrene, kidney disease, or advanced heart disease
- Post–heart attack or post-stroke patients who have not yet been medically stabilized
- Severe headache of unknown origin
- High blood pressure that is not controlled by medication
- Fever
- Aneurysm
- Intoxication
- Most viral infections
- Measles and other immediately contagious diseases

Local Contraindications for Massage Therapy

The following are commonly accepted local contraindications:

- Frostbite
- Local contagious skin condition
- Local skin irritation of unknown origin
- Open wound, sore, or ulcer
- Recent radiation or recent burn
- Undiagnosed lump
- Acute arthritic flare-up
- Fracture

Contraindications for massage therapy are a concern for more than massage therapists. In 2003, Mitchell Batavia, a physical therapist and PhD in pathokinesiology, performed an analysis of 10 years' worth of literature on contraindications for therapeutic massage. Batavia's work was exhaustive and thorough, and he found little of concrete value and no consensus:

- Of the sources, 24% did not list infection or neoplasm (cancer) as a contraindication.
- Of the sources, 28% failed to list open wounds.
- Of the sources, 33% did not mention bleeding, bruising, or anticoagulation disorders.
- Of the sources, 48% failed to mention any problems at any state of pregnancy or labor.

Massage therapists recognize that *not all massage is safe for all clients*, and that *there are conditions and patients that require no touching*. But as with most rules, this one is not carved in stone. Given sufficient skill level, expertise, and sometimes supervision, an advanced massage therapist can approach many medical conditions that would be beyond the scope of the beginning therapist.

ASSIGNING CLIENT HOMEWORK

Therapy sessions range from 30–120 minutes, yet many clients have been living with chronic conditions for weeks, months, or years. It is not feasible to diminish all pain and restore range of motion in the miniscule amount of time a therapist works in a single session or series of sessions. By the time the client climbs on the massage table, his muscles are so hypertonic, the condition is so entrenched down to the cells of his muscle, and his neuromuscular patterns are so embedded that table work can only scratch the surface of his pain. Inherent in the intelligent massage therapist's work is the appropriate suggestion of self-care assignments, or client "homework."

Self-care might include the application of heat, rolling the ankles while watching TV or reading, or taking deep breaths whenever the client arrives at a red light when driving. It is up to the therapist and the client to devise appropriate homework assignments that fit into the client's lifestyle and that will ultimately move him toward full functioning, independent of the massage therapist's work.

Offering client self-care instructions ties in subtly with scope of practice. The safe and therapeutic use of exercise bands or exercise balls is not usually included in a massage therapist's basic curriculum. A seemingly innocuous handout and verbal instruction on the use of a large medicine ball could result in serious damage if the client has an undiagnosed lumbar spine disc abnormality. Yet some homework assignments involve offering the client a copy of a reputable, relevant published article. Extensive continuing education training by the massage therapist is necessary for responsibly assigning many client self-care suggestions (see Chapter 5).

SUBJECTIVE, OBJECTIVE, ASSESSMENT, AND PLAN (SOAP) CHARTING AND DOCUMENTATION

The treatment of clinical conditions includes meticulous documentation of techniques used, as well as the client's response to those techniques. Massage therapists who choose to address medical conditions must keep some form of charting or documentation from session to session. In addition to the following listed reasons, a chart may be subpoenaed for evidence in a court of law, it may be requested by the patient's physician, and it may be used as evidence to prove progress by an insurance company for fee coverage. Appropriate, detailed charting is therefore important for the following reasons:

- Providing a record of techniques used
- Keeping a record of the client's responses to techniques used
- Helping the therapist remember a client's personal details (e.g., a sick child, an upcoming wedding)
- Reminding the therapist of the client's self-care homework assignments
- Providing a record of progression or digression and the level of pain
- Proving efficacy when insurance companies ask for therapeutic results
- Serving as a record of care when the physician asks for massage treatment details and effects
- Providing a historical record if the client discontinues care and returns in the future

Massage therapy charting is based on the common SOAP nursing protocol of documentation, with the acronym representing subjective, objective, assessment, and plan. These four components are briefly reviewed subsequently, and examples of SOAP notes can be found online at http://thePoint.lww.com/Versagi.

The actual paper chart can take any form. Specially tailored medical charts are available to purchase online, or a very simple one-sheet SOAP chart with the letters S, O, A, and P spaced out evenly down the left margin can be created. The point is for the massage therapist to document her work in an acceptable format that will serve many purposes.

Subjective

A subjective statement is one that reflects the client's or patient's point of view; it does not have to be factual or provable. Here are examples of subjective notes:

- "I have a headache today."
- Client states lower backaches.

- "My doctor said I have fibromyalgia."
- Patient states she has been nauseous for several days and thinks she may be pregnant.

None of these statements is provable; all are opinions. There are two options for charting subjective notes: (1) quoting directly from the patient's words, which requires the use of quotation marks; and (2) paraphrasing what the client said, which simply requires "client states" or "patient states" in front of the note.

Objective

Objective notes reflect what the massage therapist observed and palpated, as well as the techniques she used. Here are typical examples of objective notes:

- Client's left superior trapezius hypertonic. Therapist performed effleurage, petrissage, digital kneading, and more effleurage to the area.
- Patient has an unusual quarter-sized mole below the right scapula that has reddened edges; therapist did not massage directly over the area.
- Client's musculature at the occipital ridge very hypertonic; deep digital massage along mastoid processes and up into the head and scalp.
- Patient appeared agitated, did not stop talking throughout the session, and jumped several times when therapist approached the body.

Therapists must be careful to describe observations in detail and to assess what must be done without crossing the line into diagnosing, which is clearly outside the therapist's scope of practice.

Assessment

Although massage schools differ in their teaching philosophies about the documentation of assessment, with confusion arising when the student believes she is to assess *the condition*, the standard medical practice of *assessing the results of the treatment* is the standard used in this text. The documentation here reflects the results of the various techniques that have been applied. What happened to the muscles? What response did she have? What did the client say? Continuing with the previous examples:

- Client's left superior trapezius became less hypertonic; client stated she could move more easily and is in less pain.
- Patient's response was one of concern for the unusual mole found by therapist.
- Client stated, "That head massage was the best part of the whole thing." Stated headache lessened somewhat.
- As a result of patient agitation, therapist lowered lights, played music more softly, and sat by the table until patient's agitation passed. Asked permission to continue.

Plan

The plan includes the next steps for both the therapist and the client or patient. What will be asked of the client or patient as a result of this session? Will there be homework? When is she coming back? Is the therapist suggesting the client see a physician? Using the previous examples to complete the chart:

- Therapist assigned doorway stretches to be performed three times daily; stretches demonstrated by therapist and performed by client successfully.
- Therapist strongly suggested patient call her dermatologist for a checkup. Therapist to ask whether appointment was made at next massage session.

- Therapist suggested a talk therapist for client's continual sources of stress.
- Patient said she doesn't enjoy massage as much as she thought she would and will not return.

IN SUMMARY

This book reminds the therapist of the fundamental knowledge she gained during her massage therapy education and will support her as she steps into the realm of attempting to relieve pain. As the therapist prepares her plan to treat common medical conditions, she uses her knowledge to:

- Understand the clear distinction between "relaxation" and "clinical" or "therapeutic" massage
- Apply her expertise based on her initial massage therapy training, her personal continuing education strengths, and her knowledge of cautions and contraindications
- Discriminate the use of her skills by practicing well within her scope of practice
- Prepare detailed documentation appropriate for a responsible member of a health care team
- Assign client homework based only on her level of expertise

With these parameters soundly in mind, the therapist can now move on to a deep understanding of the physiologic effects of what she is doing with her hands.

Review

1. Explain the difference between relaxation and therapeutic massage.
2. Explain the different physiologic effects of light and medium massage pressure.
3. List four absolute contraindications for massage therapy.
4. List four local contraindications for massage therapy.
5. Explain the acronym "SOAP" and describe the components of each.

BIBLIOGRAPHY

Andrade CK, Clifford P. *Outcome-Based Massage: From Evidence to Practice*, 2nd ed. Baltimore: Lippincott Williams & Wilkins, 2008.

Batavia M. Contraindications for therapeutic massage: do sources agree? *Journal of Bodywork and Movement Therapies* 2004;8:48–57.

Roberts L, NeuroMassage of Santa Cruz County: Holistic Neurotherapy for Children and Adults. Roberts' website. Available at: http://www.neuromassage.com/frame-main.html. Accessed November 26, 2005.

Roberts L. Poster presentation: To investigate the effects of applying different levels of massage pressure on muscular tension. Presented at the 2004 American Massage Therapy Association, National Convention, Nashville, TN.

Vanderbilt S. Moderate vs. light pressure in massage: new studies from Touch Research Institute. *Massage & Bodywork* 2005;April/May:134–136.

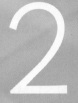

Physiologic Effects of Basic Massage Strokes and Techniques

THE IMPORTANCE OF MOVING BLOOD

Blood is so important that the massage therapist takes great effort to move it and to increase its presence in areas of hypertonicity (tightness). Without the movement of blood, there can be no therapy, no healing, no health—no life. Instead, pain, stagnation, disease, and accumulated waste products in tissues result. Stroking, for example, usually initiates profound parasympathetic (relaxing) effects on the body by aiding the release of hormones and other calming chemicals in the brain.

By increasing circulation, the massage therapist supports the following important physiologic processes:

- Cellular oxygenation
- Healing and proper functioning of cells, tissues, muscle, and bone
- Removing waste products
- Regulating body temperature
- Fighting disease
- Moving hormones to their target organs

By reviewing the physiologic effects of specific massage techniques, and truly understanding how they can profoundly affect the body, the therapist gains the knowledge for starting to treat specific conditions. This knowledge is, of course, combined with an understanding of the client's or patient's health or medical condition itself, which is covered in Part II of this book. We will describe the most commonly used massage strokes and techniques and outline their physiologic effects on the body. The goal for the massage therapist is to reflexively understand, "If technique A is performed on the body, then result B can be expected."

While technique is clearly important, massage is an art; different hands and intentions produce different results. The physiologic effects described in the succeeding text bring together science and art, with the understanding that varying levels of skill and focus produce different results.

STROKING

The movement that makes a cat purr, a dog's tail thump, and a baby sleep is an intuitive starting point to explain stroking. Stroking is the *unidirectional* (for our purposes), slow, not deep but not feathery, noninvasive, gliding, careful, usually slow drag of the full hand on the body (Figure 2-1).

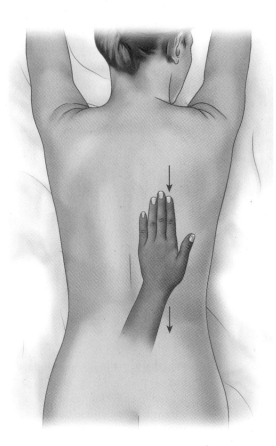

FIGURE 2-1 **Stroking. The client is lying prone while the therapist's slightly open, flattened hand strokes her back, applying only the weight of the hand itself.**

The specific physiologic effects of stroking include:

- Sedation
- Decreased pain perception
- Decreased anxiety and distress
- Decreased nausea and temporarily decreased spasticity if applied over the spine
- Rehabilitation of nerve afferent transmission
- Decreased sympathetic nervous system activity

Stroking alone has been used on premature infants to soothe them and to increase their weight gain and activity level, as well as to increase alertness and improve body tone. For people of all ages, the slow-stroke back massage is effective in decreasing blood pressure and reducing heart rate.

EFFLEURAGE

Effleurage can be thought of as "stroking with depth." The lighter and faster effleurage is performed, the more stimulating its effects; the deeper and slower the stroke, the more relaxing. It is often used as an introductory or parting stroke during a massage session. It is also used to apply lubricant, and as a transition technique either between strokes or when moving from one body part to another. The therapist uses the whole hand with fingers gently closed, conforming to the body, or uses the ulnar surface of the forearm. Long, flowing, moderate-to-deep pressure is delivered to a broad surface of the body (Figure 2-2).

The specific physiologic effects of effleurage include:

- Increased venous return
- Increased lymphatic drainage and decreased edema
- Strengthened immune function

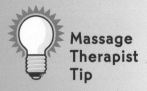

Massage Therapist Tip

Different Names for the Same Stroke

You may notice that strokes sometimes have different names, depending upon the textbook or article you're reading. "Lifting and rolling" may be the same stroke we call "skin rolling." "Myofascial spread" is another term for fist kneading. A stroke's name depends on the author, the country, and the therapist's educational background. The intent, however, is the same—to have an effect on the body with specific actions. No matter what the strokes are called, your job is to know when to use them based on their physiologic effects.

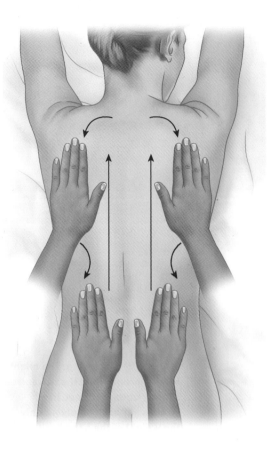

FIGURE 2-2 **Effleurage. Slightly deeper than stroking, effleurage is used to apply lubricant and as a transition technique between strokes.**

- Localized warming and tissue softening
- Enhanced hormone release
- Initial increased heart rate and blood pressure followed by decreases in both

PETRISSAGE

Petrissage "goes for the muscle." Leaving behind superficial or broad work, the therapist uses petrissage to firmly grasp either individual muscles or groups of muscle to affect underlying tissues. Relying on previous tissue warming (effleurage is always used prior to this technique), petrissage begins the serious business of mobilizing and softening tissue. This stroke is performed rhythmically as the therapist squeezes and releases muscle tissue. Maintaining full hand contact, she grasps the muscle belly firmly with the palm of the hand, forcing the tissue up into the slightly arched fingers. Tissues are pumped with the one-hand or two-hand cephalic (toward the head) movement as the muscle is gripped, squeezed, and then released.

Various forms of petrissage include the following:

- *Knuckle kneading:* The knuckles are used to deeply move the tissue.
- *Digital kneading:* The fingers are used to deeply move the tissue.
- *Fist kneading:* The entire balled fist is used to deeply move the tissue.
- *Wringing:* The tissue (normally part of an extremity) is grasped as if wringing out a large sponge, and pressure with two hands is applied in opposite directions.
- *Skin rolling:* The skin is plucked up off the underlying muscle and rolled along to move the superficial fascia from deep fascia (Figure 2-3).

The desired results of petrissage include deep, lasting, warming effects on blood and muscle. The intelligent use of these techniques forms the basis of therapeutic massage.

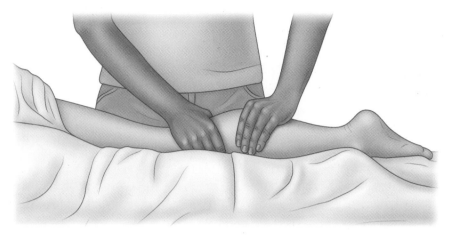

FIGURE 2-3 **Petrissage. The therapist firmly grasps the client's calf muscle with the full palm of her hand. She makes deep contact while lifting the muscle away from the bone.**

The specific physiologic effects of petrissage include:

- Movement of cellular waste products
- Decreased muscle tension
- Decreased muscle hypertonicity
- Pain relief
- Increased joint range of motion (ROM)
- Increased connective tissue extensibility and loosening
- Localized tissue warming

TAPOTEMENT

The techniques described thus far are intended to sedate, relax, or at least not stimulate the body. By moving into tapotement, the therapist recognizes the necessity of periodically stimulating the body for either a localized or a systemic effect.

Tapotement includes the following techniques:

- *Tapping:* Using alternating quick, loose wrists, the therapist taps the fingertips on the skin, snapping the fingertips back quickly to affect superficial tissue only (Figure 2-4). Tapping is most effective when used directly on the skin.
- *Pincement:* Using alternating loose wrists, the therapist plucks the skin between thumbs and fingertips wherever ample skin allows for lifting (Figure 2-5). The technique is superficial only and is applied directly to the skin.
- *Hacking:* Using alternating quick, loose ulnar sides of the hands, the therapist applies as much pressure as the client will allow (Figure 2-6). Hacking can be performed directly on the body or through sheets.
- *Cupping/clapping:* With semirigid, cupped hands but loose, alternating wrists, the therapist creates a little cup with each hand as it strikes the anterior, lateral, and posterior surfaces of the thoracic cavity (Figure 2-7). The technique is performed directly on the skin or through sheets, and the therapist is careful not to invade the breast tissue.
- *Pounding:* With soft but clenched fists and quick alternating wrists, the therapist pounds the body with the soft ulnar surface with gently closed hands (Figure 2-8). Pounding is performed directly on the skin or through sheets.

The specific physiologic effects of light tapotement include:

- Increased nervous system stimulation
- Increased muscle tone
- Rehabilitation of sensory nerve transmission

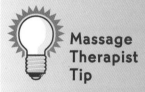

Massage Therapist Tip

Tapotement Intensity

When applying tapotement, always gently alert your client that you are about to begin this sometimes startling technique. Begin lightly as an introduction to the body, increase intensity as your stroke reaches its full, committed vigor, and then ease off before exiting the body with care.

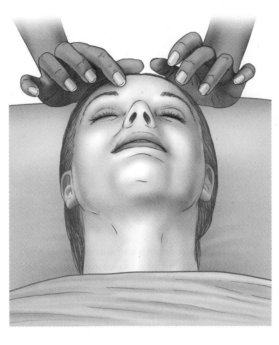

FIGURE 2-4 **Tapping. The therapist uses her fingertips to lightly tap the client's forehead.**

The specific physiologic effects of heavy tapotement include:

- Local numbing
- Increased local circulation
- Increased muscular blood flow
- Increased sympathetic nervous system activity
- Increased muscle tone temporarily, followed by muscle relaxation
- Loosening of mucus in the lungs
- Desensitization of a local area of skin

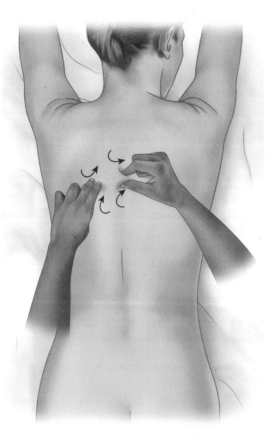

FIGURE 2-5 **Pincement. The therapist uses a twisting and plucking technique to move the superficial tissue.**

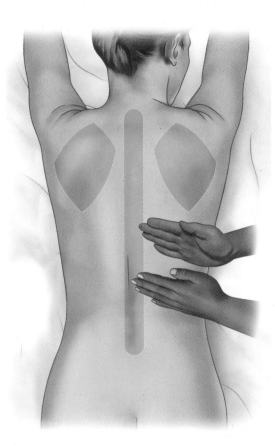

FIGURE 2-6 Hacking. Loose, flexible wrists allow the ulnar side of the therapist's hand to intermittently strike the client's back. Remember to stay away from bony prominences, as indicated by the shaded areas.

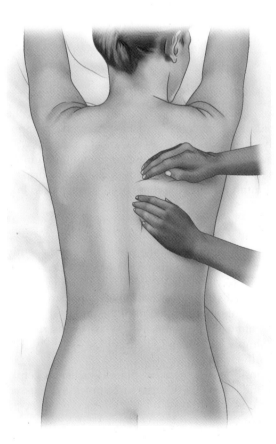

FIGURE 2-7 Cupping. Firmly cupped hands and loose, flexible wrists create a popping sound if cupping is properly performed to the posterior thoracic cavity.

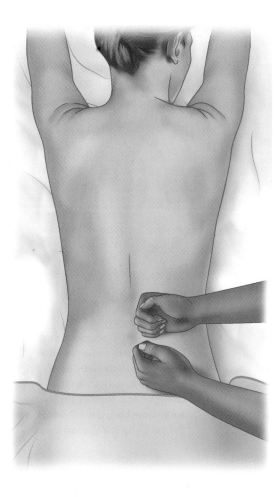

FIGURE 2-8 Pounding. Gently held fists and loose, flexible wrists intermittently strike the client's gluteal region.

ROCKING

Perhaps as natural as the act of stroking, rocking, too, can easily be applied at the beginning or end of a session. Without the advantage of a rocking chair, the therapist is limited to rocking the body in only one plane. Therefore, she must be careful with the rate and depth of rocking to avoid agitating the body and reversing the calming intention. Rocking is one technique that can be incorporated at any point during a session when the massage therapist intuitively feels the client needs to be placed into a deeper state of relaxation.

Rocking can be performed with the client lying supine or prone:

1. With the client in the supine position, the therapist places her hands gently and slightly laterally to the anterior superior iliac spine (ASIS). The body is nudged from side to side by the force of the therapist's alternating hands, creating a rocking motion. The client's body does not move more than an inch or two from side to side. The rhythm is continued until the therapist feels as if the client's body has, itself, almost unconsciously taken over the rocking process, at which point she simply continues to help nudge the body. The stopping point is reached intuitively.
2. With the client in the prone position, the therapist places her hands gently and slightly laterally to the gluteus medius, and the same process discussed previously is followed (Figure 2-9).

It is difficult to rock an adult at any other point of the body without either invading personal space or causing vertigo.

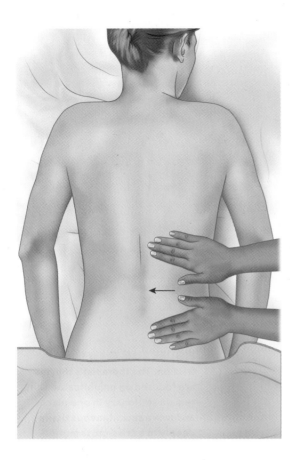

FIGURE 2-9 Rocking. The therapist's hands gently placed along the bilateral gluteus medius push each other to create a rocking motion.

The specific physiologic effects of rocking include:

- Muscle relaxation
- Increased parasympathetic nervous system activity
- Increased feeling of well-being
- Improved balance

CROSS-FIBER FRICTION

Used with discretion and intelligence, this technique is highly effective. If the technique is used without focus or knowledge, the therapist can irritate the tissues and the person, in which case the client will never return and the therapist will have failed in the attempt to help. "Do no harm" is worth remembering in the context of using cross-fiber friction.

Cross-fiber friction can be performed at the point where a muscle turns into tendon (at the origin or insertion of muscle on bone), in the middle of the muscle belly itself, anywhere along the muscle mass, on and around scar tissue, at any location where muscles are deeply layered in the body, and at places where superficial muscles lie directly against bone. The therapist performs cross-fiber friction using the tips of her thumbs, an elbow, or a knuckle. Here is the basic technique:

1. The therapist identifies a small, localized, focused area of tissue.
2. Using her thumbs or fingertips, the therapist begins rubbing "across the grain" of the muscle fiber using no lubricant and *without moving over the skin* (Figure 2-10). She focuses on the client's level of discomfort, paying close attention to body language indicators for pain beyond "good hurt." Communication with the client is essential.

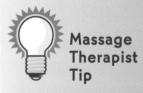

Massage Therapist Tip

Cross-Fiber Friction and Medication

When considering whether to use cross-fiber friction, be aware of your client's medications. If she is taking high doses of pain medication, she may not be able to accurately report her pain level, and you could inadvertently bruise her by moving beyond acceptable limits of tissue tolerance.

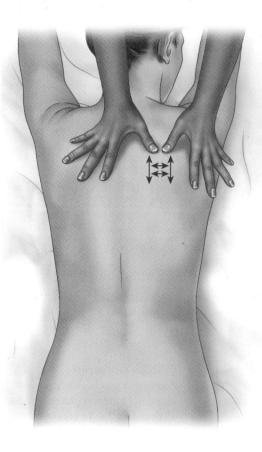

FIGURE 2-10 **Cross-fiber friction. The therapist's thumbs are focused on unlubricated skin, remain stationary in one place, and move subcutaneous tissue deeply in a criss-cross motion.**

3. The back-and-forth cross-fiber friction is continued until a localized area of hyperemia (redness) is noted on the skin; until the desired region, tendon, or muscle has reached an acceptably decreased level of hypertonicity (tightness); or until the client requests stopping the technique.
4. Cross-fiber friction is always preceded by effleurage and petrissage to warm and prepare the tissue. It is also always followed by effleurage and petrissage to "clean out" the effects of this aggressive but effective technique.

The specific physiologic effects of cross-fiber friction magnify the effects of friction. The physiologic effects of both include:

- Breaking down existing soft tissue adhesions, as well as those about to be formed through injury, surgery, or inactivity
- Breaking down the erratic formation of scar tissue; repeated treatments can re-align the collagen fibers to create a more normal, mobile muscle fiber direction
- Increased connective tissue extensibility
- Localized hyperemia, followed by a localized inflammation and healing
- Temporary analgesia
- Decreased hypertonicity

The mechanism by which the massage therapist creates a localized reaction to which the body is forced to respond proves to be one of the most valuable tools in treating many conditions. After the body suffers a localized insult, it *attempts to heal*. The insult can be a fresh injury around which a scar is forming, or an older injury around which scar tissue has already formed, or perhaps merely a localized area of hypertonicity that has set up the pain-spasm-pain cycle (see Chapter 3). Whatever the cause, this injured, disorganized tissue needs the body's resources to heal.

In order for soft tissue to heal, it is necessary to increase the blood supply to the injured area. Cross-fiber friction creates a localized area of hyperemia, leading to a localized area of inflammation so the healing can begin. An example of this process is the body's response to a simple splinter. The splinter, a mild irritant, within a day or two is encased in a small reddened, pus-filled area surrounding the offending matter (phagocytes doing their job). The body recognized the splinter as an irritant and responded by sending blood and special chemicals directly to the area. This is the physiologic effect of cross-fiber friction, which the massage therapist can create by sending blood to a specific region that requires attention.

The medial epicondyle (bony landmark at the medial, anterior surface of the antecubital fossa) and a case of epicondylitis are an appropriate example:

1. The tender area is precisely identified by the therapist and the client.
2. The therapist's thumb begins to rub in a perpendicular direction at several spots along the tendons that insert the muscle onto the bone.
3. Because of the friction, blood vessels are dilated and the blood supply to the area is increased.
4. Because of the depth of the therapist's work (she is working to the point of "feel good" pain), she causes minor tissue damage.
5. Whenever the body experiences tissue damage, no matter how small, chemicals are sent to the area to dilate blood vessels and affect local pain receptors.
6. The local increased blood circulation speeds healing by transporting more healing chemicals to the area.
7. While the therapist works, the client first identifies pain and then notices the pain slightly decreases because the friction reduces the activity of local pain receptors, thereby allowing the therapist and the client to work "through the pain."
8. The chemicals in the blood facilitate tissue repair and a reorganization of the collagen fibers, producing more efficient muscle fiber function.

USING HEAT AND COLD

The effective application of heat and cold is a complicated issue for massage therapists. Some massage schools do not teach these therapies, believing they are not within the therapist's scope of practice. Other schools teach the use of hot and cold packs to address superficial tissues, with the understanding that it is only the physical therapist who has all the tools to substantially affect the body's deeper tissues by alternating hot and cold therapies.

To the extent that the massage therapist has been trained, hot or cold applications should be moist, not dry, for the most effective therapeutic use. The length of application varies depending on the reference used and on the patient's tolerance. The techniques listed as follows assume that hot or cold is applied externally and locally—not by submersion. Here are some safety guidelines.

Heat Application

Heat can safely be applied for 15–20 minutes, as long as the therapist observes both the local area of hyperemia and the patient's level of tolerance. The specific physiologic effects of the application of heat include:

- Increased local skin temperature
- Increased local vasodilation and blood flow to the skin and muscles directly below
- Increased local cellular metabolism and nutrient supply
- Increased local oxygenation
- Decreased pain perception because of decreased nerve conduction velocity
- Reduced muscle tone and decreased spasm from reduced sensitivity and firing rate in the muscle spindles
- General sense of sedation and relaxation

Because of the simultaneous comforting, relaxing, and mildly therapeutic effects on both the entire body and the localized tissue, the therapist will be able to

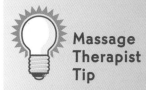

Massage Therapist Tip

The Application of Heat

A rice pack or electric heating pad is not considered a therapeutic application of heat. Heat is most effective when applied in a moist form—either a microwaved gel pack, a hot water bottle, or a compress made from a hot wet towel. *Do not place these applications directly on the client's skin;* lay them over a thin sheet of cotton, such as a pillowcase.

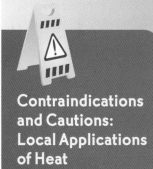

Contraindications and Cautions: Local Applications of Heat

If, for multiple reasons, a client cannot accurately report the effects of a heat application, that client represents a contraindication for this modality. Examples are unconsciousness, inebriation, infancy, old age, and the intake of high doses of pain or mood-altering medications. Further, patients with an acute injury, a circulatory pathology, or an active, systemic infection would represent a contraindication. For a patient who presents with a local skin compromise, such as an open wound or a rash of unknown origin, the therapist can safely apply heat to unaffected surfaces of the body.

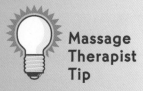

Massage Therapist Tip

The Application of Cold

It is normal for a patient receiving a local application of cold to experience first the sensation of cold, then a tingling or itching feeling, then a dull aching or burning sensation, and followed finally by numbness. You should inform your patient that the "therapy isn't working" until he experiences all of these phases. When he finally reaches the point of numbness, and this might take encouragement on your part for him to leave the pack in place, it is time to remove the pack for 30 minutes before reapplying the cold therapy.

Contraindications and Cautions: Local Application of Cold

The contraindications and cautions listed previously for the local application of heat hold true for the local application of cold. In addition to those are the patient's hypersensitivity or allergic reactions to cold (itching, hives, sweating), her possible compromised local circulation or circulatory insufficiency, and any statements indicating she is experiencing a whole-body chilling.

comfortably use heat during many of the protocols outlined in this book. The effects of heat will help the therapist "get into" the body on both a psychological and a physical level.

Cold Application

Just as there are times when the massage therapist wants to increase circulation to a localized area of the body, it is often appropriate to decrease a local inflammatory process, or to try to slow down or decrease swelling. Following are guidelines for the general application of cold. (The distinction is made between "cold" and "ice" here because most massage therapy schools do not teach the application of "ice pops" or "ice massage," but rather the application of frozen gel packs, which are merely very cold, but are not ice.)

The specific physiologic effects of the application of cold include:

- Activation of the pain-gating mechanism in the spinal cord, thereby decreasing perceived pain in the area and allowing localized therapeutic work to be performed (see Chapter 3)
- Reduced nerve conduction velocity
- Reduced local temperature of skin and muscle
- Duration of local effects up to 45 minutes after prolonged application
- Decreased local blood flow, initially, from vasoconstriction
- Increased blood viscosity resulting in less bleeding of the injured tissue, decreased inflammation, and decreased swelling and edema
- Decreased pain and muscle spasm
- Stimulation from brief application and analgesia from prolonged application

Cold packs can be locally applied safely for 5–20 minutes "on," with a rest period of 30 minutes "off." The therapist's cues from the patient for the beginning of the "off" phase would be words like "numb" and "painful" in reference to the effect of the cold.

PASSIVE AND ACTIVE RANGE OF MOTION

If you remember the Tin Man from *The Wizard of Oz*, it's easy to understand the relationship between continuous joint movement and the lack of joint pain. The Tin Man stood in the middle of a field, frozen solid, barely able to use his jaw muscles from years of disuse. He painstakingly called, "Oil . . . oil" to Dorothy and the Scarecrow as they walked by. When "oil" was applied to each of his joints, the immediate sigh of relief and movement let us know the oil had done the trick. And so it is with the "oil"—synovial fluid—in the joints of the body that facilitates smooth, pain-free joint movements. The more body movement, the more synovial fluid is released in the joints.

Further discussion about effective ROM exercises is found in Chapter 5. The specific physiologic effects of ROM exercises include:

- Controlled stimulation to joint mechanoreceptors (nerve signals monitoring and directing movement)
- Decreased sensitivity of joint sensory nerve receptors, with passive movement
- Increased synovial fluid production
- Increased lymphatic and venous return

IN SUMMARY

Massage therapists often erroneously believe they can do very little when confronted with the chronic pain associated with many medical conditions. Nothing is further from the truth. The following allow the therapist to have a profound effect on pain and discomfort:

- Increasing local circulation, which supports important physiologic processes, such as cellular oxygenation, removal of waste products, and moving hormones to target organs
- Stroking to sedate or quiet the nervous system
- Using effleurage transitionally or to apply lubricant
- Employing petrissage to move the deep muscle tissue
- Stimulating either the entire body or specific regions with tapotement
- Rocking the body as a means of sedation or to induce calm
- Breaking up adhesions and scars with the use of cross-fiber friction
- Applying heat or cold therapeutically and safely

The next chapter discusses the physiology of pain and moves the therapist one step closer to treating conditions.

Review

1. List the physiologic effects of increasing local circulation.
2. List specific physiologic effects of stroking.
3. List specific physiologic effects of effleurage.
4. List specific physiologic effects of petrissage.
5. List various forms of tapotement.
6. List specific physiologic effects of rocking.
7. Explain and demonstrate cross-fiber friction.
8. When is heat appropriately applied? Describe safe application.
9. When is cold appropriately applied? Describe safe application.

BIBLIOGRAPHY

Klein MJ, Wieting JM. Superficial Heat and Cold. EMedicine article, Topic 201. Available at: http://www.emedicine.com/pmr/topic201.htm. Accessed April 1, 2010.
Solkoff N, Yaffe S, Weintraub D, et al. Effects of handling on the subsequent development of premature infants. *Developmental Psychology* 1969;1:765–768.
Solkoff N, Matuszak D. Tactile stimulation and behavioral development among low-birth-weight infants. *Child Psychiatry and Human Development* 1975:33–37.
Versagi C. Hands of Peace. *Massage Magazine.* November/December 1999;68–77.
Wible J. *Pharmacology for Massage Therapy*, Baltimore: Lippincott Williams & Wilkins, 2005.
Yates J. *A Physician's Guide to Therapeutic Massage*, 3rd ed. Toronto: Curties-Overzet Publications, 2004.

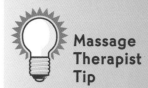

Massage Therapist Tip

Range-of-Motion Exercises

Active ROM is movement performed by the client, without your help. You observe as your client performs requested movements. When your client's joint movements are completely dependent upon your assistance, *passive* ROM is being performed. In either method, ROM is never performed beyond the point of a little client discomfort and should never be forced.

3

The Physiology of Muscular Activity and Pain

THE PAIN-SPASM-PAIN CYCLE

Knowledge of muscle physiology, pain perception, and the role of emotions is fundamental as the skilled massage therapist attempts to relieve pain. The pain-spasm-pain cycle is an invaluable tool with which the therapist can critically think through the client's pain status. Understanding this cycle is so central to the therapist's effective use of the massage protocols in Part II of this text that we will take time to discuss a typical demonstration of how myofascial pain is created in the body. Equipped with this knowledge, the therapist can use her wide array of skills to learn how best to interrupt the cycle to help eradicate, or at least decrease, myofascial pain.

How the Cycle Works

Figure 3-1 shows the step-by-step progression soft tissue undergoes when hypertonicity is not addressed.

Hypertonicity

Overused or underused muscles become hypertonic, or tight. Blood normally flows freely in and out of the moving muscle. Hypertonicity slows the free movement of oxygenated fresh blood in and metabolic waste products (like lactic acid and metabolites) out. When this happens, the client feels slight discomfort. No real pain has developed at this point.

Ischemia

With prolonged hypertonicity, local circulation (and therefore oxygen) decreases, causing a condition known as ischemia (lack of oxygen). Oxygen debt is accompanied by the beginning of the sensation of pain. Prolonged ischemia leads to more severe pain, resulting from the retention of metabolites. Normal, moving healthy muscle needs a constant supply of fresh oxygenated blood to function properly. Once the nutrients in blood are metabolized in the muscle tissue, waste products are produced, which must be washed out. This normally occurs through muscular activity. In the absence of adequate muscle movement, or upon physical exertion, wastes, such as carbon dioxide and lactic acid, accumulate. Lactic acid creates hydrogen ions, which stimulate the pain receptors (nociceptors) in the muscle.

Spasm

Ill equipped to handle the buildup of waste products, the muscle now begins to spasm. Metabolites have not yet moved out of the muscle, so the pain continues.

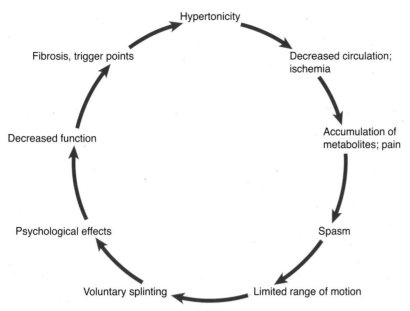

FIGURE 3-1   The pain-spasm-pain cycle. Simple hypertonicity leads to painful trigger points unless the cycle is broken.

Decreased Range of Motion

If the client is experiencing pain and spasm, the natural result will be a decreased range of motion (ROM) at the proximal joint. Compensation in other muscles occurs as he tries to adjust his body to the localized pain.

Voluntary Splinting

At this point, the client will "guard" a joint, a compensatory action known as voluntary splinting, or muscle splinting. Splinting protects the affected muscle from movement, which he has learned causes pain.

Emotional and Psychological Manifestations

Physical pain takes its toll on the psyche, and now the client's pain gains emotional and psychological components. These manifestations, combined with the pain in movement, lead to a further decrease in function. The client must adapt either his movement or his daily functioning.

Fibrosis

With prolonged muscle disuse, compensation, and splinting, tissue changes occur and the process of fibrosis, the development of excess connective tissue, begins. Fibrosis further restricts movement. As healthy muscle tissue is replaced by fibrotic tissue, the client is unable to move and function normally.

Trigger Points

The presence of fibrotic tissue embedded in normal muscle tissue creates trigger points. This is the stage at which many clients will seek help.

Continuation of the Cycle

Having moved from mild stiffness and irritation to pain to spasm to voluntary splinting, the client's movements are now accompanied by radiating pain beyond the initial point of hypertonicity. He experiences more hypertonicity, and the cycle continues.

A Classic Example of the Pain-Spasm-Pain Cycle

Taking a common example of a client, let's call him Sam, who spends one intensive week working on a major project, we can see how the previous physiologic explanation quickly becomes clear:

- *Monday, 11:00 a.m.:* Sam has been seated, hunched over his computer screen, since 8:00 a.m. He notices a mild discomfort in his superior trapezius, rubs his shoulders unconsciously, but continues to work without addressing the impending problem. *(Hypertonicity)*
- *Wednesday, 8:00 a.m.:* Sam's stress level has risen, he's not making his deadline, and he's clenching his jaw. He notices a mild burning sensation at his superior trapezius and in the middle of his back. Throughout the day, he grabs at his shoulder and rolls his neck but keeps on working. *(Decreased circulation and ischemia)*
- *Thursday, 6:00 p.m.:* Sam has not slept much, probably is not hydrating properly, and continues to put in long days, hunched in front of the screen. The discomfort in his shoulder has progressed to a noticeable, distracting pain. He continues to ignore the problem. *(Accumulation of metabolites and pain)*
- *Friday, 6:30 a.m.:* When Sam gets out of bed and reaches to turn off the alarm clock, his superior trapezius spasms and burns, finally getting his conscious attention. *(Spasm)* He notices while taking his shower that his shoulders aren't as mobile as they used to be, and he can't reach to dry his back. *(Limited ROM)*
- *Friday, 12 noon:* Sam's coworkers ask him why he's "holding himself" when he reaches for his cup of coffee, and he realizes he's adjusted his movements because he's in so much pain. *(Voluntary splinting)* At this point, because of his pain, his choice not to address it, and his overall stiffness, he becomes grouchy. *(Psychological effects)*
- *Saturday morning:* Sam sleeps in, but when he rolls out of bed, he notices his shoulder movement is accompanied by stabbing pain. Shaving is difficult for him. *(Decreased function)* When his wife tries to rub his painful shoulders, she tells him she feels "knots" deep in his muscle. *(Fibrous trigger points)*

Unless Sam addresses the causes of the hypertonicity, the pain-spasm-pain cycle will continue. In order to relieve pain, *the cycle must be broken—and it can be broken at any point.* The painful region needs movement, increased blood flow, stretching, and strengthening. If the massage therapist can address even one component of the pain-spasm-pain cycle, she has a good chance of stopping, or at least reducing, myofascial pain.

Breaking the Cycle

There are many ways to break this cycle, medications and surgery being the two most dramatic. Massage therapy, however, is a simpler, noninvasive method that takes longer but that can have profound long-term effects not only on the body but on the mind as well. Table 3-1 outlines the various pain relief techniques available to all levels of massage therapists. Part II of this book is dedicated to the use of massage skills in treating specific conditions; Table 3-1 is simply a taste of things to come. (For the specific physiologic effects of each stroke listed in the table, see Chapter 2.)

THE GATE CONTROL THEORY OF PAIN

Understanding myofascial pain is only one component of clinical massage. A thorough understanding of the patient's *perception of pain* is also essential. The concept of pain and where exactly it is perceived in the body or brain have mystified scientists for a long time. Although scientists understood that nerve endings that respond to pain are different from those that respond to gentle touch, no one was sure what role the brain or spinal cord played in how pain is perceived. The gate control theory of pain is widely

TABLE 3-1	Techniques for Breaking the Pain-Spasm-Pain Cycle
Cycle Component	**Pain Relief Technique**
Hypertonicity	ROM exercises, application of heat, effleurage-petrissage-effleurage, kneading, vibration
Decreased circulation	All of the previous
Accumulation of metabolites	Application of heat followed by deep effleurage-petrissage-effleurage, contrast (hot-cold-hot-cold) therapy, deep kneading.
Pain	All of the previous, compassion
Spasm	Very localized, deep kneading followed by effleurage-petrissage-effleurage; application of heat; rocking; localized deep vibration; cautious stretching; calming, careful work.
Limited ROM	Application of heat, ROM exercises, effleurage-petrissage-effleurage, kneading, vibration, encouragement
Voluntary splinting	Therapist assesses this mechanism and watches for compensatory patterns that are developing. Massage to compensating muscles, not simply the localized area of pain or injury.
Psychological effects	Compassion, increased listening skills, understanding that the client is more than her physical pain, asking sufficient questions to determine the extent of the "terrible triad"
Decreased function	Keen observation and assessment to determine functional impairment, followed by the use of all previous techniques as appropriate
Fibrosis	Manual assessment to determine where normal muscle fibers have moved into an abnormal state of fibrosis; all previous techniques as appropriate
Trigger points	Initial warming of distal tissue, followed by warming techniques to exact trigger point location, followed by heat application, effleurage-petrissage-effleurage and kneading, proximal joint ROM, and client self-care homework assignments

accepted as a comprehensive explanation of how the brain perceives pain and—for the massage therapist's purposes—how the perception of pain can be decreased.

In 1965, Canadian psychologist Ronald Melzack and British physiologist Patrick Wall proposed the gate control theory. However, before discussing the science, let's consider another simple example. If a client is having a bad day to begin with and slams his toe into the corner of his desk at work, it will really, *really* hurt. He might utter a few expletives, rub the spot, and go on with his day, more irritated than before the minor injury. What if the same client just found out he won the lottery? In his rush to tell the world, he slams his toe—just as hard, at exactly the same spot—but he barely notices it; in fact, the injury doesn't even slow him down on his way to the phone. A few days later, he notices a bruise and wonders where it came from.

The physiologic explanation of what happened to this client is the gate control theory of pain (Figure 3-2). Melzack and Wall suggested that there is a gating mechanism in the *spinal cord* that closes in response to normal stimulation of fast-conducting "touch" nerve fibers and then opens when slower-conducting, higher-volume, and high-intensity sensory signals of "pain" are received. The two scientists determined that signals of "pain" and "touch" could be intermittently sent and not sent to the brain, depending on input received by the spinal cord. In other words, *whatever is going on in the periphery of the body combined with whatever is going on in the brain itself will determine pain perception*. Figure 3-3 diagrams the gate control theory, using music and touch as examples.

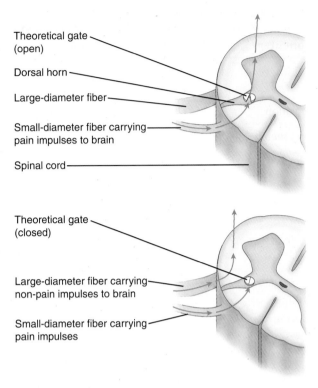

Theoretical gate (open)

Dorsal horn

Large-diameter fiber

Small-diameter fiber carrying pain impulses to brain

Spinal cord

Theoretical gate (closed)

Large-diameter fiber carrying non-pain impulses to brain

Small-diameter fiber carrying pain impulses

FIGURE 3-2 The gate control theory of pain. The brain has a gating mechanism that controls how many stimuli it can receive.

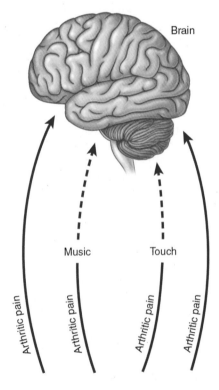

Brain

Music   Touch

Arthritic pain   Arthritic pain   Arthritic pain   Arthritic pain

FIGURE 3-3 The massage therapist can use the brain's gating mechanism to reduce her client's pain perception.

The scientific world quickly accepted this theory because it explains many previously misunderstood concepts of the emotional, psychological, and cultural components of pain. The application of this knowledge for the practicing massage therapist is profound: *She can directly alter her client's perception of pain.*

When the client is experiencing pain and that pain is the only message going to his brain, the therapist has the opportunity to "block" his pain perception by adding "touch" signals to the "pain" signals in his nervous system. The touch signals in the therapist's toolkit—heat, rocking, deep work, effleurage, petrissage, vibration, music, candles—are literally sending so many messages to the client's brain that he (according to the gate control theory) has to block *something* out, and some of what gets blocked out is his *perception of the physical pain.*

SLAYING THE DRAGON

An ancient concept of Japanese warfare is a metaphor for effectively treating a painful site. If there is a dragon across the field and a warrior wants to slay it, if she yells loudly and runs straight for the dragon, she will probably not meet with great success in her attempts to slay the dragon. If, however, she is contemplative, careful, strategic, and perhaps sneaks up to the side or behind the dragon, she has a better chance of victory. So it is with treating pain in the body.

If a hasty therapist begins her treatment by digging into the client's exact point of pain, the client will wince and *pull away*. But if she starts farther away from the point of pain—even going to the extent of relaxing the client by massaging the hands first—the body relaxes and the local pain is much more receptive to treatment. The body, in all of its wisdom, does not take a liking to being invaded. Slaying the dragon is an easy concept of pain treatment that simply means: *When a localized area of pain is identified, start somewhere else; don't treat the immediate point of pain first.* Simple dragon-slaying examples include:

- Massaging the shoulders for 5 minutes before treating a tension headache
- Working on the gluteus maximus before approaching lumbar spine area pain
- Softening and warming the superior trapezius before working on burning pain in the rhomboids

These techniques are respectful and dignified approaches to treating the body with care and compassion.

THE PAIN SCALE

Therapists need a measuring tool to indicate the level of the client's initial pain and the point when that pain has decreased. Used by nurses, physical therapists, chiropractors, physiatrists, and many other medical professionals, the 0–10 pain scale is commonly applied in massage therapy as an effective method of assessing before- and after-treatment myofascial pain (Figure 3-4). The patient is asked to verbally indicate his level of pain, with 0 representing no pain at all and 10 indicating the worst pain imaginable. The therapist then documents the patient's pain on a SOAP chart (see Chapter 1) at the beginning of the treatment (under subjective) and after the treatment (under assessment). Periodic questioning of the regional severity of the pain by the therapist, and accurate reporting of the client's responses, will, over time, give a clear picture of whether the therapy is effective.

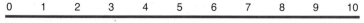

```
0    1    2    3    4    5    6    7    8    9    10
```
No pain...mild discomfort............pain cannot be ignored.........unbearable pain

FIGURE 3-4 The pain scale is a simple tool to determine the location, presence, and decrease of pain.

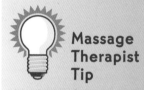

Massage Therapist Tip

Adapting the Pain Scale for Children or Non–English-Speaking Clients

Not all of your clients will understand your questions about their pain "on a scale of 0–10." Children, stroke patients, and clients who don't understand or speak English will find it difficult to communicate about pain unless you simplify the measuring tool. Many hospitals use a "smiley to frowney face" chart that they create on a card or piece of paper for these patients (Figure 3-5). The "no hurt" face corresponds to 0 and the "hurts worst" face corresponds to 10. Through body language and facial expressions indicating pain, show your client the chart and draw a line with your finger from the happiest face to the saddest face. Point from the card to your client and then back again with a questioning look on your face. Most clients will understand and point to their "level of pain" on the card. You can then have a reasonably accurate method of determining pain increase or decrease, which you then document.

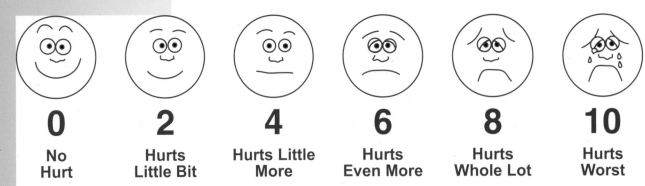

FIGURE 3-5 The Wong-Baker FACES™ Pain Rating Scale is one way of measuring pain in children and adults with communication challenges. Copyright 1983 by the Wong-Baker FACES™ Foundation, www.WongBakerFACES.org. Used with permission.

Here are two examples of effective charting using the 0–10 pain scale:

- Client states pain is at a 5 on a scale of 0–10, and he points to the left lumbar spine region.
- Patient states pain is at an 8 on a scale of 0–10, indicates that the pain is shooting down his hamstrings and into the bottom of the foot.

Chronic and Acute Pain

Massage therapists treat chronic pain. A client does not stop off at the massage therapist's office after a car accident; therapists are not first responders. Chronic pain treatment is well within the massage therapist's scope of practice, yet defining "chronic" is often a challenge. Many massage schools and medical theories attempt to place a timeline on when pain is considered "chronic" and when it is "acute." For the purposes of this book, the common medical definition of the terms will be our reference point.

Chronic pain is an unpleasant sensation or discomfort that lasts over a long period (such as 3 or 6 months) and often does not have one easily defined cause. Examples of chronic pain are arthritis, trigger points, tension headaches, and diabetic neuropathy. Acute pain has a sudden onset and often is associated with a specific medical event. Examples of acute pain include the pain associated with appendicitis, labor pains, and a fall or accident.

The therapist must remember, however, that it is not up to her to determine whether pain is chronic or acute. The client or the physician will describe or label the chronic or acute nature of the pain.

EMOTIONS AND PAIN PERCEPTION: THE TERRIBLE TRIAD

Volumes have been written about the effect of emotions and cultural inclinations on the perception of pain. Overall health, mood, self-esteem, attitude, and feelings of being loved all affect an individual's perception of physical and emotional pain.

Scientists have studied the effects of chronic pain on more than the body and have identified that irritability and depression often accompany chronic pain. This cycle can lead to a state called the "terrible triad" of suffering, sleeplessness, and sadness. In her role as a health care professional, the massage therapist has an obligation to understand that she is treating many levels of the client's pain, and she must use all her available tools to attend to the client's mind, spirit, and body.

Why a Horse's Pain is Different than Ours

While staying at a friend's horse farm, I once witnessed a dramatic example of how the human emotional response to pain adds significantly to our perception of that pain and how deeply we suffer. Walking with my friend early in the morning on our way to feed the horses, we noticed that one of the stall doors had been kicked open and a horse had escaped during the night. Looking out in the field, we saw the escapee standing very still next to a large fencepost. Upon approaching the horse, we noticed that about a 12-inch flank of flesh had been peeled back and was bleeding badly. My friend surmised that the horse had, in the dark, run into a fencepost and cut himself open. As I watched her assess the damage and determine that she had better call the vet, I marveled at how the horse just stood there. I don't know what I expected him to be doing, hopping up and down or making some sort of fuss perhaps, because I knew he had to be in pain. But he just stood there, blinking and allowing my friend to probe the wound.

When I mentioned how amazed I was that the horse didn't seem to be in very much pain, her response opened a whole new world of understanding about pain and suffering. "He's in a lot of pain," she said. "He just doesn't have an emotional reaction to the pain the way we humans do." Her simple explanation helped me to understand how our emotions determine not only our perception of the pain but also the level to which we choose to suffer.

IN SUMMARY

Most common medical problems are accompanied by some level of soft tissue pain. A massage therapist who understands both the physiology of pain and the effects of basic massage techniques can effectively become a part of the client's solution. Helping to effectively reduce pain includes:

- Assessing the client's stage in the pain-spasm-pain cycle
- Understanding the emotional, cultural, and psychological components of pain
- Determining the wise use of mechanisms to block pain signals to the brain
- Utilizing the appropriate massage therapy techniques at the appropriate time

The next chapter discusses medications your clients might be taking, and how these substances affect both your treatment and your client's response.

Review

1. Explain the pain-spasm-pain cycle and its relevance to the massage therapist.
2. What is ischemia?
3. What is fibrosis?
4. Explain the gate control theory of pain and its relevance to the massage therapist.
5. Explain the concept of slaying the dragon; offer two examples the therapist might use during a massage session.

BIBLIOGRAPHY

About.com. Senior Health. Pain's "Terrible Triad." Available at: http://seniorhealth.about.com/library/conditions/blchronicpain2.htm. Accessed December 28, 2010.

Association of the British Pharmaceutical Industry. Target Pain: Pain and Pain Research and the Pharmaceutical Industry. January 2003. Available at: http://www.abpi.org.uk/publications/publication_details/targetPain. Accessed April 1, 2010.

Chek P. The Healing Power of the Pool. Available at: http://www.personalpowertraining.net/art%20healing%20pool%20power.html. Accessed April 1, 2010.

Darling LM. The Gate Control Model Opens a New Era in Pain Research. Biomedical Library. Available at: http://www.library.ucla.edu/libraries/biomed/his/painexhibit/panel6.htm. Accessed November 22, 2005.

Hendrickson T. *Massage and Manual Therapy for Orthopedic Conditions*, 2nd ed. Baltimore: Lippincott Williams & Wilkins, 2009.

McMahon S, Koltzenburg M. *Wall and Melzack's Textbook of Pain*, 5th ed. London: Churchill Livingstone, 2005.

Melzack R, Wall PD. Pain mechanisms: a new theory. *Science* 1965;150:971–979.

4

Medications for Common Medical Conditions

WHY KNOWLEDGE ABOUT MEDICATIONS MATTERS TO THE MASSAGE THERAPIST

An oversimplification or rigid interpretation of the massage therapist's scope of practice might lead her to believe that the medications her client is taking do not concern her. Further thought will dispel this thinking, leading her to realize that a full understanding of every medication taken by a client leads to safe, intelligent, and holistic care, and that inquiring about every medication is well within the massage therapist's scope. Two commonplace examples can clarify this point.

Most post-stroke or post-cardiac event clients take anticoagulants. Because of the blood-thinning effects of these medications, these clients bruise easily with the slightest bump against a table or kitchen counter. Given this knowledge, a therapist would decrease her pressure during massage because of the risk of further bruising the client. In addition, knowing that a client is taking antiseizure medication would provide invaluable direction for a therapist who would then avoid all overstimulating, percussive, or abrupt modalities in an attempt to maintain central nervous system (CNS) equilibrium.

Once a healthy curiosity about medications replaces any potential hesitation a therapist might have, it becomes clear that knowledge about many common medications should accompany all good care plans.

BEING AWARE OF "CHASING SYMPTOMS" THAT ARE MEDICATION SIDE EFFECTS

A quick glance at the medications table that follows reveals that often similar side effects manifest with very different classes of medications. For example, headaches and constipation—two symptoms effectively treated by massage therapy—are common medication side effects. A client may be taking medications that, either individually or in combination, will cause symptoms that the therapist might believe are of musculoskeletal origin. Although the therapist would continue to try to treat, let's say, both the headaches and the constipation, the therapist and the client should understand that these symptoms will recur, no matter how stellar the massage therapy treatment, as long as the client continues to take certain medications.

WHY KNOWLEDGE OF MEDICATION ADMINISTRATION IS ESSENTIAL

The method by which a medication is administered—whether injected, delivered by patch, or rubbed on the skin, for example—directly affects the performance of the massage. A corticosteroid injection into the elbow joint given within the last 24 hours, which is intended to quiet tennis elbow inflammation, would be a local massage therapy contraindication. The medication's effectiveness is intended for a very *localized effect*, and massaging the area might cleanse the joint of the much-needed medication. Similarly, a local Betaseron injection into the belly fat of a patient with multiple sclerosis (MS) must be left undisturbed because this site can be easily irritated and will be sore. This is not a case of the possibility of sending the medication through the body too quickly, as with corticosteroids. Knowing about and avoiding an adhesive patch containing pain-relieving medication is another example of the therapist's "need to know" regarding drug administration methods.

Clients will often offer drug administration information to the massage therapist. For example, "My doctor injected my left knee with a steroid this morning, can you still massage it?" Or, "I took my MS medication last night, just wanted you to know." Again, knowledge of the intended effects of the medication, as well as method of administration, paves the way for safe, intelligent care.

AN EXPLANATION OF GENERIC AND TRADE NAMES, CLASS, AND ACTION

In pharmaceutical parlance, a generic drug name is the general, scientific name assigned to a formula during its testing phases and throughout its final clinical trials. This term is not generally used by consumers. A trade name (or brand name) is intended for consumer use; it is more easily pronounced and is assigned to the drug by the pharmaceutical companies once the drug has passed all testing phases and is ready for marketing and safe, human consumption. Examples include the generic drug naproxen, which is sold under the trade names of Aleve, Anaprox, and Naprosyn; and the drug hydroxychloroquine sulfate, which has been simplified and branded as Plaquenil.

A medication class is a method of categorizing the drug's actions. A mere few dozen drug classes exist to corral and categorize the thousands of existing medications. Examples of drug classes include nonsteroidal anti-inflammatory drugs (such as Motrin, Advil, Aleve, Anaprox, Naprelan, Orudis, and Actron), skeletal muscle relaxants (such as Lioresal, Valium, and Flexeril), and antiparkinsonian drugs (such as Mirapex, Requip, Eldepryl, and Comtan).

A NOTE REGARDING CURRENCY

New medications are developed regularly for many of the medical conditions discussed in this book. I have attempted to represent the most common and most accurate medication usage in the following chart; however, because of the nature of ongoing medication development, newer drugs that have come to market since this chapter was written will not be reflected in this reference table. Please check online for more updated information.

Generic and Trade Names	Class	Action	Common Side Effects	Massage Therapy Considerations	Conditions (Chapter Number)
abatacept (Orencia)	Immunosuppressant	Reduces symptoms of moderate to severe RA	Dizziness, headache, mild pain at injection site	Use caution around injection site.	RA (33)
acetaminophen (Tylenol, Feverall, Anacin, Panadol)	Nonopioid pain reliever	Mild analgesic; reduces fever	Liver damage from prolonged use	Decreases pain perception; use deep massage with caution.	DDD (13), fibromyalgia (15), frozen shoulder (16), migraine headache (17), tension headache (18), RA (33) sprains and strains (37), TMJ dysfunction (40), tendinosis (41), TOS (42)
acetaminophen and codeine (Tylenol #3)	Narcotic	Relieves moderate-to-severe pain.	Dizziness, drowsiness, nausea, vomiting, headache, dry mouth	Help client on/off table.	Migraine headache (17)
acyclovir (Zovirax)	Antiviral	Kills specific viruses	Hypotension, nausea, headache	Help client on/off table.	Bell's palsy (7)
adalimumab (Humira)	Antirheumatic	Relieves signs and symptoms of RA	Increased blood pressure, headache, nausea	None.	RA (33)
amitriptyline hydrochloride (Apo-Amitriptyline, Endep)	Tricyclic antidepressant	Relieves depression	Dry mouth, constipation, drowsiness	Abdominal massage may help relieve constipation. Help client on/off table.	CFS (11), fibromyalgia (15), neuropathy (25), stress (38)
anakinra (Kineret)	Immune regulator, antirheumatic	Decreases progression of RA	Nausea, vomiting, headache		Stress (38)
apomorphine hydrochloride (Apokyn)	Non-ergoline dopamine agonist	Reduces symptoms of Parkinson's disease	Yawning, nausea, vomiting, drowsiness, flushing	Help client on/off table. Use deep-tissue massage with caution.	Parkinson's disease (27)
aspirin (Ecotrin, Empirin, Astrin)	Salicylate nonopioid pain reliever	Analgesic, reduces fever	Stomach upset, increased bruising	Decreases pain perception. Use deep massage with caution.	Ankylosing spondylosis (6), tension headache (18), stroke (39), RA (33)
azathioprine (Imuran)	Immunosuppressant	Suppresses immune response	Anorexia, pancreatitis, mouth sores, hair loss	No massage if therapist has cold/flu symptoms. If client has hair loss, no scalp massage.	RA (33)

(continued)

Generic and Trade Names	Class	Action	Common Side Effects	Massage Therapy Considerations	Conditions (Chapter Number)
baclofen (Lioresal)	Skeletal muscle relaxant	Relieves muscle spasm	Constipation, drowsiness	Deep-tissue massage is contraindicated. Abdominal massage may help relieve constipation.	CP (10)
benztropine mesylate (Cogentin)	Antiparkinson	Increases physical mobility in Parkinson's patients	Cardiac complications, dry mouth, constipation, incoherence, confusion	Abdominal massage may help relieve constipation. Place a reminder call the day before the appointment.	Parkinson's disease (27)
bisacodyl (Correctol, Dulcolax, Fleet, Feen-a-Mint)	Stimulant laxative	Relieves constipation	Nausea, vomiting, abdominal cramping	None.	Constipation (12)
bupivacaine hydrochloride (Bupivacaine)	Local anesthetic	Decreases local pain	Agitation, depression	None.	Piriformis syndrome (28)
carbidopa-levodopa (Sinemet)	Antiparkinson	Improves voluntary movement	Cardiac irregularities, dry mouth, constipation, involuntary grimacing	Abdominal massage may help constipation.	CP (10), Parkinson's disease (27)
celecoxib (Celebrex)	Anti-inflammatory	Relieves signs and symptoms of osteoarthritis and RA	Stomach upset, dizziness	Help client on/off table. Decreases pain perception. Use deep massage with caution.	DDD (13), frozen shoulder (16), RA (33)
chloroquine hydrochloride (Aralen)	Antimalarial, amebicide	Slows progression of some autoimmune diseases	Anorexia, abdominal cramps, fatigue, irritability	None.	RA (33)
cyclobenzaprine hydrochloride (Flexeril)	Skeletal muscle relaxant	Relieves muscle spasm	Tachycardia, dry mouth, constipation, drowsiness	Use deep-tissue techniques with caution. Abdominal massage may help constipation. Help client on/off table.	DDD (13), fibromyalgia (15), muscle spasm (24)

Drug	Classification	Action	Side effects	Massage considerations	Conditions
diazepam (Valium)	Benzodiazepine anxiolytic, skeletal muscle relaxant, anticonvulsant, sedative	Reduces muscle spasm, anxiety, and seizures; promotes calmness	Nausea, vomiting, constipation, physical or psychological dependence, bradycardia, drowsiness	Deep-tissue massage is contraindicated. Abdominal massage may help relieve constipation. Help client on/off table.	CP (10), CFS (11)
diltiazem hydrochloride (Dilacor)	Antianginal	Lowers blood pressure, restores normal heart rhythm	Flushing, nausea, weakness	Help client on/off table.	Raynaud's phenomenon (32)
dihydroergotamine mesylate (Migranal spray)	Cranial vasoconstrictor	Reduces symptoms of migraine headaches and cluster headaches	Nausea, vomiting, abdominal pain, anxiety, sweating	None.	Migraine headache (17)
divalproex sodium (Depakote)	Antiseizure	Treatment of acute manic episodes of bipolar disorder or seizure disorders	Drowsiness, nausea, vomiting	Help client on/off table.	PTSD (31)
docusate sodium (Colace)	Emollient laxative	Stool softener	Mild abdominal cramping	None.	Constipation (12)
doxepin hydrochloride (Sinequan)	Tricyclic antidepressant	Relieves depression and anxiety	Tachycardia, dry mouth, constipation, drowsiness	Abdominal massage may help constipation. Help client on/off table.	Fibromyalgia (15), TOS (42)
doxycycline (Doryx, Vibramycin)	Tetracycline antibiotic	Hinders bacterial growth	Nausea, diarrhea	None.	CFS (11)
duloxetine (Cymbalta)	Selective serotonin and norepinephrine reuptake inhibitor (SSNRI), antidepressant	Antidepressant, treats general anxiety disorders	Can dull thinking, slow reaction time, dry mouth, mild nausea, constipation, gas	Place a reminder call the day before the appointment. Abdominal massage may help relieve constipation.	CFS (11), neuropathy (25)
eletriptan hydrobromide (Relpax)	Antimigraine	Relieves migraine headache symptoms	Flushing, palpitations, abdominal pain, dizziness	Help client on/off table.	Migraine headache (17)

(continued)

Generic and Trade Names	Class	Action	Common Side Effects	Massage Therapy Considerations	Conditions (Chapter Number)
enfuvirtide (Fuzeon)	Anti-HIV, antiviral	Controls symptoms of HIV infection	Abdominal pain, diarrhea, constipation, peripheral neuropathy, bruising, depression	Deep-tissue massage is contraindicated. Gentle abdominal stimulation may help relieve constipation.	HIV/AIDS (19)
entacapone (Comtan)	Antiparkinson	Controls signs and symptoms of Parkinson's disease	Abdominal pain, constipation, diarrhea, anxiety, depression	Abdominal massage may help constipation.	Parkinson's disease (27)
ergotamine tartrate and caffeine (Cafergot) (suppositories)	Cranial vasoconstrictor	Relieves migraine headache pain	Nausea, vertigo	Help client on/off table.	Migraine headache (17)
escitalopram oxalate (Lexapro)	Selective serotonin reuptake inhibitor (SSRI), antidepressant	Relieves depression and anxiety	Cardiac complications, abdominal pain, indigestion, heartburn, gas, migraine, abnormal dreams, dizziness, sedation	Position for gastric distress. Help client on/off table.	Stress (38)
estazolam (ProSom)	Benzodiazepine hypnotic	Sedation	Abdominal pain, fatigue, dizziness, daytime drowsiness	Use deep-tissue massage with caution. Help client on/off table.	Insomnia (22)
eszopiclone (Lunesta)	Sedative, hypnotic agent	Promotes sleep	Chest pain, migraine headache	None.	Insomnia (22)
etanercept (Enbrel)	Antirheumatic	Relieves signs and symptoms of RA	Abdominal pain, headache, dizziness	Help client on/off table.	RA (33)
fexofenadine hydrochloride (Allegra)	Antihistamine	Relieves seasonal allergy symptoms	Fatigue, drowsiness	Help client on/off table.	CFS (11)
fluoxetine hydrochloride (Prozac)	Selective serotonin reuptake inhibitor (SSRI)	Antidepressant, relieves obsessive-compulsive behaviors	Nausea, diarrhea, abdominal pain, insomnia, constipation	Abdominal massage may help constipation. Help client on/off table.	Fibromyalgia (15), PTSD (31)
gabapentin (Neurontin)	Anticonvulsant	Prevents and treats partial seizures, relieves neuralgia	Nausea, dry mouth, dizziness, amnesia, relieves constipation	Abdominal massage may help relieve constipation. Help client on/off table. Place a reminder call the day before the appointment.	CFS (11), neuropathy (25)

Medication	Classification	Effect	Side effects	Massage considerations	Conditions
glatiramer acetate (Copaxone)	Immunomodulator	Reduces symptoms of MS	Irritation at injection site, short-term flushing, chest tightness	Do not massage day of or day after injection; caution around injection site.	MS (23)
golimumab (Simponi)	Human monoclonal antibody	Reduces joint inflammation	Immune-compromise, irritation at injection site	Use caution around injection site. No massage if therapist has cold or flu symptoms.	RA (33)
hydroxychloroquine sulfate (Plaquenil)	Antimalarial, anti-inflammatory.	Reduces inflammation	Anorexia, abdominal cramps, fatigue, irritability	None.	RA (33)
hydroxyzine embonate (Atarax)	Antihistamine, sedative, antispasmodic	Promotes calmness, reduces nausea and vomiting	Dry mouth, drowsiness	Use deep-tissue massage with caution.	Stress (38)
ibuprofen (Motrin, Advil)	Nonsteroidal anti-inflammatory drug (NSAID)	Anti-inflammatory, analgesic, reduces fever	Stomach upset, ringing in ears, headache	Decreases pain perception. Use deep massage with caution.	Ankylosing spondylosis (6), bursitis (8), carpal tunnel syndrome (9), DDD (13), DOMS (14), fibromyalgia (15), migraine headache (17), hyperkyphosis (20), ITBS (21), MS (23), muscle spasm (24), neuropathy (25), osteoarthritis (26), piriformis syndrome (28), plantar fasciitis (29), post-polio syndrome (30), sciatica (35), scoliosis (36), sprains and strains (37), TMJ dysfunction (40), TOS (42), whiplash (44)
imipramine hydrochloride (Tofranil-PM)	Tricyclic antidepressant	Relieves depression	Cardiac complications, dry mouth, constipation, drowsiness, confusion	Abdominal massage may help relieve constipation. Help client on/off table.	Neuropathy (25)
infliximab (Remicade)	Anti-inflammatory	Relieves signs and symptoms of RA	Cardiac complications, nausea, headache, dizziness, painful urination, increased sweating	Help client on/off table.	RA (33)

(continued)

Generic and Trade Names	Class	Action	Common Side Effects	Massage Therapy Considerations	Conditions (Chapter Number)
interferon beta-1a (Avonex, Rebif)	Antiviral, antiproliferative, immunomodulator	Reduces symptoms of MS	Flu-like symptoms, depression, liver problems	Do not massage day of or day after injection. Use caution around injection site.	MS (23)
interferon beta-1b, recombinant (Betaseron)	Antiviral, immunoregulator	Decreases MS exacerbations	Hemorrhage, depression, anxiety, dizziness, flu-like symptoms	Help client on/off table. Do not massage day of or day after injection.	MS (23)
ketoprofen (Oruvail, Orudis)	Nonsteroidal anti-inflammatory drug (NSAID)	Anti-inflammatory, analgesic; reduces fever	Nausea, vomiting, constipation, ringing in ears	Use deep-tissue massage with caution. Abdominal massage may help relieve constipation.	Migraine headache (17)
ketorolac tromethamine (Toradol)	Nonsteroidal anti-inflammatory drug (NSAID)	Analgesic	Stomach upset	Decreases pain perception, use deep-tissue massage with caution.	Migraine headache (17), tension headache (18)
lamotrigine (Lamictal)	Anticonvulsant	Prevents partial seizures	Nausea, vomiting, fever, dizziness, headache, depression	Help client on/off table.	PTSD (31)
lidocaine topical (LidoCream, Lidoderm, Xylocaine)	Local anesthetic	Blocks pain nerve signals	Mild skin irritation, redness	Do not massage over patch.	CFS (11), piriformis syndrome (28)
lorazepam (Ativan)	Benzodiazepine anxiolytic, sedative, hypnotic	Relieves anxiety, promotes calmness and sleep	Dry mouth, drowsiness, restlessness	Use deep-tissue massage with caution.	Stress (38)
magnesium citrate (Milk of Magnesia)	Saline laxative	Soothes upset stomach, relieves constipation	Abdominal cramping, nausea	None.	Constipation (12)
methylcellulose (Citrucel)	Bulk-forming laxative	Encourages peristalsis and bowel movement	Nausea, vomiting, abdominal cramping	None.	Constipation (12)
methylprednisolone (Medrol)	Anti-inflammatory, immunosuppressant	Reduces inflammation, suppresses immune response	Serious cardiac complications, peptic ulcer, psychotic behavior, euphoria, insomnia	Use only gentle, non-stimulating massage modalities. No massage if therapist has cold or flu symptoms.	RA (33)

Drug	Classification	Action	Side effects	Massage considerations	Indications
metoclopramide hydrochloride (Reglan)	Antiemetic, gastrointestinal stimulant	Prevents or minimizes nausea and vomiting from chemotherapy or surgery	Nausea, anxiety, fatigue	Help client on/off table.	Migraine headache (17)
mexiletine hydrochloride (Mexitil)	Ventricular antiarrhythmic	Decreases pain of diabetic neuropathy	Cardiac complications, nausea, dizziness	Help client on/off table.	Neuropathy (25)
mitoxantrone hydrochloride (Novantrone)	Antineoplastic	Hinders cancer cell growth, reduces MS symptoms	Cardiac complications, abdominal pain, headache, bruising	Use only the gentlest massage modalities.	MS (23)
naproxen (Aleve, Anaprox, Naprelan, Naprosyn)	Nonsteroidal anti-inflammatory drug (NSAID)	Anti-inflammatory, analgesic, reduces fever	Stomach upset, ringing in ears, headache	Decreases pain perception. Use deep massage with caution.	Ankylosing spondylosis (6), bursitis (8), carpal tunnel syndrome (9), DOMS (13), fibromyalgia (15), migraine headaches (17), neuropathy (25), osteoarthritis (26), TMJ dysfunction (40), tendinosis (41), whiplash (44)
natalizumab (Tysabri)	Immunomodulator	Reduces symptoms of MS	Headache, fatigue, depression, joint pain	Caution around injection site.	MS (23)
nevirapine (Viramune)	Antiviral	May inhibit replication of HIV-1	Nausea, diarrhea, headache, muscle pain, paresthesia	No deep-tissue massage if client experiences paresthesia or muscle pain. Help client on/off table.	HIV/AIDS (19)
nifedipine (Adalat)	Antianginal	Lowers blood pressure, prevents angina	Flushing, nausea, weakness	Help client on/off table.	Raynaud's phenomenon (32)
olanzapine (Zyprexa)	Antipsychotic	Relieves signs and symptoms of psychosis	Cardiac complications, constipation, sleepiness, anxiety	Abdominal massage may help relieve constipation. Prolonged relaxation massage is contraindicated.	PTSD (31)
oxycodone hydrochloride (OxyContin)	Opioid analgesic	Reduces moderate-to-severe pain	Nausea, vomiting, dry mouth, constipation, sedation	Use deep-tissue techniques with caution. Abdominal massage may help relieve constipation. Help client on/off table.	DDD (13)

(continued)

Generic and Trade Names	Class	Action	Common Side Effects	Massage Therapy Considerations	Conditions (Chapter Number)
paroxetine hydrochloride (Paxil)	Selective serotonin reuptake inhibitor (SSRI)	Antidepressant, relieves obsessive-compulsive behaviors	Nausea, diarrhea, abdominal pain, insomnia, constipation, sexual dysfunction	Abdominal massage may help constipation.	Fibromyalgia (15), neuropathy (25), PTSD (31)
penicillamine (Cupri-mine)	Heavy metal antagonist, antirheumatic	Unknown for RA	Anorexia, loss of taste, oral ulcerations, bruising, hair loss, thin skin (especially around pressure points)	Use deep massage with caution. If client has hair loss, no scalp massage. Position according to skin sensitivity.	RA (33)
pramipexole dihydrochloride (Mirapex)	Antiparkinson	Relieves symptoms of Parkinson's disease	Chest pain, confusion, malaise, sleep disruption, constipation, swallowing difficulty	Help client on/off table. Abdominal massage may help relieve constipation.	Parkinson's disease (27)
prazosin hydrochloride (Minipress)	Antihypertensive	Lowers blood pressure	Dry mouth, dizziness, depression	Help client on/off table.	Raynaud's phenomenon (32)
prednisone (Deltasone, Orasone, Meticorten)	Adrenocorticosteroid	Anti-inflammatory, immunosuppression	Gastrointestinal irritation, thromboembolism, euphoria, insomnia	Deep-tissue massage is contraindicated.	Bell's palsy (7), DDD (13)
pregabalin (Lyrica)	Anticonvulsant	Decreases neuropathic pain	Drowsiness, dizziness, blurred vision, easy bruising	Help client on/off table.	Fibromyalgia (15), neuropathy (25)
prochlorperazine (Compazine)	Antipsychotic, antiemetic, anxiolytic	Relieves signs and symptoms of psychosis, relieves nausea and vomiting, reduces anxiety	Dry mouth, constipation	Abdominal massage may help constipation.	Migraine headache (17), headache (18)
promethazine hydrochloride (Phenergan)	Antiemetic, antivertigo, antihistamine, sedative	Relieves nausea, prevents motion sickness, reduces allergy symptoms; promotes calmness	Nausea, vomiting, dry mouth, constipation	Abdominal massage may help constipation. Use deep-tissue massage with caution.	Migraine headache (17), headache (18)

Drug	Class	Action	Side effects	Massage considerations	Condition
psyllium (Fiberall, Metamucil, Serutan)	Bulk-forming laxative	Encourages peristalsis and bowel movement	Nausea, vomiting, abdominal cramping	None.	Constipation (12)
quetiapine fumarate (Seroquel)	Antipsychotic	Relieves signs and symptoms of psychosis	Cardiac complications, constipation, sleepiness, anxiety	Abdominal massage may help relieve constipation. Prolonged relaxation massage is contraindicated.	PTSD (31)
ramelteon (Rozerem)	Melatonin receptor agonist	Promotes sleep	Drowsiness, fatigue, dizziness	Help client on/off table.	Insomnia (22)
rasagiline (Azilect)	Dopamine agonist	Reduces symptoms of Parkinson's disease	Headache, depression	None.	Parkinson's disease (27)
rizatriptan benzoate (Maxalt)	Antimigraine	Reduces acute migraine headache with or without aura	Cardiovascular abnormalities, dry mouth, nausea, dizziness	Use deep-tissue techniques with caution. Help client on/off table.	Migraine headache (17)
ropinirole hydrochloride (Requip)	Antiparkinson	Increases physical mobility in Parkinson's patients	Cardiac complications, fatigue, hallucinations, impotence, weakness, difficulty breathing	Help client/on off table. Adjust positioning for breathing difficulties.	Parkinson's disease (27)
rotigotine (Neupro)	Dopamine agonist	Reduces symptoms of early stage Parkinson's disease	Joint pain, constipation, dry mouth, fatigue	Do not massage around patch. Abdominal massage may help relieve constipation.	Parkinson's disease (27)
saquinavir mesylate (Invirase)	Antiviral	Reduces symptoms of HIV/AIDS infection	Diarrhea, mouth sores, weakness, dizziness	Help client on/off table.	HIV/AIDS (19)
selegiline hydrochloride (Eldepryl)	Antiparkinson	Increases physical mobility in Parkinson's patients	Cardiac complications, fatigue, hallucinations, impotence, weakness, difficulty breathing	Help client/on off table. Adjust positioning for breathing difficulties.	Parkinson's disease (27)

(continued)

Generic and Trade Names	Class	Action	Common Side Effects	Massage Therapy Considerations	Conditions (Chapter Number)
sertraline hydrochloride (Zoloft)	Selective serotonin reuptake inhibitor (SSRI)	Relieves depression	Nausea, diarrhea, abdominal pain, insomnia, constipation, sexual dysfunction	Abdominal massage may help constipation.	Fibromyalgia (15), neuropathy (25), PTSD (31)
sulfasalazine (Azulfidine)	Anti-inflammatory	Relieves gastrointestinal tract inflammation	Abdominal pain, nausea, vomiting, headache, depression	Use deep-tissue massage with caution.	RA (33)
sumatriptan succinate (Imitrex)	Antimigraine	Relieves acute migraine pain	Cardiovascular abnormalities, abdominal discomfort, drowsiness	Help client on/off table.	Migraine headache. (17)
temazepam (Restoril)	Benzodiazepine hypnotic, sedative	Sedation	Diarrhea, nausea, dry mouth	Use deep-tissue massage with caution.	Insomnia (22)
tenofovir disoproxil fumarate (Viread)	Antiviral, antiretroviral	Inhibits HIV replication	Abdominal pain, anorexia, nausea, vomiting	None.	HIV/AIDS (19)
tiagabine hydrochloride (Gabitril)	Anticonvulsant	Prevents partial seizures	Abdominal pain, dizziness, drowsiness, language problems	Help client on/off table. Speak slowly.	PTSD (31)
tramadol hydrochloride (Ultram)	Synthetic analgesic	Relieves moderate-to-moderately severe pain	Nausea, constipation, sedation	Use deep-tissue techniques with caution. Abdominal massage may help constipation. Help client on/off table.	DDD (13), fibromyalgia (15)
triazolam (Halcion)	Sedative, hypnotic	Sedation	Nausea, vomiting, dizziness, confusion	Use deep-tissue massage with caution. Help client on/off table.	Insomnia (22)
trihexyphenidyl hydrochloride (Apo-Trihex)	Antiparkinson	Increases physical mobility in Parkinson's patients	Dry mouth, constipation, nervousness	Abdominal massage may help constipation.	Parkinson's disease (27)

Drug	Classification	Effect	Side effects	Massage considerations	Condition
venlafaxine hydro-chloride (Effexor)	Antidepressant	Decreases nausea and vomiting, relieves depression	Increased blood pressure, nausea, constipation, weakness, agitation	Abdominal massage may help relieve constipation. Use caution with stimulating techniques.	Stress (38)
warfarin sodium (Coumadin)	Anticoagulant	Reduces ability of blood to clot	Anorexia, cramps, mouth sores, headache	Consult physician before massage.	TOS (42)
zaleplon (Sonata)	Sedative, hypnotic	Sedation	Chest pain, dry mouth, abdominal pain	Use deep-tissue massage with caution.	Insomnia (22)
zidovudine (Azido-thymidine/AZT, Apo-Zidovudine, Novo-AZT, Retrovir)	Antiviral	Reduces symptoms of HIV/AIDS infection	Nausea, abdominal pain, taste alteration, weakness, dizziness	Help client on/off table.	HIV/AIDS (19)
zolmitriptan (Zomig)	Antimigraine	Relieves acute migraine pain	Cardiovascular abnor-malities, abdominal discomfort, dizziness	Help client on/off table. Use deep-tissue massage with caution.	Migraine headache (17)
zolpidem tartrate (Ambien)	Sedative, hypnotic	Sedation	Nausea, vomiting, abdominal pain, dry mouth	Use deep-tissue massage with caution.	Insomnia (22)

BIBLIOGRAPHY

Drugs.com. Available at: http://www.drugs.com.

WebMD. Available at: http://www.webmd.com.

Wible, Jean. *Drug Handbook for Massage Therapists*, Philadelphia: Lippincott Williams and Wilkins, 2009.

5

Beyond the Table: Client Homework and Referring Out

CLIENT HOMEWORK

An essential yet reasonable goal of a successful clinical massage therapy practice is for the client to reach a point of decreased pain, increased range of motion (ROM), a wide variety of stretching capabilities, and increased strength. This goal cannot be met with the therapist's solo efforts, because, ultimately, healing is up to the client. No matter how competent or skilled the therapist is, her accomplishments are minimal during the limited hour she has to work in a session. During the remaining 167 hours of the client's week, he must contribute to his own healing process. Diplomacy and a professional, compassionate approach are helpful ingredients as the therapist nudges her client toward his highest functional level.

The massage therapist can assign homework to her client in complete confidence because of the tools she gained during her massage therapy education. She takes the following knowledge "off the page" to create gentle yet effective homework assignments:

- Muscle origin, insertion, and innervation
- Joint "end-feel"
- Passive and active ROM exercises
- Lung and diaphragm function
- Musculoskeletal frame normal alignment and reasonable ROM of each joint

When this knowledge is combined with an understanding of the pathophysiology of a medical condition, self-care assignments can be given in confidence and with little risk to the client or patient.

Scope of Practice

The massage therapist must be careful not to exceed her level of training in assigning homework to her clients. Her keen awareness of the patient's medical history, combined with her own training, will ensure that no harm is done when she develops a self-care plan. Following are examples of cautions involving seemingly innocuous homework assignments:

- Suggesting to drink more water is usually safe, unless the patient is suffering from heart, lung, or kidney failure.
- Suggesting that a client with a stiff back roll backward on a large exercise ball is appropriate only if the therapist has had extensive training in the use of the exercise ball and if she is sure that the client does not suffer from any spine or disc abnormalities.

- Recommending that a client lift weights at a certain repetition and frequency is appropriate only if the therapist is also an experienced personal trainer or physical therapist (PT).
- Suggesting that a client take any supplements is completely outside the massage therapist's scope of practice.

With the previous precautions in mind, therapists can use a wide range of helpful homework assignments to achieve increased ROM, increased strength and vigor, and decreased pain.

Application of Heat and Cold

Moist heat is far more effective in transmitting warmth to the muscle belly and decreasing hypertonicity than dry heat. A microwaved gel pack, hot water bottle, or warm, moist towel is far more effective in relaxing the muscles than rice packs or beanbags, which merely produce a localized comforting effect. The therapist must never place the source of heat or cold directly on the patient's skin; packs should be wrapped in a pillowcase, for example, or placed over the sheets to protect the skin from burns or excessive reddening. Both heat and cold are usually applied on a specific area of the body before the therapist begins his work.

Heat application is used for the following therapeutic effects:

- To loosen a hypertonic set of muscles
- To relax an agitated patient
- To warm a patient who is chilled
- To increase hyperemia to a body part

The effective use of cold by the massage therapist is limited to the application of a cold pack to help stop a muscle spasm or to prepare a chronically inflamed joint for therapy. Using cold to reduce a fever or to limit a new inflammatory response is beyond the therapist's scope of practice. Cold packs (even just a bag of frozen peas) must be used judiciously, and the use of "ice pops" must be preceded by appropriate training. (Refer to the use of heat and cold in Chapter 2.)

Epsom Salts Baths and Soaks

A timeless and effective aid for sore muscles is the use of Epsom salts. The active ingredient in Epsom salts is magnesium sulfate, a substance found in most of the "healing waters" around the world. It is believed that the salts either "pull toxins out of the muscles" or seep into the muscle belly to aid in muscle function, but there is no clear evidence either way. There is no single recipe for the use of Epsom salts, but a good guideline is to instruct the client to put two heaping cups in a tub, or a half-cup in a bucket or pan, in which he is soaking a foot or hand. The therapist should suggest that the client add the salts to warm (not hot) water and to rinse off the salts after the soak or bath.

It is wise to recommend the use of Epsom salts after the client's first massage and after therapy for a strain, sprain, or mild, chronic joint inflammation. In fact, many therapists offer a plastic sandwich bag filled with Epsom salts as a part of their welcome package for first-time clients. Athletic clients can also use frequent Epsom salts baths or soaks as a regular part of their overall self-care regimen.

Range of Motion

The key to the safe assignment of ROM exercises is for the therapist to understand appropriate joint end-feel and to respect the client's perspective of pain. In a normal, healthy joint, the client painlessly moves the joint to the "end" of the anatomic and functional movement, and there is a slight—again painless—"spring" or "push back" at that point. Examples of the differences in ROM based on function and anatomy are apparent if the therapist thinks of the elbow joint and its natural end-point upon full extension, compared to the wrist with an almost 180-degree movement range.

Stretching

ROM homework assignments are appropriate when the therapist is addressing a client's joint pain that has escalated to the point of compromising and limiting her joint movement, thus placing her at risk for experiencing the pain-spasm-pain cycle, which will then set up new musculoskeletal problems. Recent injuries, such as a fall or car accident, and chronic conditions, such as multiple sclerosis and arthritis, are examples of reasons the therapist assigns extensive (yet often cautious) ROM stretches.

Since these movements can seem quite boring or rigorous, and since the therapist wants client compliance, it is best to include play, humor, or creativity in the assignment. Here are some suggestions for ROM exercises:

- *Hoola hoop:* While being fun, silly, and unique, the use (or the attempted use) of this easily acquired toy helps ROM at the hips, knees, and thoracic spine. It also certainly increases thoracic capacity as the client is busy laughing at herself.
- *ABCs:* While the client traces the entire alphabet in capital letters with any joint in the body, the joint is moved through its full range; the A to Z assignment gives her a beginning, middle, and end-point for her exercises. With a little imagination and humor, ABCs can be performed on any joint from the shoulder to the ankle to the lower jaw (Figures 5-1 and 5-2).
- *Soup can or tennis ball under the foot:* While the client watches TV or reads, she rolls a tennis ball or soup can under the sole of her foot with as much vigor and pressure as she can muster. This technique is especially effective in neuropathies and sensory and balance disorders.
- *Arm wall walking:* While the client either faces the wall or places her hip along the wall, her fingers "crawl" to the highest point she can reach. This exercise is especially effective for any breathing-related or upper extremity restrictions.

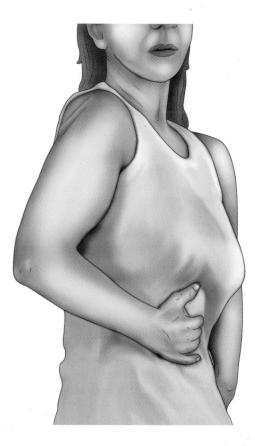

FIGURE 5-1 **Range-of-motion exercises for the shoulder. While the client places her hand on her abdomen, she traces the capital letters from A to Z in the air with her shoulder.**

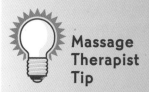

Massage Therapist Tip

Assigning More Homework than You Expect the Client to Perform

For maximum improvement, you may know that your client should perform his assigned homework exercises three times a day for 10 minutes each, for example. But you also know that most people have busy schedules and cannot or will not take the time they need for themselves. A good tip is to assign more homework than you think your client can possibly perform. Don't overwhelm him, but make it clear that your expectation is for him to judiciously take time out every day to work on himself as you have assigned. If he's serious about getting better, he will at least try to do *one set* so he can report back to you that he *did something*. The effort and the mind-set of self-care is what you are trying to teach the client; the number of reps matters less than the fact that he tried and had some success.

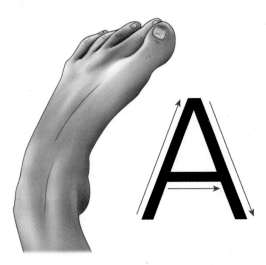

FIGURE 5-2 Range-of-motion exercises for the ankle. Making sure the movement originates at the ankle and not the knee, the client traces the capital letters from A to Z in the air using only her ankle joint.

- *Dancing:* While the client plays her favorite music, she is instructed to simply "let the music move her." Best performed without onlookers, the client is encouraged to move, sway, hop, jostle, wiggle, and stretch her joints.
- *Dish towel over and behind the head:* Holding a dish towel by both ends behind her head and shoulders, the client pulls on one end and then the other, creating a sawing motion and effectively moving the entire shoulder girdle (Figure 5-3).
- *Doorway stretches:* Standing with her feet comfortably spread apart and arms at shoulder height, the client takes a deep breath, leans through the doorway *leading with her chest* as she exhales (Figure 5-4). She reaches a comfortable end-point, takes another breath, and stretches just another inch. If her hands are moved along the doorframe alternatively from shoulder height to 6 inches below and then 6 inches above shoulder height, the entire shoulder girdle and muscles of the thoracic cavity get a highly effective stretch (Figures 5-5 and 5-6).

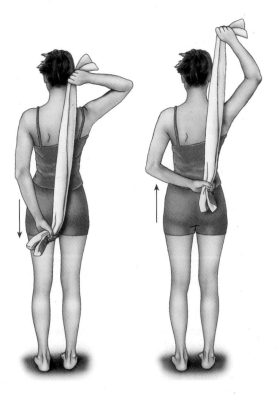

FIGURE 5-3 Dish towel stretch. Holding both ends of the towel over and behind her head, the client alternately pulls each end of the towel until she feels her shoulder blades stretch in each position.

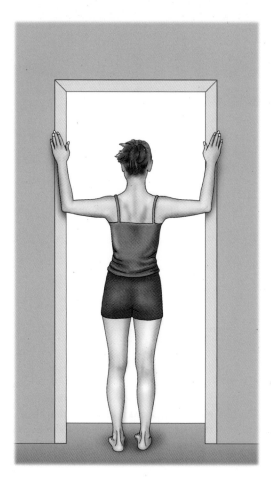

FIGURE 5-4 Doorway stretches. Starting with the arms parallel in the doorframe and the feet evenly spaced, the client exhales as she leans through the door, leading with her chest.

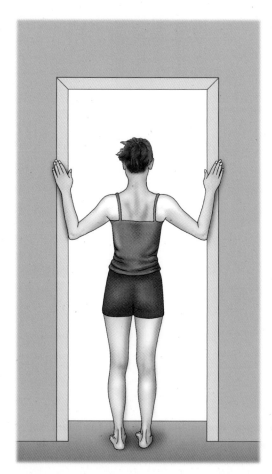

FIGURE 5-5 Doorway stretches. Moving the arms 6 inches below the first position, the client exhales as she leans through the door, leading with her chest.

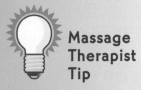

Massage Therapist Tip

True Stretching

Remember that a true stretch moves the joint slightly beyond the normal end-feel and gently past the point of comfort. When your client moves a joint only as far as she comfortably can, it's not a stretch. The true stretch is achieved when she *moves to the point of comfort, takes a big breath, and then moves that joint 1 inch farther than her comfort zone.* It's critical to help your client understand that simply moving the way she's used to is not therapy; it is that extra inch with effort that truly constitutes a stretch.

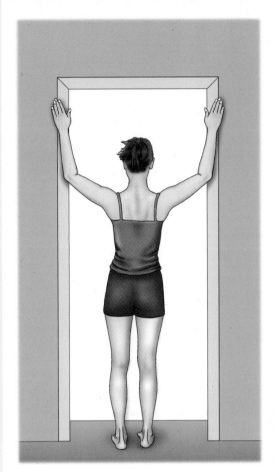

FIGURE 5-6 Doorway stretches. Moving the arms 6 inches higher than the first position, the client exhales as she leans through the door, leading with her chest.

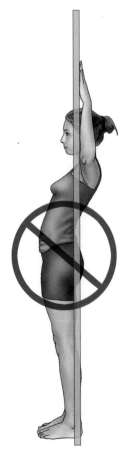

FIGURE 5-7 Doorway stretch, the wrong way. The client is at risk for lumbar spine injury if she leans through the door leading with her pelvis instead of her chest.

Strengthening

Most massage therapists are not trained in strength training. The appropriate use of exercise bands, weights, the medicine ball, and the exercise ball is best left to PTs, physical medicine physicians, personal trainers, and orthopedic surgeons. Strengthening muscles is a vital step toward many patients' complete rehabilitation, so it is a wise massage therapist who creates a working relationship with any of these specialists, for reasons discussed later in the chapter.

However, highly effective gentle strengthening exercises can be given with wisdom and in moderation as the therapist considers her client's condition. Appropriate strengthening exercises include the following:

- Performing biceps curls using a dumbbell (Figure 5-8)
- Doing push-ups while pressing against a wall instead of using the full weight of the body off the floor (Figure 5-9)
- Squeezing a tennis ball intermittently throughout the day
- Doing isometric exercises (pushing the palm of one hand against the palm of another) while standing or sitting

Deep Breathing

Many hospitalized patients eventually die not from their admitting diagnosis but from pneumonia. One of the greatest contributing factors in a cancer patient's demise is pneumonia, for example. Nursing homes are filled with aging people whose relatively robust lifestyle was ended because of a respiratory compromise. The massage therapist must take into account that any condition that restricts the movement of the thoracic cavity or the efficacy of the diaphragm must definitely be addressed with homework exercises. A condition as seemingly simple as the pain-spasm-pain cycle occurring in the rhomboids, combined with the flu season, combined with aging and a weakened immune system can spiral into pneumonia and potentially end a client's life. A massage therapist addresses breathing and its depth, the quality of the inhalations and exhalations, and the vigor with which her clients breathe in every condition she treats.

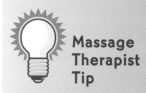
Massage Therapist Tip

Three-Part Deep-Breathing Exercises

There are three parts to effective deep-breathing exercises. Ask your client to inhale through her nose as deeply as she possibly can. You should see her chest and/or abdomen move. Then tell her to hold her breath for a few seconds, perhaps to the count of three. Then instruct her to "exhale with as much force as you can through your mouth, really blow it all out." In asking her for this final forced exhalation, she is literally moving the diaphragm up against the bottom of the lungs, helping to empty and stimulate this important organ. This should be a vigorous process, and if the client says she "feels a little light-headed," congratulate her for doing the exercise properly.

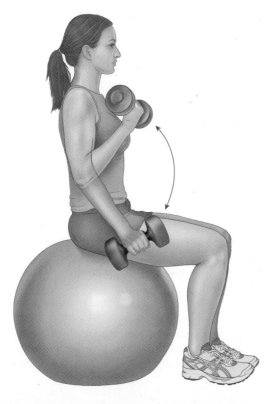

FIGURE 5-8 **Easy biceps curl. Holding a dumbbell and sitting in a comfortable position, the client curls her arm toward her chest and then extends it down toward her knee.**

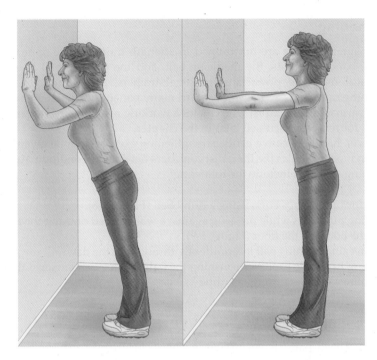

FIGURE 5-9 **Wall push-ups. With hands at shoulder height and standing a comfortable distance away from the wall, the client attempts to touch her nose to the wall and then pushes away from the wall, using only the strength of her arms.**

Again, humor and creativity contribute to patient compliance. Although physical movement is ideal to accompany deep breathing, these exercises can be performed by the weakened or bedridden patient as well:

- Add a "memory tag" to deep-breathing exercises; for example, instruct your patient to perform her breathing exercises whenever she stops at a red light while driving or using the bathroom.
- Purchase several bags of balloons, and give your patient an entire bag. (Helium balloons are best because they are harder to inflate.) Her assignment is to blow up (and allow to deflate for reuse) 10 balloons per day.
- Purchase toy flutes or harmonicas, and instruct your patient to play one of the instruments as loudly as possible frequently throughout the day.
- Instruct your patient to inhale as deeply as he can, then, holding his breath, "beat his chest like Tarzan" before exhaling forcefully.

Purposeful Walking

Simple walking can be a stretching, strengthening, ROM, and breathing exercise. It is a sublimely powerful mind-body activity that can restore confidence and strength to an otherwise enfeebled patient. The instructions are simple: The patient is told to walk as often and as far as she can every day; outdoors is preferable, but around the living room or just to the driveway mailbox will do. The walking must be done "with purpose": The head is up, the shoulders squared, the gait slightly longer than normal, and breathing is as deep as the patient can tolerate.

The effectiveness of this exercise cannot be overestimated. Patients living with chronic pain or lifelong illnesses begin to "cave into themselves," looking to the ground rather than ahead while walking. They stop swinging their arms during their gait and slowly increase the pain-spasm-pain cycle as they lose thoracic capacity, balance, and self-confidence. Purposeful walking can help reverse these tendencies.

REFERRING OUT: THE THERAPIST AS PART OF THE HEALTH CARE TEAM

There may come a time during a client's care and treatment when goals are not being met, improvement is minimal, ROM is not increasing, or pain is not decreasing. At this point, it is essential to refer out to another massage therapist or a health care practitioner in a related field. Because most people with neuromuscular problems also experience compromised joints or a spinal column issue, it is very helpful for the massage therapist to develop a working relationship with a trusted chiropractor or PT. Responsible, resourceful massage therapists surround themselves with like-minded professionals with whom they communicate regularly. This networking not only provides a resource for the massage therapist, but it also becomes a link to further care when it is time to refer out. For the massage therapist, referrals can be made to the following practitioners and specialists:

- PT
- Personal trainer
- Yoga instructor
- Registered dietitian
- Chiropractor
- Orthopedic specialist
- Physical medicine physician
- Psychotherapist
- Spiritual counselor
- Hospice physician

Referring out, however, *does not necessarily discontinue the massage therapist's care*. In fact, at this point, she may become one of several professionals caring for her client; in effect, she becomes part of a health care team. Some pragmatic ethical and professional practices can lubricate this new professional relationship. The massage therapist must:

- Receive written permission from the client to share information with the health care professional to whom she is referring
- Summarize her SOAP notes for a concise reporting to the referring physician or health care professional
- Maintain an active role in her client's care by communicating professionally yet frequently with the other professionals involved in her client's care
- Realize when it is time to discontinue massage therapy and relinquish further care to another professional who is achieving better results

Here are some guidelines for knowing when it is time to refer to another health care professional or massage therapist with advanced training:

- If the massage therapist has treated the client *once a week, every week, for 2 months*, the client is compliant and has performed all self-care assignments, and there is no improvement, it is time to refer out.
- If the client complains of pain during the performance of her homework assignment, she should stop the work immediately; the therapist should reassess the assigned self-care, and if pain persists, refer out.
- If the therapist realizes she is unqualified to treat a client who is taking multiple medications, has chronic unrelenting pain, and complains of several concurrent physical problems, refer out.
- If a client comes for massage therapy complaining of acute pain following a car accident or stroke, for example, refer out.
- If a client suffers from unrelenting, acute headaches of unknown origin, refer out.
- If a client is being treated for cancer and is receiving chemotherapy or radiation, refer out. (Cancer patients can definitely receive massage therapy, but only by therapists with specialized training.)

RESOURCES FOR HOMEWORK ASSIGNMENTS

Within the scope of this text, it's not possible to list all the possible self-care assignments that might be helpful for treating the health and medical conditions in Part II. Short homework assignments are suggested, but dozens more options are available to the massage therapist. The following Bibliography includes resources for safe and effective client self-care. It is, by no means, an exhaustive list, but it's a useful starting point.

IN SUMMARY

When a massage therapist takes on the responsibility of helping to treat medical conditions, she turns from performing solely as a therapist to becoming a cheerleader and advocate for her client, as well as an active member of a health care team. In that role, the therapist:

- Works carefully within her scope of practice while offering beneficial homework assignments
- Refers out to other, more advanced massage therapists or other health care professionals if she reaches a point of declining effectiveness in meeting her clients' goals
- Develops a professional network that serves as a professional resource for both herself and her clients
- Relinquishes care (and a summary of her documentation) for the good of her client's long-term success when she deems her work is no longer effective

The therapist can now move with confidence from reviewing her fundamental knowledge to actually using her skills to practice specific protocols.

Review

1. Describe a clinical scenario in which a massage therapist would assign the application of cold as a homework assignment.
2. Describe a clinical scenario in which a massage therapist would assign the application of heat as a homework assignment.
3. Demonstrate the doorway stretch.
4. When is a true stretch achieved?
5. Why is deep breathing an important homework assignment for many clients?
6. Give several examples of how a client might perform deep-breathing exercises during the day.
7. When is it appropriate to refer a client out to another health care professional or therapist?

BIBLIOGRAPHY

Anderson DL. *Muscle Pain Relief in 90 Seconds: The Fold and Hold Method by Dale L. Anderson, M.D.,* New York: John Wiley & Sons, Inc., 1995.

Creager CC. *Therapeutic Exercises Using the Swiss Ball,* Bolder, CO: *Executive Physical Therapy,* 1994.

Deason S. Balance Ball Fitness with Suzanne Deason (Tape and DVD). Living Arts. Four to a series: Beginners, Upper Body Workout, Abs Workout, Lower Body Workout. *Gaiam* 2002.

Natural Relief from Back and Muscular Pain: The Kates Method (DVD). Available at: www.katesmethod.com.

Miller OH. *The Stretch Deck: 50 Stretches,* San Francisco: Chronicle Books, 2002. Available at: www.chroniclebooks.com.

Weinert J, Bielawski J. *Stretching for Health: Your Handbook for Ultimate Wellness, Longevity, and Productivity,* Chicago: Contemporary Books, 2000.

Step-by-Step Massage Therapy Protocols

Ankylosing Spondylosis

Definition: A chronic, systemic inflammatory disease of the axial skeleton joints, characterized by pain and progressive stiffening of the spine.

GENERAL INFORMATION

- Etiology (cause or origin) unknown
- Chronic multisystem inflammatory condition; considered in the group of spondyloarthropathies (multisystem inflammatory disorders affecting the axial skeleton, the bones of the head, spine, sacrum, coccyx, and thoracic cage)
- Onset usually late adolescence to early adulthood
- Genetic predisposition
- Prevalence in males

Morbidity and Mortality

Exacerbations (temporary worsening of symptoms) and remissions (temporary lessening of symptoms) are common with this condition. The prognosis is good, especially with early diagnosis and ongoing management. Patients can live a productive, if limited, life, and they often continue to work following a diagnosis of ankylosing spondylosis.

A common nonskeletal concern is iritis (inflammation of the colored portion of the eye). The skeletal complications include an increased risk of spinal fracture, reduced lung volume, and in severe cases, spinal fixation in a flexed position. At this stage, the patient is unable to stand upright, lift his head, or look forward. Balance is compromised and accidents occur frequently.

PATHOPHYSIOLOGY

Ankylosing spondylosis typically begins at the sacroiliac joints with cephalic (toward the head) progression; hip and shoulder joints are affected less commonly, while peripheral joints are affected least of all. Inflammation occurs at the sites along the spine where the tendon and ligament attach to bone. This inflammation causes damage and erosion of vertebral bone tissue, leading to fusion of the spine.

Although the etiology is unknown, the presence of large macrophages (white blood cells that destroy foreign cells in the body) during the acute stage indicates a probable autoimmune response. Fibrosis, calcification, ossification (tissue turning into bone, in this case, abnormally), and stiffening of the joints are common.

The inflammatory nature of this disease is not isolated to bone and may spread to major organs, including the eyes, lungs, heart, and kidneys.

OVERALL SIGNS AND SYMPTOMS

- Chronic low-back pain extending into the buttocks and down to the heels, especially upon rising

- Increased pain with inactivity and decreased pain with movement or a hot shower
- Pain worst at rest, reduced by mild activity
- Swelling and tenderness at tendon and ligament insertions along the spine
- Reduced lateral flexion (bending to one side)
- Fatigue resulting from pain, stiffness, and decreased functionality
- Hyperkyphotic changes (abnormal posterior curvature of the spine) from fusion in cervical and thoracic regions, leading to limited ability to ambulate and look straight ahead
- Labored breathing and chest tightness from decreased thoracic range of motion (ROM) and limited expansion from costovertebral (rib-to-spine) joint movement
- Decreased temporomandibular joint (TMJ) ROM and increased pain in 10% of cases
- Immobilization of spine in late stages

SIGNS AND SYMPTOMS MASSAGE THERAPY CAN ADDRESS

- Because living with ankylosing spondylosis demands a constant repositioning of the cervical and thoracic spine, as well as an altered forward-bending walking gait, both of which produce low-back and buttocks pain, the therapist can work to relieve muscle stiffness at multiple sites.
- The pain associated with kyphotic changes that lead to stiffness due to decreased costovertebral joint ROM—if treated in early stages—can be addressed with massage therapy.
- The therapist can significantly help increase the restricted breathing patterns often associated with this condition, thereby reducing the risk of pneumonia.

TREATMENT OPTIONS

Therapeutic exercises to help maintain motion, combined with strengthening exercises to work the involved spinal extensor muscles, can be directed by a physical therapist (PT). Heat application in the form of a hot shower or hot packs can be used by the patient himself or anyone involved in his care. Swimming is excellent because of the lack of joint impact. Although pain and fatigue may lead to stasis, immobilization is not recommended, and regular lifelong exercise should be the mainstay of any therapeutic program.

Patients are strongly encouraged to maintain healthy weight, to avoid smoking, and to perform daily diaphragmatic breathing exercises.

Although there is no cure, the previous treatments and the following medications can help control symptoms and minimize the worsening of the condition.

Common Medications

- Nonsteroidal anti-inflammatory drugs (NSAIDs), such as ibuprofen (Motrin, Advil) and naproxen (Aleve, Anaprox, Naprelan, Naprosyn)
- Salicylate nonopioid pain relievers, such as aspirin (Ecotrin, Empirin, Astrin)

MASSAGE THERAPIST ASSESSMENT

The therapist must obtain an official diagnosis from the patient's physician before beginning treatment. In addition, treatment is more beneficial if, with the patient's permission, any written reports from CT scans, MRIs, or X-rays are made available to the massage therapist to help her understand the extent of the condition. (These

Thinking It Through

Because ankylosing spondylosis affects many aspects of the patient's life, the therapist must look at the whole person. To achieve the best possible outcome from massage therapy, the therapist can tactfully ask the patient about certain areas of his life.

- If he is overweight, I can recommend a dietitian to help him begin a weight-loss program.
- If he smokes, I can anatomically show how lung capacity is already compromised because of his condition, and offer information about a program to quit smoking.
- If the patient suffers from depression, I can expect to see antidepressant medication on the intake form, and I can gently suggest counseling.

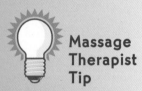

Massage Therapist Tip

Structuring—Not Removing—the Art of Massage

The step-by-step protocols in this book include suggested time durations, in addition to the use of specific techniques. As you come to know your patient's body and tolerances and what works and what doesn't, you can alter the suggested times and techniques. If you are trained in the use of other techniques and modalities, you can use every skill in your toolkit to treat patients. The protocols are presented as a springboard for starting your work.

documents are reasonable for the therapist to request and are kept confidentially in the patient's chart.)

The entire first session consists of the massage therapist's assessment, combined with patient education as the therapist and patient determine joint goals. To begin, the therapist performs gentle ROM assessments of the patient's cervical, thoracic, and lumbar spine, including lateral bending ability or limitations. Limitations and pain experienced by the patient during these movements are carefully noted. Charting should be very specific, and the use of the 0–10 pain scale is an excellent monitor of progress. If a goniometer is used (a plastic, hinged measuring device used more typically by PTs to determine degrees of joint movement), the massage therapist records ranges; if not, she estimates degrees of movement with the patient's help.

The patient takes several deep breaths while the therapist notes appropriate diaphragmatic movement (the shoulders should be relaxed, and the abdomen might extend slightly during inhalation). However, if the patient's shoulders elevate sharply during the inhalation, and if the therapist notes muscles of the neck and upper chest are involved during the inhalation, the patient is using secondary (inefficient) muscles of breathing. This indicates there is much work to be done by both the patient and the therapist.

If the patient is experiencing any vision problems or TMJ pain, he should be referred to his physician, but the therapist's work can continue.

The therapist asks the patient to lie on the table supine, prone, and side-lying, determining which position is most comfortable, which one produces labored breathing, which causes pain, and so on. Because positioning can be a major source of either discomfort or relaxation, positioning challenges should be charted for future reference, and plenty of pillows should be kept on hand.

Finally, the therapist inquires about the patient's activities of daily living (ADLs), such as brushing his teeth, getting dressed, tying his shoes, and driving. She can ask if he currently exercises. The therapist asks about the patient's profession, whether his condition affects his work, if he experiences pain during the day, and how often he might be able to perform regular stretching exercises.

THERAPEUTIC GOALS

There are two primary therapeutic goals for patients with ankylosing spondylosis: maintaining mobility and increasing lung capacity. Secondary goals are maintaining proper posture, positioning, and ROM. Alleviating as much localized pain as possible, of course, accompanies all goals.

MASSAGE SESSION FREQUENCY

Ankylosing spondylosis is a complicated condition with multiple joint and systemic manifestations; it is therefore not possible to treat *every* symptom at *every* session. This patient will present with different complaints each time. It is important to address his greatest concerns, remembering that increased lung capacity and overall mobility are paramount.

- Ideally: 60-minute sessions twice a week
- Minimally: 60-minute sessions once a week
- Infrequent, inconsistent therapy will not be effective

MASSAGE PROTOCOL

It may be difficult to imagine the effects of a condition that slowly and insidiously forces the spine to bend forward. However, your effective treatment of a person who has ankylosing spondylosis depends on your understanding of the pain caused by the infinitesimal daily muscle adjustments necessary to live with this condition.

To understand how ankylosing spondylosis affects your patient, you may choose to perform the following exercise: Slightly hunch your shoulders and angle your torso so you are leaning about 3 inches more forward than you normally walk. Now try to go about your usual daily routine—shopping, bending, and twisting—in this position. It will soon become obvious that compensating muscles of much of the rest of the body can easily be thrown into the pain-spasm-pain cycle by maintaining this position.

Getting Started

Side-lying is usually the preferred position for treating patients with ankylosing spondylosis. Pillow and bolster appropriately to maintain spinal alignment. Although this position presents a body mechanics challenge for you, the massage therapist, it is often more comfortable for the patient because of his compromised breathing and extensive spinal changes.

With the patient lying on one side, cervical spine supported with a pillow, arms supported by "hugging" another pillow, and another pillow between knees to the ankles, the protocol that follows is based on working muscles nearest you, those that are not lying on the table. You will turn the patient over to repeat the same sequence on the other side of the body.

You can lay a hot pack on the patient's back as you perform your preparatory strokes and/or throughout the entire sequence.

HOMEWORK

Give weekly written self-care instructions according to your patient's tolerance. Challenge him, but don't overtax his ability. Pick and choose from the following items over your weeks of care, and he will find his favorites. Impress upon your patient the importance of self-care and the fact that his consistent therapy will help slow the inevitable progression of this disease.

Although ankylosing spondylosis is a serious condition, humor and an element of play can contribute much-needed levity to your approach to his self-care. Homework assignments can include the following:

- "Tarzan" is a silly but helpful exercise. Beat your chest with lightly clenched fists while humming as loudly as you can (preferably not in public). This increases the exhalation of dormant air, increases lung capacity, and is just silly enough for you to remember to perform daily.
- Do deep breathing, four breaths at a time, three times a day, every day. Raise your arms overhead while inhaling deeply; hold the breath for a few seconds, and then forcibly exhale while bringing your arms back down to your sides.
- Bending your arms at the elbows, try to touch your elbows behind you. Hold for 30 seconds, head up, looking straight forward, not at the floor, then release.
- Either in bed, in the shower, or anytime during the day, perform gentle ROM exercises of every joint in your body. With a little thought, most of the exercises can be performed while driving, while sitting at a desk, while in the bathroom, or while on the phone. Be creative, be a "belly dancer," or use a hoola hoop to keep the lumbar spine supple.
- One of the most effective and simple exercises is the doorway stretch (Figure 6-1). Place one hand on either side of any doorway, stand in the doorway, legs shoulder-width apart. As you exhale, gently lean through the doorway, *leading with your chest*. When you're all the way through the door, inhale and exhale to your maximum capacity one more time. Then return to your starting position in the doorway. This stretch not only helps increase lung capacity, but it also stretches most of the chest and back muscles. (Refer to Figures 5-4, 5-5, and 5-6 for more doorway stretches.)

Contraindications and Cautions:

- Because ankylosing spondylosis is an inflammatory disease and can spread during the acute, inflamed stage (when the patient is in extreme pain, may have a fever of 100.5°F or higher, and medications are not easing the pain as usual), perform massage therapy with caution only during the subacute stage (no active signs of fever or increased pain). You must develop an ongoing professional relationship with the patient's physician or health care team and become comfortable asking about symptomatic flare-ups.

- Spinal fracture is a complication of ankylosing spondylosis, especially in the cervical spine. Any recent trauma or unusual increase in neck or back pain signals a referral to a physician.

- Unusual *increases* in movement or changes in spinal position may indicate a spinal fracture and also signal a physician referral.

Step-by-Step Protocol for Ankylosing Spondylosis

Technique	Duration
Greet the patient's body with general warming compression. (The patient is side-lying.) • Use this time to evaluate tissue and the patient's response to your touch. • Note any differences from previous treatment.	3 minutes
Effleurage, medium pressure, evenly rhythmic • Anterior, lateral, posterior thoracic region Digital muscle stripping, medium pressure, evenly rhythmic • Intercostal muscles • Work anterior, lateral, and posterior intercostals from the sternum to the posterior thoracic vertebrae • Include serratus anterior muscles, pectoralis major and minor • Watch your body mechanics; walk around the table to get at the rib cage effectively without hurting your wrists or back	5 minutes
Kneading, medium pressure, evenly rhythmic • Pectoralis major and minor • Transverse abdominis • Quadratus lumborum Digital diaphragm kneading, working as if you are trying to move that muscle away from the bottom ribs	5 minutes
Rocking, gentle, rhythmic • Thoracic cavity while the patient slowly and evenly breathes deeply • During inhalations, instruct him to stretch his arm over his head near his ear. • During exhalations, instruct him to stretch his arm as far behind himself as he can. Four inhalations and exhalations in this position. (Be careful, this will be difficult work for him; don't let him overexert.)	2 minutes
Fist or forearm kneading, evenly rhythmic, medium pressure • Gluteal muscles with pressure working medially (down toward the table, if side-lying) toward the sacroiliac joint Kneading, medium pressure, evenly rhythmic • Proximal hamstring muscles that insert up under the gluteal muscles	5 minutes
Digital kneading, medium pressure, evenly rhythmic • Sacrum, all the way from the coccyx (ask the patient's permission before working in this area) to the sacroiliac joint Finish with large kneading strokes and effleurage of the gluteal complex.	3 minutes

(continued)

Technique	Duration
Digital kneading, medium pressure • Every vertebrae starting at L-5 and working to C-2, as high as you can palpate • Work cephalically (toward the head) with medium digital pressure into the laminar grooves. Pay great attention to detail. • Follow with rhythmic light effleurage to the spine.	5 minutes
Effleurage, rhythmic, pressure to tolerance • Erector spinae complex and entire back, working off onto the posterior deltoid	5 minutes
Carefully turn the patient over and repeat the protocol on the other side. End the massage with soothing techniques, such as slow-stroke back massage, stroking the legs, quietly placing your hand on a body part, or a gentle head massage.	
Additional steps in your protocol can include the following, per your patient's request: • Medium pressure effleurage, petrissage, kneading, and final effleurage to the lower extremities • Digital kneading to the TMJ muscles • Head massage and digital kneading at the occipital ridge (for relaxation)	

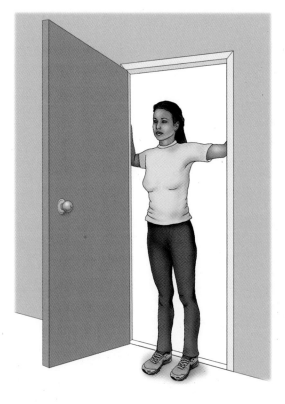

FIGURE 6-1 **The doorway stretch. Placing her hands on the two sides of the doorway, the patient exhales while leaning through the doorway leading with her chest, inhales and exhales to her maximum capacity, and then returns to her starting position.**

- Hot showers can provide relief, and hot packs can be used at work or at home. (Hot rice packs or beanbags are not effective; the heat must be moist.)
- Every time you get into your car, place your right arm behind the passenger seat and look into the back seat as far as you can stretch, holding it for 30 seconds. Your physical limitations may make you a driving hazard, and you need to be able to look over your shoulder quickly and painlessly.

Review Questions

1. What are some of the signs and symptoms of ankylosing spondylosis?
2. Besides the musculoskeletal system, what other body systems may be affected by this condition?
3. What is one primary goal of your therapeutic sessions with an ankylosing spondylosis patient?
4. What is a secondary goal in your therapy?
5. Is infrequent therapy effective? If not, why not?

BIBLIOGRAPHY

Brent LH, Kalagate R. Ankylosing Spondylitis. EMedicine article. Updated November 3, 2009. Available at: http://emedicine.medscape.com/article/332945-diagnosis. Accessed April 1, 2010.

Porth MP. *Pathophysiology: Concepts of Altered Health States*, 7th ed. Baltimore: Lippincott Williams & Wilkins, 2005:1425–1427.

WebMD, Healthwise, Inc. *Medication to reduce pain and stiffness in ankylosing spondylitis.* May 14, 2009. Available at: http://arthritis.webmd.com/tc/ankylosing-spondylitis-treatment-overview. Accessed April 1, 2010.

7

Bell's Palsy

Definition: A motor paralysis of cranial nerve VII, the facial nerve, affecting one side of the face.

GENERAL INFORMATION

- Direct cause unknown; correlations with respiratory infections, viral infections, stress, trauma, previous diagnosis of cold sore or fever blister, previous diagnosis of shingles
- Usually sudden onset without warning
- Unilateral condition
- Temporary condition, lasting from 1 week to 3 months
- Men and women equally affected

Morbidity and Mortality

More than 40,000 people in the U.S. are affected. The annual incidence is about 23–25 cases in 100,000 people. The prognosis is good; 80–90% of patients recover with no noticeable facial disfigurement. The rate of recurrence is 10–15%, in the same or the opposite side of the face.

PATHOPHYSIOLOGY

The facial nerve, which is affected by Bell's palsy, travels from the brain to a wide area of muscles in the face (Figure 7-1). This nerve controls the movement of the eyelids, the muscles around the mouth, and the muscles for tearing (eyes), chewing, and facial expression, among other actions.

Paralysis of the facial nerve is believed to result from either edema (swelling) or ischemia (temporary reduced blood flow), both of which compress the nerve against bony areas in the base of the skull where it travels from the brain to the muscles of the face. The reason for the presence of edema and/or ischemia continues to be the subject of debate.

There are usually no warning signs or symptoms. However, similar symptoms may be caused by a stroke or tumor. Therefore, the final appropriate diagnosis of Bell's palsy must be made by a physician to rule out more serious conditions.

OVERALL SIGNS AND SYMPTOMS

- Self-discovery upon waking: wet pillow from salivation (drooling), a drooping eyelid, sagging mouth, crooked smile, and an inability to completely close the eyelid
- Weakness or paralysis of one entire side of the face
- Pain around the ear on the affected side
- Inability to taste foods or a disturbance in normal taste

Thinking It Through

Before the therapist begins working on the face and eyes of any client, she must ask herself some practical questions:

- Does she wear contact lenses?
- Does she have dentures?
- Does she have any facial implants or internal fixations that should not be massaged directly?

The massage for Bell's palsy, although it begins lightly, ultimately moves "to the bone" with deep work that is highly stimulating. The therapist must be sure the client's face can safely tolerate the work.

Since the face often represents a person's sense of self-esteem and privacy, and can carry a history of abuse, it is important at the beginning of the therapeutic relationship to build trust with the client. During the initial interview, the therapist might ask:

- How do you feel about this change in your face?
- May I ask if you will be able to tolerate therapy on your face for about 30 minutes?
- Do you understand this is usually a temporary condition and that it will pass?
- Do you understand that we'll take this therapy at your pace, and we'll sit back and relax at any time?
- Do you think you'll be comfortable massaging your own face and helping me along in this process?

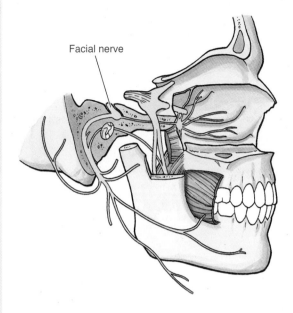

FIGURE 7-1 **The facial nerve, or cranial nerve VII. The facial nerve travels from the brain to a wide area of muscles in the face, and controls movements of the eyelids, the muscles around the mouth, and the muscles for tearing (eyes), chewing, and facial expression, among other actions. From Moore KL, Agur AMR.** *Essential Clinical Anatomy,* **2nd ed. Baltimore: Lippincott Williams & Wilkins, 2002.**

- Acute sensitivity to sound
- Inability to create normal facial expressions of eyebrow crinkling, smiling, squinting, and pursing lips
- Decreased tearing; susceptibility to corneal abrasion and dryness of the eye
- Drooling from decreased control of the muscles inside, outside, and around the mouth

SIGNS AND SYMPTOMS MASSAGE THERAPY CAN ADDRESS

- Given the transient nature of this muscular paralysis, the massage therapist can affect the condition of the facial muscles upon their return to normal functioning, but not the duration of the disorder.
- Although addressing salivation, tearing, corneal abrasion, acute hearing, and taste disturbances is beyond the massage therapist's scope of practice, every facial muscle affected by Bell's palsy—and all muscles on the opposite, unaffected side of the face—can be treated to reduce hypertonicity (muscle tightness), increase range of motion (ROM), and decrease hypotonicity (decreased muscle tone).
- Because of the understandable psychological impact of temporary facial disfigurement, the therapist can significantly help reduce the client's general stress level by performing both Swedish massage and the suggested treatment protocol.

TREATMENT OPTIONS

Because the condition is usually short-lived and the efficacy of medication continues to be debatable, treatment is often conservative and based on symptoms. Eye drops can prevent corneal damage; wearing an eye patch at night protects the eye; the client is advised to try to reduce her stress level.

Common Medications

- Adrenocorticosteroids, such as prednisone (Deltasone, Orasone, Meticorten)
- Antivirals, such as acyclovir (Zovirax)

MASSAGE THERAPIST ASSESSMENT

It is critical for the massage therapist not to proceed with client care until both stroke and tumor have been ruled out. Once the physician has made a clear diagnosis of Bell's palsy, the massage therapist performs a very simple assessment. Since conditions of the face carry a psychological component, the first massage therapy session focuses on reinforcing that the condition is temporary, and that the combined efforts of the client and therapist will probably return the client's facial muscles to normal. Warmth, compassion, humor, and hope are important components of the first assessment appointment.

With the client fully clothed and seated directly in front of the therapist, the client performs a normal set of facial ROM movements. *The therapist performs the requested movements along with the client.* Because of the location and size of the facial muscles, it is difficult to measure or assess their ROM. Instead, the therapist records the notable limitations of the unilateral muscles on the affected side compared to the muscles on the contralateral (opposite) unaffected side of the face. Movements include the following:

- Wrinkling the forehead
- Blinking the eye
- Wiggling the nose
- Squinting
- Puckering the lips
- Smiling
- Frowning
- Grimacing

THERAPEUTIC GOALS

Since there is a good chance that, left untreated, Bell's palsy would resolve in time, the massage therapist is in the unique position of being able to (1) help hasten the facial muscles' return to normal ROM and tone, (2) help ensure that the flaccid muscles' return to normal is not accompanied by disfigurement, and (3) provide a hopeful and humorous companion for the client's often frustrating return to normalcy. The therapist's goals reflect those of the client: to regain normal use and movement of the facial muscles with as little remaining disfigurement as possible.

MASSAGE SESSION FREQUENCY

- 60-minute sessions twice a week for the first 2 weeks
- 60-minute sessions once a week until complete recovery
- Exercise sessions performed twice a day by the client alone

MASSAGE PROTOCOL

After the initial assessment session, during which you write extensive SOAP notes, explain to your client why you will be working on both the affected and unaffected sides of her face. Explain that the affected side needs stimulation, increased circulation, and venous drainage, and the unaffected side is hypertonic from compensating and needs the same therapy. Finish this first session with some relaxation techniques in order to reduce the client's stress level and accustom her to your touch.

Since the facial muscles are not accustomed to deep therapy, your early therapeutic sessions will last about 15 minutes. Do not start with extensive and deep

Thinking It Through *(cont.)*

An understanding of the face's muscular anatomy is essential for the best therapeutic outcome in treating Bell's palsy. Sloppy or general work will result in a relaxed face, but not a face in which every muscle set has benefited from massage therapy. The therapist must visualize exactly what she is doing as she works by thinking, for example:

- Where does the masseter muscle begin and end? Can I find the anterior edge by slowly dragging my fingers anterior to posterior on the mandible?
- When working the temporomandibular joint (TMJ), am I following the zygomatic arch all the way to the base of the nose and then back to just in front of the ear?
- When I'm working the orbital ridge, am I being careful to stay on the outside edge and not invade the soft tissue or nerves of the orbit?
- Am I willing to work deeply to the client's tolerance without letting my own personal "face agenda" interfere with the work?

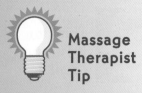

Massage Therapist Tip

Massaging Your Own Face

To overcome your own hesitation about working on a client's facial muscles too deeply, practice on your face first. Start by placing your fingertips on the zygomatic arch. Now make small circles using medium pressure. Increase your pressure until you can feel the bone beneath the skin and muscles. Continue working to this depth for 1 minute. Work slowly and with focus. Try to feel the contour of the bone and feel the muscle moving over the bone. When you remove your hands, your face will feel a slight tingling sensation that's quite pleasant. Move to various parts of your face, and repeat this process. No harm has been done. This exercise can help you overcome any hesitancy about working as deeply as you need to in effectively treating Bell's palsy.

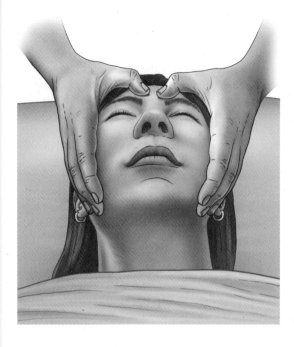

FIGURE 7-2 **Gently cradle the client's face at the beginning of this protocol.**

facial massage. Each session will include some form of relaxation massage that will consume the appropriate remaining time of your 60-minute session. Ask the client what might relax her; you might massage the hands, feet, shoulders, or abdomen. Your ultimate goal will be 30-minute sessions focused solely on the muscles of the face.

Remember, the face is "private property," and many people hold personal agendas associated with issues of the face. Approach the face with extreme care and tenderness, being careful to "invade" as little as possible. Figure 7-2 is one example of how the face can be carefully cradled before beginning the protocol.

Getting Started

As fragile, small, and circuitous as they are, the facial muscles can be stimulated and stretched, drained of and refreshed with blood, just like any other muscles of the body. Study a good diagram of the nerves, muscles, and bones of the face, and imagine these structures under your hands as you work with a gentle yet firm technique. Work to your client's tolerance—not to your level of discomfort or preconceived notion of how much pressure the muscles of the face can tolerate.

While treating conditions involving only the face and neck, it is advisable for the client to disrobe only to the extent necessary for your work. In this case, she need only remove her blouse; drape appropriately. Position your client comfortably supine (laying on her back, face up). The absence of a pillow makes it easier for you to perform your work, but the client's comfort is paramount. Seat yourself at the client's head for most of this protocol. Remember these guidelines:

- Clean hands, short fingernails, and no jewelry are essential.
- Do not use lubricant.
- Your hands must be scent-free.
- After massaging the muscles of the scalp, rewash your hands before returning to work on the face.

You will spend no more than 30 minutes focused on the facial muscles, with the remaining 30 minutes dedicated to relaxation techniques per your client's request.

Step-by-Step Protocol for Bell's Palsy

Technique	Duration
Place your hands on either side of the client's face as if to embrace it. Rest here for a moment before beginning your therapy. No pressure, just simple presence.	1 minute
Compression, light pressure, using your whole hand • Both sides of the face • Covering every inch of the face from the hairline to underneath the mandible	1 minute
Digital kneading, medium pressure, circling clockwise and counterclockwise • Entire forehead from the hairline to above the brows • Both sides of the forehead, including the temple region • Do not engage the hair or scalp (cross-contamination risk when you return to the face)	2 minutes
Digital kneading, medium pressure, circling toward the chest; small, slow circles • Work down the lateral perimeter of the face, from the temples to the medial, anterior mandible Repeat the sequence twice.	2 minutes
Digital kneading, medium pressure; tiny, slow circles performed with finger pads, not fingertips • Entire bilateral bony ridges of the orbit • Do not invade the soft tissue near the eyeball; stay on the bony ridge.	1 minute
Digital kneading; slow, small circles; medium-to-deep pressure (This is the first time "deep" pressure is applied: "go for the bone" to the client's tolerance; this work must be deep to be effective.) • Bilateral zygomatic arches • Work out to the TMJ and in to about 0.5 inch lateral to the nose	1 minute
Digital kneading, using finger pads; slow, small circles • Maxilla region below the nose (the mustache ridge) • Do not invade the nose or the mouth or touch the upper lip	1 minute
Digital kneading, using finger pads; slow, larger circles; medium-to-deep pressure • From the TMJ to the anterior middle of the maxilla	1 minute
Stop a moment. Stroke the entire face using both open hands simultaneously, moving from the midline of the face to the lateral hairline. Finish this resting period with soft compression of the entire face. Ask the client how she is doing. Reconfirm comfortable positioning.	
Digital kneading, a little faster but still very smooth; larger, deeper circles on the entire surface of the face. • From the hairline to mandible, from the base of the nose to the TMJ, all cheek muscles; include the maxilla region	2 minutes

Contraindications and Cautions:

- Do not proceed with this therapy until stroke and tumor have been ruled out by a physician.
- Bell's palsy clients experience good days and bad days based on swelling, discomfort, acute hearing, lack of sleep, eye pain or discomfort, side effects of medications, and self-image. Do not perform therapy if the face is extremely sensitive or if the client is experiencing pain. *As in all massage therapies, "no pain, no gain" is not our motto, and it certainly applies to work on the face.*
- Do not apply deep pressure near the styloid or mastoid processes at the lateral bases of the skull during the scalp massage or when positioning the client's head; allow the client's head to rest in midline, with little pressure to the base of the skull for most of the treatment. Roll the head from side to side only when absolutely necessary. The facial nerve exits the brain at a small hole near the base of the skull behind the earlobe, and pressure on this area can further inflame or compress an already agitated nerve.

(continued)

Technique	Duration
Pincement or plucking. Quick, light, careful but thorough enough to displace more than superficial tissue • Start at the mandible. • Use the procedure on every part of the face that allows you to grasp a little muscle or skin; even try to engage the small thin muscles of the forehead. • Do not use pincement around the eyes or nose.	2 minutes
ROM and gentle resistance of all facial muscle actions • Ask the client to wrinkle her forehead by raising her eyebrows; return to normal. • Place your fingertips along the superior ridge of the forehead just below the hairline. • While providing very gentle resistance against the movement of the frontal muscle, ask the client to wrinkle her forehead again and gently push against her movement. Return to normal. Repeat 5 times.	2 minutes
Ask the client to close her eyes; ever so gently place two fingertips on her closed eyelids. Apply no pressure to the eyeball. (Make sure she is not wearing contact lenses.) • Ask her to try to open her eyelids while you apply the gentlest of resistance pressure, not allowing the eyelids to open completely, not applying any pressure to the eyeball. Repeat slowly 5 times.	2 minutes
Ask the client to grimace, teeth gritted, mouth slightly open, pulling the platysma (superficial muscle of the neck) very tight. • Massage the entire mandibular ridge with deep, large circles on the bone, while she holds this position.	2 minutes
Allow the client to rest from these exercises, and gently massage the face with large, slow, progressively deeper circles. Stroke the face when the therapy is finished. Massage the superficial muscles of the neck lightly and massage the superior trapezius. (Remember to apply no pressure to the occipital ridge; a contraindication for this work.) You are taking focus away from the face for a moment and allowing the client to take a break.	2 minutes
Scalp massage, deep to tolerance, digital kneading of all muscles of the scalp (being careful not to apply pressure behind the earlobes). End with "scrubbing" the hair by using quick, "washing" movements of the entire surface covered by hair. Be careful not to tug the hair.	4 minutes
Sit the client up on the side of the table and stand in front of her. • Demonstrate (or review) the AEIOU exercises you want her to perform several times throughout the day. • Teach (or review) how to deeply and thoroughly massage every bony ridge of her face and all major muscles. • Teach (or review) the plucking (pincement) of all the muscles of her face. • Teach (or review) how to massage the muscles of her neck.	5 minutes
Inform the client that the therapeutic face work has ended, and ask her which area of her body she would like to have massaged, simply for relaxation, for the remaining 30 minutes.	30 minutes

HOMEWORK

A E I O U

Unlike many self-care assignments that require space, privacy, and the right time of day, one of the most effective exercises your client suffering with Bell's palsy can perform is a simple exaggerated enunciation of the vowels A E I O U. This exercise can be performed anywhere, anytime—although probably not in a crowd or when being observed too closely by coworkers. It is fun and silly enough to add a little humor to this otherwise psychologically devastating temporary condition.

Explain the homework exercise to your client as follows, while demonstrating every move with your own face:

- Remember when you learned the vowels A E I O U in school? I want you to overenunciate each one very slowly while stretching every single muscle in your face and holding the position for several seconds at a time. (*At this point, you demonstrate, so she can see how humorous the exercise can be. Exaggerate each move.*)
- Open your eyes and mouth wide for the "AAAAAAAA."
- Grimace to the point of (feigned) horror and show all your teeth for the "EEEEEEE."
- Open your mouth and eyes wide for the "IIIIIIIII."
- Furrow your brow, pull the muscles tight over your cheekbones, and open your eyes wide for the "OOOOOOOO."
- Purse your lips, thrust your jaw forward, and look devilish for the "UUUUUUU."

Then, place your client in front of a mirror; stand behind her, also looking in the mirror, and ask her to perform the exercises again. She will begin to feel how the stretches affect every muscle of the face and will undoubtedly understand the value of performing this easy exercise frequently throughout the day. If she's performing the exercises correctly, her facial muscles will feel as if she has been working them out.

More Homework Assignments

It is essential that your work be accompanied by exercise sessions the client performs twice a day. In addition to the previous exercises, you can give her the following, which can be done in any combination:

- Purchase a package of helium balloons (they are tougher to inflate), and blow up several throughout the day.
- When washing your hair, apply more than the usual amount of vigor to your entire scalp.
- Allow the water to hit your face for a longer time while showering.
- Splash alternating warm and cold water on your face during the normal face-washing routine.
- Try whistling throughout the day.

Review

1. What are some signs and symptoms of Bell's palsy?
2. Can you begin therapy on this condition without a physician's clearance?
3. What is the condition's typical duration, and is recurrence normal?
4. What is the duration of treatment on the client's face, and which techniques can be used effectively?
5. Name some homework exercises for the client, and explain why self-care is important for this condition.

BIBLIOGRAPHY

Monnell K, Zacharia S. Bell's Palsy. EMedicine. Available at: http://www.emedicine.com/neuro/topic413.htm. Accessed April 1, 2010.

Premkumar K. *Pathology A to Z: A Handbook for Massage Therapists*, 3rd ed. Baltimore: Lippincott Williams & Wilkins, 2010.

Rattray F, Ludwig L. *Clinical Massage Therapy: Understanding, Assessing and Treating over 70 Conditions*, Toronto: Talus Incorporated, 2000.

Werner R. *A Massage Therapist's Guide to Pathology*, 4th ed. Philadelphia: Lippincott Williams & Wilkins, 2009.

8

Bursitis

Definition: Inflammation of a bursa, a small fluid-filled sac that cushions and lubricates the areas in and around joints.

GENERAL INFORMATION

- History of progressively worsening local tenderness; decreased, painful range of motion (ROM); redness or swelling; inflammatory disease, such as rheumatoid arthritis
- Pain lasting from a few days to a few weeks
- General bursitis: secondary to fracture, dislocation, trauma, or tendonitis
- Septic (infective) bursitis: from bacteria introduced into the joint after a traumatic injury or a systemic spread of microorganisms
- Superficial bursitis: over a bone, just beneath the skin (as in prepatellar bursitis); deep bursitis: embedded in the joint, sometimes lodged between complicated joints (as in the multiple bursae located in the shoulder girdle)
- Most common in the elbow, knee, shoulder, and hip

PATHOPHYSIOLOGY

Bursae are jelly bean–shaped, flexible, fluid-filled sacs containing synovial fluid; they ensure the smooth pain-free movement of bone around bone (Figure 8-1). There are about 160 bursae in the body. Trauma, overuse, sustained pressure, or bacteria can disrupt the functioning of the bursae. As inflammation sets in, the sacs swell and small surrounding hemorrhages sometimes occur; the normally noninvasive sacs then push against surrounding tissue, causing pain and more inflammation. As the adjacent muscles receive the pain signal, they initiate small spasms in an attempt to brace (splint) the now painful joint. This cycle of inflammation and pain-spasm-pain must be halted or the condition will worsen. Diagnosis is made by physical examination after ruling out other possible joint conditions, such as arthritis, tendonitis, or sprains, and after a history taking of all activities.

OVERALL SIGNS AND SYMPTOMS

Acute and chronic bursitis can occur either superficially or deep, and each has a distinct set of symptoms.

Acute bursitis:

- Local inflammation, swelling, and heat
- Deep, burning pain; often referred pain during rest and activity
- Restricted ROM accompanied by muscle spasm and voluntary splinting

71

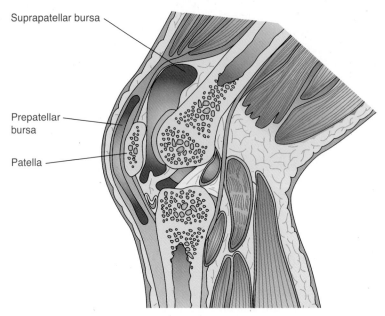

FIGURE 8-1 **Bursae are fluid-filled sacs that contain synovial fluid to cushion joint movement. From Porth CM.** *Pathophysiology Concepts of Altered Health States,* **7th ed. Philadelphia: Lippincott Williams & Wilkins, 2005.**

Chronic bursitis:

- Local dull, aching pain; or tenderness, usually with activity or when pressing on the bursa
- Restricted ROM but not as severe as in acute bursitis
- Muscle spasm and voluntary splinting
- Local warmth and swelling (less likely than acute bursitis)
- Adhesions, low-grade inflammation, and fibrosis

SIGNS AND SYMPTOMS MASSAGE THERAPY CAN ADDRESS

- Joint pain results in restricted ROM, forcing the client into compensatory patterns. The pain-spasm-pain cycle of the muscles surrounding the affected joint, as well as the stiffened compensating muscles, can be treated to reduce painful symptoms, decrease hypertonicity, and remove accumulated cellular waste products.
- Localized inflammation, if it is low grade, can be addressed effectively with cryotherapy (cold packs).

TREATMENT OPTIONS

The physician managing bursitis may be an orthopedic surgeon or a physical medicine physician, both of whom may refer the client to a physical therapist (PT).

Most cases of bursitis can be treated at home by a regimen of rest, ice application, over-the-counter (OTC) pain relievers suggested by the physician, and gentle exercises and stretching to prevent stiffness. Typically, these steps will reduce pain and tenderness and the bursa will heal.

Septic bursitis, however, is treated with antibiotics. With more persistent or puzzling forms of bursitis, the physician might perform a needle aspiration (inserting a hollow needle into the bursa to draw fluid out) to determine whether the condition is septic or aseptic, local or systemic. Needle aspiration is often followed by bandage compression of the joint.

Ultrasound treatments performed by a PT are commonly used for chronic bursitis. Corticosteroid injections into the joint may be used to reduce inflammation if no infection is present. Surgical excision of the bursa is reserved for severe cases that do not respond to other treatments.

A challenge to the healing process, especially for the athlete or the worker who depends on a certain activity for his livelihood, is the necessary change or eradication of the offending behavior that created the bursitis in the first place.

Common Medications

- Nonsteroidal anti-inflammatory drugs (NSAIDs), such as ibuprofen (Motrin, Advil) and naproxen (Aleve, Anaprox, Naprelan, Naprosyn)

MASSAGE THERAPIST ASSESSMENT

Clients sometimes say, "Oh, it's just my bursitis acting up again," but rather than using potentially harmful assessment techniques that may be outside the therapist's scope of practice, it is best to begin the treatment of joint pain with a sound diagnosis from a physician. It is then safe to proceed with ROM evaluations of both the affected and the contralateral joints (joints on the other side of the body), while taking detailed notes. Watching for compensatory movement, painful facial expressions, limitations in ROM, the therapist also notices whether the client is voluntarily or involuntarily holding the joint or limb (splinting).

THERAPEUTIC GOALS

The pain, inflammation, and muscle spasm bursitis causes can certainly be addressed by clinical massage. The therapeutic goals must take into consideration decreased ROM, the pain-spasm-pain cycle, and the fact that the person is probably irritated, frustrated, and facing a possible change in lifestyle, or at least the temporary or permanent loss of a favorite sport or activity.

Although the ultimate goal is to restore full, painless ROM and strength, this cannot be accomplished with massage therapy alone. The massage therapist's work is often accompanied by prescribed physical therapy, appropriate medications, and the client's performance of persistent, cautious self-care.

MASSAGE SESSION FREQUENCY

Acute bursitis:

- When pain is severe, 30-minute sessions twice a week on the affected joint, followed by 30 minutes of relaxation massage, including careful work of the entire affected limb.
- Once pain and severity lessen, continue to have weekly sessions as mentioned previously until all symptoms resolve.

Chronic bursitis:

- With the presence of fibrosis, adhesions, and trigger points, 45-minute sessions once a week on and around the affected joint and affected extremity, followed by 15 minutes of relaxation massage.
- Once fibrosis, adhesions, and trigger points are resolved, continue to have weekly sessions as mentioned previously until full ROM and flexibility return.

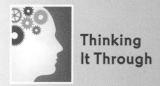

Thinking It Through

Before treating bursitis, the massage therapist should ask herself these questions:

- Do I have a firm diagnosis from a physician, or has the client self-diagnosed?
- How exactly will I use my hands and fingers, and why? While massaging over joints, in the area of released metabolites and waste products, in which direction should I "clean out" the debris using effleurage?
- While softening surrounding fascia, what are the most effective techniques I can use without creating pain?
- How will I alter my direction and depth to avoid creating drag or pressure on the affected joint?
- Does the client intend to return to the offending activity (if the bursitis was created by repetitive activity or pressure)? How can I best counsel him to consider changing his activity or behavior?

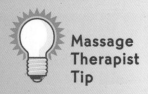

Massage Therapist Tip

Using Caution with Treatment Options

There are many theories about how to work a trigger point out of a muscle belly. The techniques vary in the level of aggressiveness, the therapist's body part used (I have seen one massage therapist apply his heel to the belly of gastrocnemius muscle), and the overall approach. Treating trigger points is covered in Chapter 43, and hands-on practice is essential to ensure no harm is done to the client. It is best to err on the side of caution until expertise in these techniques is achieved.

MASSAGE PROTOCOL

The following protocols will focus on acute bursitis and chronic bursitis of the knee, but each explanation is applicable to bursitis occurring anywhere in the body.

Getting Started: Acute Bursitis

Comfortable, pain-free, and sometimes creative positioning, bolstering, and pillowing are necessary to ensure the safe treatment of acute bursitis. Therapeutic work is combined with relaxation massage techniques to distract and relax the client.

Be willing to hear "war stories" about the occurrence of the bursitis: what brought it on, how much your client enjoyed playing tennis, or how miserable the working conditions are tiling those roofs in August. Always remember that there is a person and an interesting story attached to every condition.

Getting Started: Chronic Bursitis

Initial client positioning is important in treating chronic bursitis, but it does not present as great a challenge as with cases of acute bursitis. Make sure both cold packs and hot packs are accessible. Direct therapeutic work is alternated with relaxation techniques, although clients with chronic bursitis can tolerate longer, deeper, and more detailed work.

HOMEWORK

Acute Bursitis

Self-care is essential in order to halt further injury and complications. Make the following suggestions to your client:

- Rest, ice, elevate, and take the anti-inflammatory and pain medications prescribed by your physician.
- Although rest is essential, don't completely immobilize your limb; this can initiate a pain-spasm-pain cycle.
- Move your limb well within your pain tolerance, and don't completely immobilize it unless, of course, instructed to do so by your physician.

Chronic Bursitis

Remind your client that the work you and he accomplish on the table is only part of his rehabilitation process. Here are some homework assignments to help him regain strength and mobility:

- Use wringing and kneading techniques on the tissues surrounding your painful joint. Remember to push the tissue *toward* your affected joint.
- Use hot packs alternated with cold packs to help move waste products out of the surrounding tissue (this is called contrast therapy).
- Perform pain-free ROM exercises of your entire limb, and especially to the joints above and below your knee (hip and ankle).
- Stroke deeply your entire leg (toward your heart) when you have completed your localized work.

Reiterate that once the pain has subsided, he should not return to the same harmful activity, or at least be willing to modify it. He must change his movement patterns that caused the bursitis in order to avoid painful recurrence.

Step-by-Step Protocol for   Acute Bursitis of the Knee

Technique	Duration
Lightly place a cold pack on the client's knee, allowing him to help with exact placement. Leave the pack in place for the next few steps. Watch the clock and remove the pack after about 10 minutes, or when the client has reached his tolerance.	
Have the client take some deep breaths to help relax him and oxygenate the muscles.	2 minutes
Effleurage, light pressure, using your entire hand. Lubricate the limb appropriately. • Entire lower extremity from the foot to the groin • Get the client used to your touch; help him relax and nonverbally assure him that your work will not hurt	3 minutes
Compression and effleurage, light pressure, centripetal direction, using full, open hands, no knuckles or fists • Gastrocnemius muscle from the Achilles tendon to the popliteal fossa • Tibialis anterior and medial portion of the soleus muscle Positioning may include a slightly bent knee, placed on a pillow to allow you access to both the front and back of the leg.	4 minutes
Compression and effleurage, light pressure, working toward the knee (not centripetally), using full, open hands, no knuckles or fists • Quadriceps complex • As much of the hamstring complex as you can comfortably (for the client) access Remove the cold pack.	5 minutes
Effleurage, light pressure, with full, open hands • The entire lower extremity, anterior and posterior surfaces	3 minutes
Petrissage, light pressure • Gastrocnemius muscle belly • As much of the soleus as you can grasp	3 minutes
Petrissage, light pressure Entire quadriceps • Adductors and hamstrings	4 minutes
ROM, gentle, active (the client performs the movement), pain-free • At the ankle • At the knee • At the hip	3 minutes
Effleurage, light pressure • Entire lower extremity, as the client takes a few, final, deep breaths	3 minutes (Total first half of the protocol = 30 minutes)
Reposition the client comfortably and offer him relaxation Swedish techniques according to his preference, making sure to include deep, appropriate work to the contralateral lower extremity, which may be compensating.	30 minutes

Contraindications and Cautions

- In acute bursitis, techniques that pull tissues surrounding the affected joint are *locally* contraindicated, because they worsen the condition.
- Septic bursitis is a *systemic* contraindication.
- Never "drag" or pull tissue away from the affected bursa. Instead, perform deeper, more invasive techniques *toward* the affected area, not always cephalically, as in typical massage therapy.
- If you feel warmth or swelling or notice redness, proceed no further; consult the client's physician.

Step-by-Step Protocol for	Chronic Bursitis of the Knee
Technique	**Duration**
Place a moist hot pack on the client's thigh, hamstring, or gastrocnemius (not the knee). Leave the pack in place for the next few steps, watching for any skin reddening and client discomfort.	
Have the client take some deep breaths to help relax him and oxygenate the muscles.	1 minute
Effleurage, medium pressure, using small circling motions rather than a straight line from the foot to the groin. Avoid placing a drag on the tissues of the knee joint. • Begin proximally at the quadriceps muscles • Move to the hamstring muscles • Then massage the tibialis anterior and medial soleus • End with the gastrocnemius	5 minutes
Petrissage, medium pressure, assuring that your direction now is toward the knee, not cephalic • Begin proximally at the quadriceps muscles • Move to the hamstring muscles • Then to the tibialis anterior and medial soleus • End with the gastrocnemius	8 minutes
Digital kneading, light-to-medium pressure, using your fingertips • The knee joint and tissue surrounding the patella	5 minutes
Skin rolling, nonaggressive to the client's tolerance, but engaging sufficient tissue to bring blood to the area • 2–3 inches both proximal and distal to the knee joint	4 minutes
Cross-fiber friction, nonaggressive to the client's tolerance, using your thumb and/or fingertips • All muscle attachments around the knee joint	4 minutes
Place a cold pack on the knee to reduce any inflammation the previous techniques might have created.	Leave on for 5 minutes
With the cold pack in place and before moving ahead with further techniques to the affected side: effleurage, petrissage, compression techniques to the client's tolerance • Entire unaffected limb	10 minutes
Return to the affected limb and remove the cold pack. Passive ROM, slightly beyond the client's tolerance. • Hip joint • Knee joint • Ankle joint	5 minutes
Active ROM, slightly beyond the client's tolerance; make sure the client is not holding his breath. • Hip joint • Knee joint • Ankle joint	5 minutes
Close the session with relaxation techniques to the shoulders or anywhere the client requests.	13 minutes

Review Questions

1. Where can bursitis occur in the body?
2. What are the various types of bursitis that can occur?
3. What is different about the directional work when treating bursitis?
4. Are hot packs or cold packs used in treating acute bursitis?
5. Is it appropriate to perform therapy for the full 60 minutes when treating either acute or chronic bursitis? If not, why not?

BIBLIOGRAPHY

Chang E. Bursitis. Emedicine article, Topic 74. Available at: http://www.emedicine.com/emerg/topic74.htm. Accessed April 1, 2010.

Premkumar K. *Pathology A to Z: A Handbook for Massage Therapists*, 3rd ed. Philadelphia: Lippincott Williams & Wilkins, 2010.

Rattray F, Ludwig L. *Clinical Massage Therapy: Understanding, Assessing and Treating over 70 Conditions*, Toronto: Talus Incorporated, 2000.

Scheumann D. *The Balanced Body*, 2nd ed. Philadelphia: Lippincott Williams & Wilkins, 2002.

WebMD, A-Z Health Guide from WebMD: Health Topics. Bursitis. Available at: http://www.webmd.com/hw/muscle_problems/tn3727.asp. Accessed April 1, 2010.

Werner R. *A Massage Therapist's Guide to Pathology*, 4th ed. Philadelphia: Lippincott Williams & Wilkins, 2009.

9

Also known as:
CTS

Definition: A compressive disorder of the median nerve in the wrist.

Carpal Tunnel Syndrome

GENERAL INFORMATION

- Usual cause: repetitive stress injury (RSI) from repeated wrist flexion (e.g., assembly line duties, computer keyboard work, playing an instrument, hobbies that include repeated handwork)
- Associated systemic conditions: diabetes, hypothyroidism, pregnancy, alcoholism, obesity, and rheumatoid arthritis
- Slow onset
- Duration of weeks or months, or lifetime
- Progressive; either chronic or acute
- Irreversible neuropathy possible if repetitive patterns are not halted
- Higher prevalence in middle-aged females

PATHOPHYSIOLOGY

Located at the anterior base of the wrist, the carpal tunnel is surrounded by carpal bones and covered by the transverse carpal ligament, a tight band that is also called the flexor retinaculum (Figure 9-1). Contents of the carpal tunnel include the median nerve and nine tendons and synovial sheaths (tubes of tissue that lubricate tendons) of the anterior forearm flexor muscles. Originating in the brachial plexus (located in the posterior neck), the median nerve travels distally to end by passing through the carpal tunnel (Figure 9-2). The median nerve is essential for normal hand function. It supplies sensory (feeling) fibers to the thumb, index finger, middle finger, and half of the ring finger, and motor (movement) fibers to muscles that allow thumb movement.

A syndrome is a group of simultaneously occurring symptoms that often result from different causes. In the case of CTS, debate continues between Occupational Safety and Health Administration (OSHA) and the American Society for Surgery of the Hand regarding whether there is truly a direct link between repetitive hand movements and the development of the disorder. As inflammation occurs, symptoms manifest from increased pressure in the normally very tightly packed carpal tunnel. Pain is due to nerve ischemia (temporary lack of oxygen and blood to a localized area), rather than from direct damage to the median nerve itself.

Acute CTS can develop after a fracture or trauma, such as a crush injury, or when chronic CTS remains untreated. Chronic CTS, also termed fibrotic CTS, can result from an abnormal bony growth or a slowly growing tumor that increases pressure within the carpal tunnel.

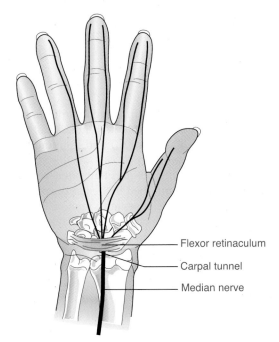

FIGURE:9-1 **The carpal tunnel. Located at the anterior base of the wrist, the carpal tunnel is surrounded by carpal bones and covered by the transverse carpal ligament. From Bickley LS, Szilagyi P.** *Bates' Guide to Physical Examination and History Taking,* **8th ed. Philadelphia: Lippincott Williams & Wilkins, 2003.**

Flexor retinaculum

Carpal tunnel

Median nerve

OVERALL SIGNS AND SYMPTOMS

Acute CTS:

• Pain and inflammation that impair daily activities and interrupt sleep

Chronic CTS:

• Moderate pain and inflammation; daily activities and sleep still possible
• Burning and tingling
• Nighttime positional exacerbations resolved upon waking and handshaking

SIGNS AND SYMPTOMS MASSAGE THERAPY CAN ADDRESS

• Shortened, hypertonic forearm muscles that have lost flexibility and strength can be effectively treated with traditional massage therapy techniques, along with range-of-motion (ROM) and stretching exercises.

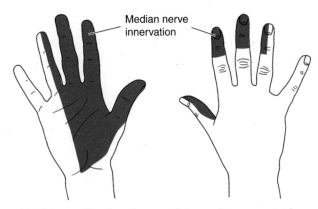

Median nerve innervation

FIGURE 9-2 **The distribution of the median nerve in the hands.**

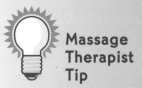

Massage Therapist Tip

Peripheral Nerves, Both Sensory and Motor

The pathophysiology of any peripheral neuropathy is more easily understood by visualizing a peripheral nerve as two differently colored, interwoven pipe cleaners—let's say red and green. The red pipe cleaner carries sensory nerves, which enable us to *feel* the cold of a glass of soda. The green pipe cleaner carries motor nerves, which let us *hold* the glass of soda in a sufficient grip without dropping it. Remembering that peripheral nerves are *both* sensory and motor helps us not only understand and treat peripheral neuropathies, but also explain symptoms to a client who is experiencing difficulty with both feeling and strength.

- Lack of oxygen and blood supply to the median nerve and surrounding tissue can be increased with localized massage techniques and the application of heat.

TREATMENT OPTIONS

All treatment options focus on relieving pressure on the median nerve in order to increase local blood circulation. Rest, nighttime wrist immobilization, anti-inflammatory pain medications (nonsteroidal anti-inflammatory drugs [NSAIDs]), and stopping the offending activity is the normal treatment.

A nocturnal wrist splint can decrease the nerve compression that often occurs with wrist hyperflexion during sleep. Clients must be cautioned in the use of splints, because the initial success rate can be as high as 70%, but relapses are common. Moreover, since the condition manifests over a period of months or years, it will take time for symptoms to decrease. In addition, damaged nerve tissue typically takes longer to heal than muscle or bone.

Localized corticosteroid injections with added lidocaine can have an initial very high response rate, but the improvements significantly decline after 1 year.

Surgery involves either an open or an endoscopic release of the transverse carpal ligament. It is the treatment of last resort, and most physicians will allow a full year of unresolved symptoms, failed attempts at other treatment options, and serious compromise of daily activities before recommending surgery. According to some sources, surgical release of the carpal tunnel has a very high success rate, while other sources cite that numbness may persist despite complete surgical release.

Common Medications

- NSAIDs, such as ibuprofen (Motrin, Advil) and naproxen (Aleve, Anaprox, Naprelan, Naprosyn)

MASSAGE THERAPIST ASSESSMENT

Although it is outside the massage therapist's scope of practice to diagnose CTS, the condition can be confirmed and symptoms can be assessed by using provocative tests, which can recreate symptoms.

- *Phalen wrist flexion test:* The client either rests her elbows on a table or raises her arms to chest height; she then places the backs of her hands together and holds the position for 60 seconds. If numbness, tingling, or burning pain occurs along the median nerve path, it is considered a positive test for CTS.
- *Tinel test:* The therapist aggressively taps on the palmer surface of the client's wrist. If symptoms become evident, the test is positive for CTS.

A strong word of caution is necessary here. Since CTS is commonly self-diagnosed by clients resisting a visit to the physician, the massage therapist must remember that many CTS symptoms mimic other serious conditions, including neck and/or shoulder injuries. Her assessment skills are appropriately used to determine treatment efficacy rather than to diagnose. When in question, it is best to consult a physician before proceeding with treatment.

THERAPEUTIC GOALS

A mantra often repeated by one of my massage therapy instructors was: "A nerve in pain is a nerve screaming for oxygen." Although massage therapy cannot heal CTS,

Thinking It Through

It is common to see wrist braces or stabilizers worn during the day by the general public. Upon questioning, the massage therapist will often find that the person has chosen to self-treat by wearing the brace and has not received an official physician's diagnosis of CTS. Often, the thinking is this: "My friend used it and she had carpal tunnel, and she said it seemed to help." At this point, the therapist, while not moving beyond her scope of practice, might think through the following and offer appropriate advice:

- Wrist braces and stabilizers are intended for nighttime use to prevent wrist hyperflexion that often occurs during sleep.
- Immobilized muscles (from the use of a splint or brace) become hypertonic, and if left immobilized, the pain-spasm-pain cycle begins. How would it help to immobilize an area of the body already at risk for pain and hypertonicity by further immobilizing it?
- Effective therapy for this overuse syndrome is stretching, deep massage, and warming techniques that will return blood to the area. The root of most nerve pain is a localized decrease in blood supply. Does splinting bring blood to the area or diminish the circulation?

common techniques can definitely decrease symptoms. It is therefore a reasonable goal for a compliant client with chronic CTS to expect reduced localized nerve pain, increased flexibility, and reduced pain in the flexor muscles. It is not reasonable to create massage therapy goals for acute CTS.

Because CTS symptoms manifest over a period of months or years, a few massage therapy sessions can provide only palliative relief. There is no quick fix. Truly successful therapy takes time, patience, change in movement patterns, and referring to and working with other health care professionals.

MASSAGE SESSION FREQUENCY

- 60-minute sessions once a week, with the first half-hour focused on the forearm, wrist, and hand until symptoms subside, and the second half-hour focused on the neck and shoulders
- Twice-a-week sessions if the client cannot perform self-care techniques, or refuses to do them

MASSAGE PROTOCOL

The preponderance of (real or self-diagnosed) CTS has reached an alarming rate in the U.S., and you will certainly encounter clients with CTS frequently throughout your career. As important as your work will be in helping alleviate symptoms, your ability to educate your client about the anatomy of the brachial plexus and carpal tunnel can lead to self-care compliance—and may help her avoid surgery. Showing the client a simple anatomic drawing of the brachial plexus—its origin, path, and endpoint—can help her understand that *her tight and hunched shoulders, sleeping patterns, or overworked forearm muscles* could be the cause of her symptoms. With the tendency of so many clients to move quickly to surgery in order to relieve symptoms, your intelligent and careful anatomic explanation, combined with skillful care, can help your client save money and avoid the inherent risks of surgery.

Getting Started

The following protocol is based on treating unilateral, chronic CTS. Wrist, hand, and forearm muscles are the focus of your work. Even with a firm diagnosis of CTS, the client's entire upper extremity and neck need to be addressed. The brachial plexus, from which the median nerve descends, originates in the neck, and a compression or impingement anywhere along the route from neck to fingers causes symptoms that mimic CTS.

Have hot packs readily available. If your practice allows, hydrotherapy techniques, in which the client's hand and forearm are submerged in a tub of warm water and the client is asked to perform gentle ROM movements of the wrist and fingers, can be quite helpful in preparation for your protocol.

Position the client supine, adding an extra pillow or two, as she will be in this position for about 30 minutes. Place a hot pack on the affected forearm and wrist. Use lubrication for this protocol.

HOMEWORK

Self-care is essential for your client if she hopes to recover. A combination of exercises, a change in work style and the way she uses her hand, and physical therapy are all essential for complete recovery. You will need to be diplomatic and persuasive to help your client comply with self-care techniques. Remember that unless she reverses the repetitive patterns, she remains at risk for increased symptoms in the

Thinking It Through *(cont.)*

- If the self-treating client insists that it "reminds her not to use the wrist," she is better reminded that a lifetime of hand movement retraining will serve her much better than a temporary, improperly used splint that could cause damage and will ultimately become discarded.

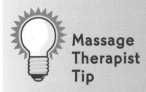

Massage Therapist Tip

Avoiding CTS Yourself

You, the therapist, are at risk for developing CTS. While performing massage, remember not to hunch your shoulders, lean too far forward, or apply too much pressure while leaning onto your hyperflexed wrist. Get adequate hydration. Rest between massages, and warm up and stretch your own forearms and shoulders before and in between every massage. A successful or growing massage practice can be halted by painful hand symptoms. You can use the techniques outlined in the following step-by-step protocol to take care of yourself and help you enjoy a long and pain-free career.

Contraindications and Cautions:

- When any massage technique or pressure used directly on the client's wrist elicits pain, all work must immediately stop.

- Although you will not work on a client who has acute CTS, there is a fine line between chronic and acute symptoms. If the condition is unstable enough to produce exacerbations during normal pressure on the median nerve, avoid that area completely. A decision must be made between client, physician, and massage therapist about whether to continue therapy.

Step-by-Step Protocol for **Chronic Carpal Tunnel Syndrome**

Technique	Duration
Effleurage, petrissage, compression, medium pressure • The entire *unaffected* upper extremity • Start proximally at the deltoid • Work down to the forearm and then the fingers and wrist • Remember, you are "slaying the dragon" by beginning on the least painful limb and getting the body used to your approach	3 minutes
Effleurage, petrissage, compression, medium pressure • The entire *affected* upper extremity. (The remainder of this protocol will focus on the *affected* extremity.) • Remove the hot pack when you approach the forearm. • Perform no special techniques at this point; simply warm the tissue and prepare it for deeper, more aggressive work.	3 minutes
Slow stroking, moderate pressure, using your fingertips • Fingertips to antecubital fossa (the bend in the arm)	1 minute
Compression, starting light, watching the client's reaction for any signs of discomfort and then advancing to medium pressure • The entire forearm, wrist, palm, and fingers	2 minutes
Muscle stripping, medium pressure • Use your fingers and imagine you are trying to separate the flexor muscles by firmly using a raking technique. • Work wrist to antecubital fossa. • Repeat slowly, multiple times. • Make sure you use sufficient lubricant to avoid irritating or pulling the skin too tautly.	5 minutes
Effleurage, medium pressure • Wrist to antecubital fossa	1 minute
Wringing, medium pressure • Wrist to antecubital fossa • Pretend you are literally trying to "wring out" the muscles of the forearm by gripping them firmly and moving your closed fists, which are gripping the forearm in opposite directions.	2 minutes
Cross-fiber friction, deep work to the client's tolerance • Focus on the carpal tunnel itself by approaching the flexor retinaculum of the wrist. • Use your thumbs to cross-fiber friction the fully extended wrist. • Now, ask the client to hyperflex the wrist and perform cross-fiber friction. • Finally, ask the client to hyperextend the wrist and perform cross-fiber friction. • Remember, stop immediately if the client experiences pain during your work.	5 minutes

(continued)

Technique	Duration
Effleurage, deep pressure • Wrist to antecubital fossa	1 minute
Digital and/or knuckle kneading, deep pressure • The palm of the hand, paying particular attention to the thenar eminence	2 minutes
Digital kneading, deep pressure • Each finger and thumb	2 minutes
Compression, deep pressure • Fingers, thumb, palm, and forearm	1 minute
Effleurage, deep pressure • Wrist to antecubital fossa	1 minute
Stroking, light pressure • Using your fingertips • Fingers to antecubital fossa, spending a few extra seconds in the antecubital fossa for this final step	1 minute (30 minutes total)
You have now completed the specific therapy for the localized symptoms of CTS; however, the entire cervical spine region, base of the skull, superior trapezius, and shoulder region must be addressed for the remaining time. • Use deep effleurage, petrissage, kneading, and compression techniques to the client's tolerance. • Grasp and nudge the scapula purposefully and carefully. • Digitally knead around the entire perimeter of the scapula. • Digitally knead deep into the laminar grooves of the cervical spine. • Digitally knead into the base of the entire occipital ridge. • Petrissage and effleurage often and with depth to tolerance.	30 minutes
If time allows, perform some softening and relaxing techniques to the unaffected shoulder.	
If you are treating bilateral CTS, your time will be completely consumed with work of the upper extremity, and extra time will have to be scheduled for the essential work on the shoulders. One option is to see the client 2 times per week, focusing on one upper extremity during each appointment.	

future, and perhaps an irreversible neuropathy. Homework assignments can include the following:

- Stretch to warm up your hands and forearms before beginning your daily activities. *(Show her simple self-massage techniques of her forearms, with deep work to her tolerance, making sure she performs effleurage in the cephalic direction.)*
- Periodically stretch your wrists and forearms by interlacing your fingers and palms together at about chest height. Then, with your fingers still interlaced, open your palms away from your chest and straighten your arms out in front. This will place your wrists in a hyperextended position and will stretch the ligaments.

- Allow ample time to rest your arms and hands during the day. If this is not possible, be sure to rest your arms at night.
- If you experience wrist pain at the end of a day, apply ice to your wrist for 10–15 minutes every hour. Place the ice only on the wrist and not on the forearm muscles, as this will restrict needed blood flow in that area. Simply rubbing an ice cube over your wrist will work, too.
- Do doorway stretches if your symptoms originate in your neck. *(Refer to Figures 5-5 and 5-6.)*
- Perform simple ROM exercises while driving or talking on the phone to prevent forearm and wrist stiffening.

Review

1. What are some of the common causes of CTS?
2. What are the main symptoms of chronic CTS?
3. Describe the path of the median nerve and how it innervates the upper extremity.
4. Describe treatment options for CTS that are used before surgery is considered.
5. What are some techniques you can use to avoid developing CTS yourself?

BIBLIOGRAPHY

Ashworth NL. Carpal Tunnel Syndrome. EMedicine article, Topic 21. April 8, 2005. Available at: http://www.emedicine.com/pmr/topic21.htm. Accessed May 5, 2010.

Field T, Diego M, Cullen C, et al. Carpal tunnel syndrome symptoms are lessened following massage therapy. *Journal of Bodywork and Movement Therapies* 2004;8:9–14.

Fuller DA. Carpal Tunnel Syndrome. EMedicine article, Topic 455. July 2, 2004. Available at: http://www.emedicine.com/orthoped/topic455.htm. Accessed May 5, 2010.

Lowe W. Assess and Address: Carpal Tunnel Syndrome. *Massage Magazine.* January/February 2004;114–120.

Norvell JG, Steele M. Carpal Tunnel Syndrome. EMedicine article, Topic 83. March 28, 2006. Available at: http://www.emedicine.com/emerg/topic83.htm. Accessed May 5, 2010.

Premkumar K. *Pathology A to Z: A Handbook for Massage Therapists*, 3rd ed. Baltimore: Lippincott Williams & Wilkins, 2010.

Scheumann D. *The Balanced Body*, 3rd ed. Baltimore: Lippincott Williams & Wilkins, 2006.

WebMD. A-Z Health Guide from WebMD: Carpal tunnel syndrome [Article]. Available at: http://www.webmd.com/hw/carpal_tunnel/hw213311.asp. Accessed May 5, 2010.

Werner R. *A Massage Therapist's Guide to Pathology*, 4th ed. Baltimore: Lippincott Williams & Wilkins, 2009.

10

Cerebral Palsy

Also known as:

CP

Definition: A collective term for nonprogressive disorders of the central nervous system (brain and spinal cord) affecting motor function; occurs during fetal development, at birth, or within 3 years of age.

GENERAL INFORMATION

- Specific causes: maternal illness and/or infection, seizure disorders, Rh incapability, genetic disorders, premature birth, low birth weight, brain damage early in life, lack of oxygen (before, during, or after birth)
- Results from damage to, or abnormal development of, motor areas of the brain (usually the basal ganglia and the cerebrum); responsible for muscle tone, muscular control, and movement activities
- No evidence for myth about cerebral oxygen deprivation at birth causing CP ("cord wrapped around the neck")
- Associated musculoskeletal conditions: extreme muscular hypertonicity, abnormal muscular movements, skeletal deformities, and contractures
- Incidence: two to four cases for every 1000 live births
- No relation between CP and mental retardation (erroneous assumption)

PATHOPHYSIOLOGY

There are four types or categories of CP:

- *Spastic CP:* Extreme muscle stiffness, accompanied by jerky or awkward movements; accounts for 70–80% of all cases
- *Athetoid CP:* Weak, involuntarily writhing muscles; accounts for 10–20% of all cases
- *Ataxic CP:* Problems with balance, coordination, depth perception, and fine motor control; accounts for 5–10% of all cases
- *Mixed CP:* Any combination of the previous symptoms

OVERALL SIGNS AND SYMPTOMS

Because normal child development varies widely, delayed milestones, such as head control, rolling over, reaching out with both hands, sitting without support, and crawling and walking, can easily be misinterpreted as nonproblematic. As the child ages, the signs and symptoms of CP become more obvious:

- Stiff or spastic muscles
- Painful muscles secondary to constant hypertonicity and spasticity
- Abnormally relaxed muscles, or jerky or slow muscular movement
- Unusual or awkward positions of the limbs, primarily a "scissoring" of the lower extremities (legs crossing each other) and severely hyperflexed wrists

- Seizures
- Compromised swallowing and chewing
- Hearing loss and vision problems
- Toileting difficulties
- Compromised respiratory system

SIGNS AND SYMPTOMS MASSAGE THERAPY CAN ADDRESS

Massage therapy cannot directly affect the pathophysiology of CP. Instead, the work affects secondary musculoskeletal signs and symptoms.

- Hypertonicity and the resulting pain-spasm-pain cycle can be treated to reduce the perception of pain, decrease tight muscles, and remove accumulated metabolites.
- Compromised breathing muscles are approached with detailed work to the thoracic cavity and careful resisted breathing techniques.
- Massage therapy can address decreased range of motion (ROM) and the potential for contractures with careful stretching techniques.

TREATMENT OPTIONS

CP cannot be cured. The extent to which the signs and symptoms can be managed depends on the severity of the original causes and the level and timing of therapies. It takes a multidisciplinary medical, rehabilitative, and integrative medicine team to manage long-term symptoms. Therapy is never completed because the lifelong baseline of the muscles is extreme hypertonicity.

Physical therapy is essential for maintaining the patient's muscle control and increasing ROM, while preventing debilitating contractures. A PT can provide braces, crutches, a wheelchair, gym equipment, weights, balls, and resistance bands. An occupational therapist (OT) can use tools to help the patient perform the activities of daily living (ADLs).

Since the fine muscles of the mouth and face are often affected, a speech therapist will likely be part of the health care team to address speech, chewing, facial expressions, and swallowing challenges. Pneumonia is a major risk for the CP patient; therefore, a pulmonologist (a specialist in lung disorders) is also often engaged in the care.

In many cases, an orthopedic surgeon will perform a series of surgeries as the patient grows. Specific spinal cord nerves may be cut to reduce spasticity and aid in mobility. A small pump that releases a spasticity-reducing drug may be surgically implanted into the abdominal wall. If irreversible contractures occur, reconstructive surgery can release the contractures, stabilize joints, and improve limb function. In addition, surgery can lengthen permanently shortened tendons created by years of spasticity.

COMMON MEDICATIONS

- Antiparkinson medications, such as carbidopa-levodopa (Sinemet)
- Skeletal muscle relaxants, such as baclofen (Lioresal)
- Skeletal muscle relaxants and anticonvulsant sedatives, such as diazepam (Valium)

MASSAGE THERAPIST ASSESSMENT

During the early childhood stages of CP, there is an intense flurry of multidisciplinary teamwork, experiments with surgery and rehabilitation equipment, and medication successes and failures. With multiple PT, OT, speech therapy, and surgical

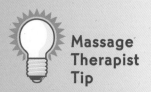

Massage Therapist Tip

Seeing the Real Effects of CP

It is almost impossible to truly comprehend the challenges an adult living with CP faces. To gain an understanding, follow and observe the patient for several hours. Discovering how he has to manipulate his body to get from the wheelchair to the front seat of the car, and seeing the challenges in something as simple as brushing his teeth, changing his clothes, or using the toilet, will make your therapeutic plan specific, detailed, and based on the real-life needs.

If logistics make visiting his home impractical, you can sit quietly and deeply concentrate for several minutes on how your own life might be compromised by the physical limitations and pain level manifested by your CP patient.

appointments and procedures, it is unusual for a parent to think beyond traditional care. This doesn't mean children with CP cannot be successfully treated with massage therapy. Early, focused weekly sessions can reduce spasticity and prevent contractures. However, given the lack of medical insurance coverage for massage therapy and the high medical costs of managing this condition, massage therapy is usually the last concern of struggling parents.

It is the adult CP patient who has survived being bound to a wheelchair, has endured reconstructive surgeries, has relatively controlled levels of pain and muscle spasm medications, and is now trying to live a limited but productive life who can be profoundly affected by massage therapy.

The history the therapist takes during the first session, with either the child or the adult CP patient, will include the cause (if known), the specific type of CP, past surgical procedures, past and present successful and unsuccessful therapies, medications, traumas or falls, communication skills, and pain level. Beyond the physical intake, the therapist also attempts to assess the client's emotional, social, and psychological adjustment to living with this challenging condition.

After taking the oral history and making copious notes, the therapist performs an assessment of full-body active and passive ROM. She asks how the patient's limitations affect his ADLs. Here are some examples of helpful questions:

- Do you crawl to the bathroom in the middle of the night, instead of getting into your wheelchair?
- Do you use crutches at home and your wheelchair in public?
- How do you get into and out of the bathtub or shower?
- Can you dress yourself and use the toilet by yourself?

THERAPEUTIC GOALS

Since CP affects multiple body systems and compromises almost all muscular activity, in general, the therapeutic goals must be the patient's goals. If he wants to improve wrist ROM in order to brush his teeth more efficiently, for example, that activity becomes the massage therapist's greatest priority. A CP patient will present with a different level of spasticity and a new challenge at each session. His spasticity depends on factors such as the weather, his emotional agitation, his level of psychological comfort with the therapist, or whether a new muscle relaxant has been prescribed.

As trust develops, the therapist not only attends to the patient's immediate needs, but also gradually convinces him of the importance of preventing contractures and of increasing, or at least maintaining, his lung capacity. CP does not kill the person living with the condition; secondary events, such as pneumonia or a hospital infection contracted after treatment for a fall, are usually responsible. His chances of dying of pneumonia or a respiratory infection can be significantly reduced by intelligent and focused massage therapy, combined with his own diligent self-care. Resisted breathing exercises, for example, can significantly decrease the risk of pneumonia (Figure 10-1).

MASSAGE SESSION FREQUENCY

Weekly sessions are essential because of the cumulative effects of the therapeutic work, and the surprising speed with which the muscles return to a hypertonic state. Sessions must be long enough to accommodate the time-consuming positioning challenges and the amount of time it takes to warm the muscles before real therapy can begin. Therefore, hourly sessions are not adequate. Of course, time and budget constraints may prohibit the necessary frequency, in which case the therapist must encourage the CP patient to schedule sessions as frequently as his lifestyle will permit.

- Ideally: 90-minute sessions once a week
- Moderately effective: irregular 60-minute sessions

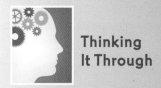
Thinking It Through

Since the body affected by CP responds readily and strongly to many external factors, before your patient arrives, ask yourself the following questions:

- Could today's weather changes have caused him pain?
- How can I check on his emotional state? Will his journal accurately reflect his emotions and bodily responses this week?
- If he's not recording his exercises and pain levels in his journal, how can I help him comply?
- If he's agitated or depressed, how will that most likely affect his body and our session today?
- Am I completely calm, warm, and open, and is the room physically prepared for him to get on the table?

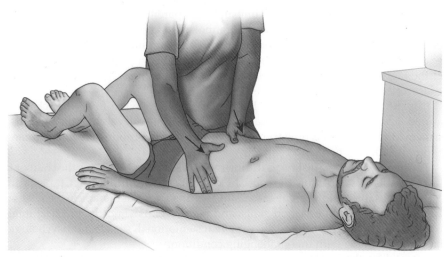

FIGURE 10-1 **Resisted breathing technique. While applying gentle pressure to either side of the rib cage, with evenly spaced wide-open hands, apply gentle downward pressure on the rib cage (toward the table, not down toward the toes), while asking the patient to take three full deep breaths against your resistance.**

MASSAGE PROTOCOL

The following protocol can be adapted to your patient's tolerance, pain level, and the timeframe in which you have to work. Pick and choose from the techniques according to your therapeutic goals for each session.

Getting Started

Positioning your patient on the table is your first challenge. You may need help from his partner or personal aid. Be sure to have plenty of pillows and bolsters on hand to position him comfortably. Do not expect this client to lie in a normal prone, side-lying, or supine position; you will have to accommodate for contracted limbs and breathing difficulties.

The placement of the body on the table, combined with pre-session small talk and bolstering, are enough to cause a spasm. Expect this, wait for it, and slowly stroke the body using medium pressure; talk to him soothingly, and the spasm will subside.

All therapy must be performed slowly, carefully, and to medium depth only. Do not use any stimulating techniques, such as muscle-stimulating devices, or light feathering or effleurage, that trigger the central nervous system. It cannot be emphasized enough—all work on the body of a patient with CP must be slow, even, rhythmic, just the right depth, not startling, and with full cooperation of the conscious patient.

Ask the patient where he would like you to begin. Only he knows the physical challenges he has experienced this week, so you will need to be flexible. The following protocol is based on therapy for an adult spastic CP patient, with work focused on upper extremities, lower extremities, the back, and the anterior chest and breathing muscles.

Begin your sessions with the application of heat. Because of extreme hypertonicity, blood circulation to the muscles will be compromised and the body will frequently be cold. (Winter is a particularly challenging time for CP patients.) Use the standard precaution of asking for feedback, but remember that this patient is taking pain medications and muscle relaxants and may not be able to accurately report sensation.

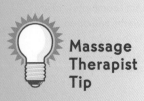

Massage Therapist Tip

Responding to a Spasm

When a spasm occurs, stop what you're doing. Keep your hands on the muscle that is in spasm. Slowly "ride out" the spasm, if the patient allows, by staying on the muscle, simply holding it firmly, not applying any pressure, but not coming off the body. It is important to keep contact with the body. The spasms will decrease in number and intensity—it will take weeks, though—as the body accustoms itself to being touched in this way. *It is important to maintain contact with the body during the spasm, but not to "force" any movement; just stay with it.* The spasm will calm, and the therapy can continue.

Step-by-Step Protocol for | Cerebral Palsy

Technique	Duration
Firmly place a hot pack anywhere on the body requested by the patient. Leave the pack in place for the next few steps. Watch the clock and remove the pack after about 10 minutes.	5–10 minutes
Begin with the patient positioned supine and hold the foot. Allow the body to become accustomed to your touch. Compression, medium pressure, very rhythmic • Dorsal, plantar, and lateral surfaces of the entire foot • Squeeze the foot between your hands	1 minute
ROM, slow moving to end-feel (the normal "end" of his ROM, not stretching beyond the normal "springiness" at the end of normal joint movement) • Toes • Ankles	2 minutes
Digital kneading, slow, medium pressure. Warm lubricant in your hands; cold lubricant can cause a spasm. • Around the malleoli • Repeat ROM at the ankle	1 minute
Effleurage, medium pressure, rhythmic • Follow the path of the tibia both medially and laterally, from malleoli to knee. • Work on as much of the gastrocnemius as can be reached with the patient supine. Have him bend his leg at the knee if he can.	1 minute
Kneading, using the heel of your hand, slow, rhythmic, medium pressure • Follow the path of the tibia; focus laterally on the tibialis anterior, from the lateral malleolus to the knee.	2 minutes
Effleurage, slow, medium pressure • Anterior leg	1 minute
Compression and digital kneading, slow, medium pressure • Knee and all surrounding tissues	1 minute
Compression, even, slow, medium pressure • Adductors • Quadriceps • Iliotibial (IT) band	2 minutes
Effleurage, long, slow, medium pressure • Adductors • Quadriceps • IT band	3 minutes
Petrissage, slow, even, medium pressure • Adductors • Quadriceps	2 minutes

Contraindications and Cautions

- Beware of redness over bony prominences and avoid massaging areas that have broken down because of poor circulation (e.g., heels, coccyx, and elbows). Be sure that the patient and caregiver are aware of broken or compromised skin.

- Understand the patient's method of communication. High-dose pain medication, combined with possible speech challenges, could result in your unintentionally treating the patient beyond his pain tolerance.

- Because of facial muscle hypertonicity, combined with high-dose pain medications, CP patients often appear to have intellectual disabilities. Do not speak to them in an elevated tone or assume limited mental capacity until this is proven to be the case.

- Before applying significant pressure to the chest wall during resisted breathing exercises, make sure the patient does not have osteoarthritis or osteoporosis.

(continued)

Contraindications and Cautions: (cont.)

- The hands of most people with CP are often contracted in unusual positions from decades of compensatory activity or nonuse. A wrist may be in complete contracture, in a state of immovable hyperflexion. Before proceeding with ROM exercises, know the patient's "normal" hypertonicity (which can be improved with therapy) and whether the joint is permanently contracted (a position not alterable with therapy).

Technique	Duration
Friction, medium pressure, performed with the palm or heel of the hand or forearm. • IT band	1 minute
ROM, slow, purposeful, moving joint to end-feel and not beyond, with the body well supported • Toes, ankle, knee, hip	5 minutes
Effleurage, slow, medium pressure • Entire lower extremity Stop and rest. Perhaps reposition the hot pack. No body contact for a minute. Wait to begin contralateral work.	1 minute bilateral At this point, your protocol has lasted ~23 minutes.
Repeat the protocol to the contralateral lower extremity	Approximate duration for bilateral lower extremity work = ~45 minutes.
Digital kneading and compression, medium pressure, rhythmic • Hand	1 minute
ROM, slowly, moving to end-feel • Wrist, fingers, and thumb	2 minutes
Digital kneading, slow, medium pressure • Fingers, palm, and the back of the hand	2 minutes
Effleurage, medium pressure, rhythmic • Follow the path of the wrist flexors (anterior surface of the forearm) from wrist to antecubital space (bend in the arm) • Follow the path of the wrist extensors (posterior surface of the forearm) from wrist to elbow	3 minutes
Muscle stripping, medium pressure (Use caution; this work can set off a spasm.) • Anterior wrist flexors and posterior wrist extensors	2 minutes
Digital kneading, medium pressure • Around the elbow joint, paying attention to the insertion points of all muscles but be careful not to press the medial nerve	1 minute
Compression, medium pressure, rhythmic • Biceps • Triceps • Work all the way up to the axilla and pectoralis major	2 minutes
Effleurage, slow, rhythmic, medium pressure • Biceps • Triceps • Work all the way up to the axilla and pectoralis major	3 minutes

(continued)

Technique	Duration
Petrissage, slow, evenly rhythmic, medium pressure • Biceps • Triceps • Work all the way up to the axilla and pectoralis major	3 minutes
ROM, slow, purposeful, moving joint to end-feel and not beyond, with arm well supported • Fingers, wrist, elbow, and shoulder	3 minutes
Effleurage • Upper extremity Stop and rest. No body contact for a minute while waiting to move to the contralateral upper extremity and repeating this same protocol.	1 minute bilateral At this point, your upper extremity work has lasted ~23 minutes.
Repeat protocol to other side.	Approximate duration for bilateral upper extremity work = ~45 minutes.
Place your hands on either side of the rib cage and gently rock your client's chest from side to side. He will probably be very stiff. This movement will be unusual for him; don't force it. You are trying to get the chest wall acclimated to touch and movement. Have him take two or three full deep breaths, as deep as he can tolerate. Inhalation is important, but so is *forced exhalation*. The attempt at forced exhalation may make him cough or laugh, which may send him into a spasm; be patient. Both laughter and coughing are good for respiratory vigor.	5 minutes
Digital muscle stripping, slow, even, medium depth and pressure • Lean over the body, reach underneath him as far as you can, try to find the spaces between the ribs in which the intercostal muscles are nestled, beginning at the posterior surface of the rib cage and pull upward and medially, ending at the sternum. • Below the 10th–12th ribs, along the surface of the diaphragm. • Repeat on the other side.	5 minutes
Two-handed effleurage, alternating hands with broad sweeps. Slow, gentle work that progresses to slow deeper work. • Over entire anterior and medial surface of the rib cage	3 minutes
While applying gentle pressure to either side of the rib cage, with wide-open hands, evenly spaced, apply gentle downward pressure (toward the table, not down toward the toes) on the rib cage while asking him to take three full deep breaths against your resistance. Stop if this causes a spasm.	3 minutes Total ~16 minutes

(continued)

Technique	Duration
Turn him to either a comfortable side-lying or prone position. *Note:* The back of a person with lifelong CP will be hypertonic to a level you probably have not experienced; decades of unrelenting hypertonicity will have produced a contorted back that will not easily yield to massage therapy. Have patience; be thorough and be gentle; the muscles will release in time; it can take months.	Allow about 5 minutes for repositioning.
Compression, evenly rhythmic, medium pressure • Back, from the base of the neck to the sacrum	3 minutes
Effleurage, rhythmic, medium pressure, using flat open hands or a soft forearm • Trapezius, latissimus dorsi, rhomboids, teres major/minor, erector group, and all back muscles	5 minutes
Note: It may take months before the back muscles have relaxed into any measure of normal tone that would let you use techniques such as petrissage. When and if that occurs, move carefully into the next level of the back, understanding that this "peeling of an onion" technique may take as long as a year to finally reach the erector spinae group.	
To finish the massage, ask your patient where he would like you to spend the last few minutes. Rubbing his head? Returning to his feet?	7 minutes Total: about 15 minutes on his back

HOMEWORK

Keeping a Journal

If your patient is committed to improving his muscle tone and breathing capacity, ask him to begin a "pain, spasm, and victory journal." Have him carry a small notebook in which he (or his caregiver) regularly answers the following questions:

• What is my level of pain? *(Explain the 0–10 pain scale so you are both using the same reference.)*
• Which events caused pain or spasms today?
• Were there any changes in medication level? Why?
• Were there any unusual emotional stressors today?
• Did the weather affect my pain and mobility?
• How often did I perform my deep-breathing exercises?
• Did I notice any small improvements in mobility or ADLs?
• Is there anything else I would like my therapist to know at our next session?

Although this seems like a lot of work for both you and the patient, in time it will reveal patterns or cycles in the onset of pain or spasm. The journal will show whether he is consistently responding to certain weather conditions; it will make clear that he always gets spasms when his in-laws visit, for example. This knowledge will help keep him accountable to his therapy and allow you to determine future therapeutic goals.

Other Assignments

Here are some recommended homework assignments:

- Inhale and exhale deeply three times every day.
- Purchase a bag of multisized balloons, and blow up at least three a day.
- Roll a volleyball or softball under your feet while watching TV or reading.
- Try to grip a small towel or washcloth with your toes.
- Perform slow, gentle ROM exercises of every joint in your body every day.

Review Questions

1. What are some of the causes of CP?
2. What other health care specialists might also help a person living with CP?
3. Why must you be particularly cautious in the use of depth and heat for these patients?
4. What are some external factors that might cause a spasm before and during your massage therapy session?
5. Can a contracted joint be improved by massage therapy?

BIBLIOGRAPHY

Ratanawongsa B, Hale K. Cerebral Palsy. EMedicine article. Available at: http://www .emedicinehealth.com/cerebral_palsy/article_em.htm. Accessed December 5, 2010.
Rattray F, Ludwig L. *Clinical Massage Therapy: Understanding, Assessing and Treating over 70 Conditions*, Toronto: Talus Incorporated, 2000.
Thorogood C, Alexander M. Cerebral Palsy. EMedicine article, Topic 24. Available at: http:// www.emedicine.com/pmr/topic24.htm Accessed May 5, 2010.
Versagi C. Medical Massage Therapy. *Cerebral Palsy Magazine*. 2003;1:7–9.
Werner R. *A Massage Therapist's Guide to Pathology*, 4th ed. Philadelphia: Lippincott Williams & Wilkins, 2008.

11

Chronic Fatigue Syndrome

Definition: A complex disorder characterized by profound fatigue and impaired short-term memory that are not relieved by sleep or rest and that worsen with physical or mental activity.

GENERAL INFORMATION

- Cause unknown
- Onset usually in middle age, although sometimes in adolescence; can be related to the aftermath of a serious immune system disease
- Duration from 2 years to decades
- Affects people of every age, gender, ethnicity, and socioeconomic background
- Prevalence is two to four times higher in women than men

Morbidity and Mortality

The multisystem effects, unknown origin, and similarity to other autoimmune disorders combine to make an accurate estimate of people with CFS almost impossible. Estimates range from tens of thousands to 500,000 to as high as one million people in the U.S. affected annually. Contributing to the wide range of occurrence is the finding of the Centers for Disease Control and Prevention (CDC) that perhaps only 20% of those who have the disorder are actually diagnosed and reported.

The severe, unpredictable nature of the condition results in serious lifestyle changes, psychological adjustments, loss of self-esteem, and decreased financial security.

Prognosis is difficult to determine because some patients suffer for years, yet others recover more quickly if the condition is identified and treated early. Most CFS patients do improve very slowly, sometimes in response to a medical treatment regimen, but just as often, the condition resolves with the passage of time.

PATHOPHYSIOLOGY

A syndrome is a group of simultaneously occurring symptoms that often result from different causes. There may be a few precursors for the existence of CFS that relate to immunosuppression, but there is no single "CFS pathogen" that can be identified in a lab test. CFS can begin after a bout of cold, hepatitis, bronchitis, or flu in adults or infectious mononucleosis in teenagers. Also, patients who have experienced a sustained stress-inducing life event are predisposed to manifest CFS within a short time after apparent resolution of the crisis. However, these findings are confused by the fact that CFS also occurs for no obvious reason.

Because immune function is directly related to the endocrine and nervous systems, this trilogy of systems is the arena for medical experts who are trying to determine the etiology of CFS. And, because CFS so frequently mimics other conditions, a final, confirmed diagnosis takes the path of ruling out (via medical tests) other possible related conditions, including multiple sclerosis, HIV infection, mononucleosis, Lyme disease, thyroid conditions, cancer, depression, and bipolar disorder.

CFS can be migratory, meaning that it moves from one point in the body to another, often unpredictably. However, the presence of multiple trigger points is not indicative of CFS. Although they are migratory, inexplicable trigger points are an indicator of fibromyalgia. While these two conditions share some symptoms and an unclear cause, a muddy etiology, each has its own distinct diagnostic criteria.

Because CFS shares similar symptoms with other immune system disorders, diagnosticians insist on a rigorous "four of eight symptoms" guideline. This guideline further designates mental confusion and/or short-term memory loss, combined with profound fatigue not relieved by rest, as the two most important requisites for making a final diagnosis. Indeed, if the patient has all the attendant physical manifestations but is not experiencing cognitive difficulties (short-term memory loss or problems concentrating or finding the right word while speaking), a final diagnosis of CFS cannot be made.

OVERALL SIGNS AND SYMPTOMS

Although 20–50% of CFS patients also complain of abdominal pain, bloating, chest pain, chronic cough, diarrhea, dizziness, dry eyes or mouth, irregular heartbeat, jaw pain, morning stiffness, depression, tingling sensation, and weight loss, a final diagnosis of CFS is made if a patient experiences four out of eight of the following symptoms, with deep fatigue and cognitive difficulties as the two "mandatory" symptoms:

- Fatigue not relieved by sleep or rest
- Impaired short-term memory, inability to concentrate
- Joint pain not accompanied by redness or swelling
- Muscle pain
- Weakness
- Persistent, sometimes daily, headache
- Tender neck or axillary lymph nodes
- Postexertion fatigue lasting more than 24 hours

SIGNS AND SYMPTOMS MASSAGE THERAPY CAN ADDRESS

- Because the immune system is severely compromised and sleep does not provide its normal healing properties, massage techniques that move the immune, nervous, and endocrine systems toward a parasympathetic (deeply restful) state will be beneficial.
- The patient is unable to exercise her muscles to the level that would allow normal toxin release; moderate petrissage and kneading can relieve the muscles of their toxic load.
- Gentle joint range-of-motion (ROM) movements, accompanied by muscle and joint massage, can help alleviate the perception of joint pain.
- Head and shoulder massage can help reduce headaches.

TREATMENT OPTIONS

Since there is no cure, treatment options range from strict medical regimens, to experimental alternative protocols, to doing nothing. No uniformly effective treatment exists.

A multidisciplinary team of health care professionals, starting with an infectious disease physician and including a physical therapist, massage therapist, dietitian, and psychotherapist, aims for symptom relief. The team attempts to help the patient adjust to a (relatively) stress-free life structured around carefully planned daily activities. The patient is instructed to prioritize tasks and to try to minimize mental and physical exertion.

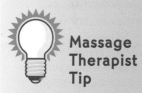

Massage Therapist Tip

Listen, Listen, Listen

People with CFS have a story to tell. They have seen multiple physicians, have had many inconclusive lab tests, and have been told by well-intentioned friends that they are "just tired" or "it's all in your head." One of the keys to helping your patient feel accepted and comfortable is to simply listen to her story. Listen deeply without giving your own story in return, without offering advice, without assuring that you can help—because your contribution to this condition may be minimal. Just listen with a compassionate heart.

Light exercise, combined with gentle stretches and strengthening routines, is strongly suggested. Walking is the ideal light exercise, and it can be modified by starting with only a few minutes per day and building gradually to a level that does not cause undue fatigue.

Diet modifications include avoiding stimulants, such as caffeine or sugar, and avoiding depressants, such as alcohol.

Overall, the health care team will counsel "moderation in all things" when attempting to treat CFS. The previous treatments, and the following listed medications, can provide periodic symptomatic relief of pain, anxiety, depression, and fatigue.

Common Medications

Recent experiments with low doses of hydrocortisone have met with some success, although the attendant risk of possible adrenal suppression may outweigh the benefits of increased energy.

- Antihistamines, such as fexofenadine hydrochloride (Allegra)
- Tricyclic antidepressants, such as amitriptyline hydrochloride (Apo-Amitriptyline, Endep)
- Anticonvulsants, such as gabapentin (Neurontin)
- Tetracycline antibiotics, such as doxycycline (Doryx, Vibramycin)
- Benzodiazepine anxiolytics, skeletal muscle relaxant sedatives, such as diazepam (Valium)
- Local anesthetics, such as lidocaine topical (Lidocream, Lidoderm, Xylocaine)
- Selective serotonin and norepinephrine reuptake inhibitor (SSNRI) antidepressants, such as duloxetine (Cymbalta)

MASSAGE THERAPIST ASSESSMENT

An overly zealous ROM intake assessment, combined with a well-intentioned comment about "looking on the bright side," could do real physical or psychological harm to a patient who has CFS. Before attempting to treat someone with multiple complaints, the massage therapist must obtain an official medical diagnosis. She should be aware of the diagnostic mimicry of fibromyalgia and other autoimmune disorders. The therapist must be sure not to rely on the patient's self-report and self-diagnosis. Once a confirmed diagnosis is made, the therapist can perform a full intake to determine her patient's symptoms. Then, with the patient's guidance, they can both determine reasonable treatment goals.

THERAPEUTIC GOALS

With a condition as complicated and mercurial as CFS, it is difficult for both the therapist and the patient to develop consistent goals, such as reduced pain or increased ROM. Since the patient's primary concern is how the fatigue and cognitive difficulties are affecting her life, perhaps the underlying therapeutic goal should be to perform any technique that will help move her into a parasympathetic state.

All therapists come to the table with their own toolkit of skills, and this full array of talent should be offered to the patient before each session so she can choose what she believes will help the most. On a day when headaches, for example, are distracting and irritating, the patient and therapist may choose to focus on the head and neck only. On a day when anxiety is high, she might need simply a moderate whole-body effleurage, followed by the opportunity to fall asleep on the table and be left until she awakes.

Long-term, measurable goals of "improvement" may be unreasonable or impossible to achieve. This is not to undervalue the benefit of helping a patient achieve a parasympathetic state, but the therapist should use caution in trying to develop the same kind of measurable goals as when treating less complicated conditions.

Thinking It Through

A patient who is dealing with the complex issues of CFS can easily overwhelm a massage therapist who is not familiar with treating multisymptomatic conditions. Before beginning treatment, the therapist might consider the following:

- What is my patient's chief complaint today?
- Is she comfortable with my focusing on that one area of pain for the entire session?
- If the patient cannot decide where to start because she is experiencing so much discomfort, would a whole-body Swedish massage be the best treatment?
- Am I thinking through every technique to ensure I avoid triggering even a minor stress response?

MASSAGE SESSION FREQUENCY

Since the success of medication and medical treatment is so spotty with CFS, estimating the efficacy of massage is solely based on the accumulative effect of helping the person reach a deeply relaxed state.

- Ideally: 60-minute sessions once a week
- Minimally: 60-minute sessions every other week
- Irregular sessions will provide little real accumulative physiologic benefit

MASSAGE PROTOCOL

When treating orthopedic and soft tissue conditions, you have a good idea of your beginning, middle, and end-point for a successful plan. Unfortunately, with CFS, your challenge is much more subtle, and your protocol may change mid-session based on your patient's response. Deep breathing is a gentle tool you can use throughout the session. This is not taking a big breath and holding it, as we sometimes do when addressing trigger points (see Chapter 43). While treating CFS, you are always gentle, thoughtful, and carefully watching a patient who could be moved to the stress response by the simplest of requests. Long, smooth, medium pressure using your forearm could be more relaxing for cleaning out the biceps femoris than possibly jerky petrissage. Silence, stillness, and sleep are the surest indicators that you have helped her immune system heal, if only temporarily.

Getting Started

Be well-prepared for your CFS patient, and try to anticipate her needs. Make sure the lights are low and the music is soft, because she'll probably have a headache; provide extra blankets, because she might chill easily; have extra pillows so none of her joints are strained, and so that even while side-lying, she'll feel like she's floating on a cloud; have a cup of water readily available for her dry mouth, and offer sips throughout your session. A visual image that might help you is to view each patient as if she is a porcelain doll to be attended to with great care and gentleness.

A patient with CFS may fall asleep or choose to remain in one position for the entire session. Therefore, side-lying or supine may be the best starting point.

The following protocol assumes the patient has requested focused work on her head and upper shoulders and prefers to remain supine for the entire session.

HOMEWORK

This is not the time for aggressive or even mildly energetic homework assignments. Because your patient is in pain, many of her joints ache, she has a headache, and sleep offers no respite, she may be inclined to limit all activity and simply sit. But that's the worst thing she can do. The immune and lymphatic systems work best with movement—even the slightest movement—and if she chooses immobility, she'll have many more complications down the road. Encourage her to keep moving and to maintain an exercise journal.

As mentioned, the typical CFS patient is probably being seen by a team of health care professionals. However, you can make the following suggestions if she is relying on you for guidance in her activities. Start by explaining that although you realize she's in pain and it's hard to even think about moving, these exercises will only benefit her in the long run.

- At night when you're watching TV or reading, get a small soup can and do a few biceps curls—not to exertion, but just to keep your arm muscles strong and moving. Begin with three curls and increase gradually if it feels okay.

Contraindications and Cautions

- If your patient's normally subtle symptoms turn into an active infection accompanied by fever, do not treat.

- While your patient may complain of deep muscle pain, the use of deep massage, cross-fiber work, or trigger point work is not appropriate and may set off an inflammatory response.

- Although a 60-minute session should be well-tolerated, gently check in with your patient (either verbally or using your keen observation skills) slightly more frequently than normal to determine if she is truly relaxed.

- As tempted as you may be to offer advice or a pep talk about how much she's going to improve, it is not wise to make even the slightest promise about the improvement of a condition as mercurial and unrelenting as CFS. Just be with her in the moment.

- If you apply a hot pack to a painful joint, be sure to reduce the amount of time the pack is on the body to avoid triggering an inflammatory response.

Step-by-Step Protocol for	Chronic Fatigue Syndrome
Technique	**Duration**
Compression, light pressure, using your whole hand, moving slowly • Entire anterior surface of the body • Start at the feet, work up one leg, include the side of the body, move to the arm and shoulder; move to the other shoulder and arm, down the side of the body, down the contralateral leg and back to the other foot.	2 minutes
Stroking, medium pressure, using your whole hand, making slow, big clockwise circles • Abdominal region, including the area below the rib cage and above the pubic region	2 minutes
Stroking through the hair, using full fingers, making sure not to tug any strands • Work the entire region of the scalp. • Work both left and right sides of the scalp, repositioning the head side to side slowly and carefully, pausing in the middle before rolling the head to the other side.	3 minutes
Digital kneading, medium pressure, entire surface of the scalp • Start at the forehead hairline, move to above one ear, move to the back of the head, work down to the occipital ridge. • Hold the head firmly but gently in your nontreating hand as you roll the head to the side to allow for thorough work on the occipital ridge. Repeat the sequence on the other side of the head.	4 minutes
Digital kneading, slightly more firm than medium but not invasive • The occipital ridge with the head cupped evenly in both of your hands • When the patient is ready (an intuitive understanding on your part), move the mandible toward the ceiling by sliding your fingers into the occipital ridge and pressing your fingertips toward the ceiling. Allow the head to rest in your hands and the patient's chin to point toward the ceiling until you feel a release of the cervical muscles. Rest here for a minute and then return the head to its normal, resting position on the table.	4 minutes
Effleurage, light pressure, as you apply lubricant One side of the superior trapezius	1 minute
Effleurage, medium pressure • All regions of the superior trapezius working up to the occipital ridge and out to the acromion process and around the top of the deltoids • Aim most of your strokes *away* from the head to avoid increasing cranial pressure and exacerbating the headache. Repeat the sequence on the other side.	3 minutes

(continued)

Technique	Duration
Digital kneading, medium pressure • Along the pectoralis major region just below both clavicles • Work both sides of the pectoralis major simultaneously, moving medial to lateral in small, distinct circles	2 minutes
Effleurage, medium pressure • Both sides of the neck • Both sides of the shoulders • Both sides of the pectoralis major	3 minutes
Effleurage, light pressure, as you apply lubricant • One arm, starting proximally (near the armpit), working cephalically (toward the head)	1 minute
Effleurage, petrissage, effleurage, medium pressure • The entire arm • Including attentive, not flimsy, work to the hand Repeat the last two sequences on the other arm.	4 minutes (5 minutes)
Effleurage, light pressure, as you apply lubricant • One leg, starting proximally (near the top of the thigh), working cephalically	1 minute
Effleurage, petrissage, effleurage, medium pressure • The entire leg • Including attention, detailed, work to the foot Repeat the last two sequences on the other leg.	5 minutes (6 minutes)
Compression, light pressure, using your whole hand • Entire anterior surface of the body • Start at the feet, work up one leg, include the side of the body, move to the arm and shoulder; move to the other shoulder and arm, down the side of the body, down the contralateral leg, and back to the other foot	3 minutes
Stroking, over the covers, medium pressure • Entire anterior surface of the body, aiming toward the feet, not toward the head	3 minutes

- Whenever you go to the bathroom, try doing one wall push-up on the back of the bathroom door to help your biceps and your core stay strong.
- If you are fond of walking, go outside for a few minutes every day and really try to stride and take some full, deep breaths. You'll be helping prevent pneumonia, stimulating your lymphatic and immune systems, and getting some vitamin D. Walking can help you feel better than being stuck inside. If the weather isn't cooperating, walk around the house to music.
- Isometric contractions are good muscle strengtheners. Push your palms together as hard as you can until you feel a little wobbly. Then stop and repeat that one or two times. This exercise helps keep your arm and chest muscles strong.
- Sit at your kitchen table in a strong, stable chair. Stand up and sit down a few times in a row. This helps with balance, leg strength, and back strength and provides a little cardiovascular exercise as well.

- Be sure to write in your journal how many times you repeat all the exercises to chart your progress.
- Remember, never work to exertion; you're not aiming for "no pain, no gain" workouts.
- Don't forget: Immobility will only make your symptoms worse down the road.

Review

1. Name the eight most common diagnostic symptoms associated with CFS.
2. Which two symptoms are mandatory for a CFS diagnosis?
3. What common autoimmune disorders mimic CFS?
4. What is your main goal during your treatment of patients who have CFS?
5. List some massage contraindications for CFS.

BIBLIOGRAPHY

American Academy of Family Physicians. Chronic Fatigue Syndrome. Available at: http://familydoctor.org/online/famdocen/home/common/pain/disorders/031.printerview.html. Accessed May 6, 2010.

Centers for Disease Control and Prevention. Chronic Fatigue Syndrome: Basic Facts. Available at: http://www.cdc.gov/print.do?url=http://www.cdc.gov/cfs/cfsbasicfacts.htm. Accessed May 6, 2010.

CFIDS Association of America. Chronic Fatigue and Immune Dysfunction Syndrome (CFIDS). Available at: http://www.cfids.org/about-cfids/treatment.asp?view=print. Accessed May 6, 2010.

Cunha BA. Chronic Fatigue Syndrome. WebMD. Available at: http://www.emedicine.com/med/topic3392.htm. Accessed May 6, 2010.

Generosa A. Living with Chronic Fatigue Syndrome. MedicineNet.com website. Available at: http://www.medicinenet.com/script/main/art.asp?articlekey=77094. Accessed December 5, 2010.

Hitti M, Chang L. Chronic Fatigue Syndrome Linked to Hormones. WebMD. Available at: http://www.webmd.com/chronic-fatigue-syndrome/news/20080118/chronic-fatigue-stress-hormone-linked. Accessed December 29, 2010.

Massage Magazine. The Pain from Fibromyalgia Is Real, Researchers Say. Available at: http://www.massagemag.com/News/2006/January/Fibromyalgia.php. Accessed May 6, 2010.

MedicineNet.com. Chronic Fatigue Syndrome. Available at: http://www.medicinenet.com/script/main/art.asp?articlekey=321&pf+3&page=1. Accessed May 6, 2010.

Rattray F, Ludwig L. Clinical Massage Therapy: Understanding, Assessing and Treating over 70 Conditions, Toronto: Talus Incorporated, 2000:988–990.

Werner R. A Massage Therapist's Guide to Pathology, 4th ed. Philadelphia: Lippincott Williams & Wilkins, 2009:421–424.

12

Constipation

Definition: Fewer than three bowel movements per week; a symptom rather than a disease.

GENERAL INFORMATION

- Dietary causes: insufficient fiber and too much animal fat (e.g., cheese, eggs, meat)
- Activity-related causes: sedentary lifestyle and aging
- Medical causes: third-trimester pregnancy, surgery, stroke, hypothyroidism, diabetes, postural abnormalities, colon cancer, hyperkyphosis, multiple sclerosis
- Medication causes: antidepressants, narcotic pain relievers, iron supplements
- Psychological or psychiatric causes: severe anxiety, depression, obsessive-compulsive disorder, eating disorders, physical or sexual abuse
- Onset usually secondary to changes in diet, fluid intake, activity level, or lifestyle, and/or compromising medical conditions
- Higher prevalence in rural, cold, mountainous states and among women, non-Whites, those who are economically disadvantaged, and all adults more than 65 years old

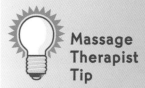

Massage Therapist Tip

Red Flags and Open Communication

When you and your client review his medications list, watch for antidepressants, anticonvulsants, narcotic pain relievers, or frequent antacid use. These are red flags signaling that he probably is constipated. Rather than wait for him to broach the topic, you can diplomatically inquire, "Are you constipated?" Most clients will not mention this condition out of embarrassment, or because it is not common knowledge that massage therapists can be of help. Your relaxed and open attitude can help break the ice.

PATHOPHYSIOLOGY

Most (secondary) constipation is temporary and not serious. The myth that a "daily BM is a sign of health," combined with a belief that stool should pass frequently and with no discomfort, has persisted to such an extent that Americans annually spend $725 million on laxative products and make 2.5–4.0 million visits to their physicians complaining of frequent constipation. In fact, normal bowel movement (BM) frequency ranges from three times a day to three times a week.

There are two basic categories. Functional constipation is a secondary result of easily recognizable causes, such as diet, exercise, medications, or medical conditions. Idiopathic constipation is due to a more serious medical condition or blockage, such as pelvic floor dysfunction, descending perineum syndrome, or retrosigmoid obstruction.

It is important to review the basic anatomy and physiology of digestion and the colon before discussing the pathophysiology of this condition. Although a small amount of carbohydrate breakdown begins in the mouth, most food digestion begins in the stomach. Once the stomach processes and liquefies the food, usable components of the digested mass are absorbed into the bloodstream through the walls of the small intestine. Still in a predominantly fluid state, unusable food debris moves to the colon (also called the bowel or large intestine) before exiting the body.

The colon has three major sections: ascending, transverse, and descending (Figure 12-1). The fecal matter moves around the bowel loop slowly and continuously, aided by the efficient, forward-pulsing, smooth muscular action of peristalsis. As the food mass leaves the small intestine and moves up the ascending colon, some water in the stool can be absorbed back into the body, if needed. By the time the stool reaches the S-shaped curve of the sigmoid colon, however, no extra fluid is available to aid the transit from the

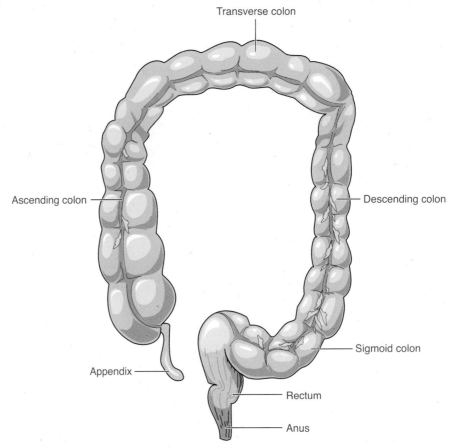

FIGURE 12-1 **The three main sections of the colon. The descending colon runs down the left almost lateral abdominal cavity, the transverse colon runs just under the diaphragm, and the ascending colon runs along the right almost lateral abdominal wall. Modified from LifeART image. Philadelphia: Lippincott Williams & Wilkins.**

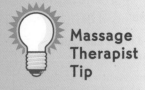

Massage Therapist Tip

What Is an Impaction?

If a large amount of stool becomes lodged in the rectum, an impaction can occur. This impacted fecal mass is too large for normal passage through the anal opening. The person may experience watery mucus or a small amount of liquid stool and therefore believes he is having diarrhea. This material, however, is only the small amount of waste that is forced, through straining, out the anus around the perimeter of the impaction. If this leakage is accompanied by a lack of BM and an extremely uncomfortable sensation of rectal fullness, the person should see a physician quickly to resolve this serious blockage.

sigmoid to the rectum and out the anal canal. The easy passage of waste out of the body depends on sufficient dietary fiber, bulk in the stool, and peristalsis.

The average transit time for food to pass through the digestive system, from the mouth at the time of ingestion to the rectum at the time of evacuation, is 24–48 hours. If food remains in the body for much longer, more water is absorbed through the walls of the colon, the feces become harder and therefore more difficult to pass, and constipation can result. If the transit time is substantially shorter, not enough water is absorbed into the body, and liquid stool, or diarrhea, can result.

When constipation seems to worsen and is accompanied by any of the following, the person should see a physician: if fecal matter significantly changes in appearance (size, shape, and color) or is accompanied by blood; if abdominal pain, fever, nausea, or vomiting accompanies the constipation; if uncontrolled leakage of stools occurs; if stools are black or darkly bloody; if rectal pain is recurrent; or if a BM is not possible without laxatives.

OVERALL SIGNS AND SYMPTOMS

- Hard, dry, marble-sized stools
- Stools that are difficult to pass
- Sensation of bloating or a too-full abdomen
- BM accompanied by excessive straining
- Feeling of incomplete or unsatisfying evacuation
- Feeling of a blocked rectal region

- Headache or feeling of malaise
- Fewer than three satisfying BMs per week

Related to the primary signs and symptoms of constipation are two sometimes alarming secondary signs. When excessive straining is necessary to pass stools, bright red streaks may appear on the toilet paper or on the stool itself, indicating a slight anal tear. Persistent straining can lead to hemorrhoids or rectal prolapse; the former can be chronic, and the latter usually resolves once straining stops.

SIGNS AND SYMPTOMS MASSAGE THERAPY CAN ADDRESS

- Functional constipation can be treated with a specific massage protocol to the entire bowel loop.
- Since the parasympathetic state supports and the sympathetic state inhibits digestion, massage therapy techniques that help the client rest and relax can be beneficial.

TREATMENT OPTIONS

Most people who have functional constipation don't need medical testing and can self-treat. Functional constipation that results from short-term medical conditions or a long-term disease is treatable with medications.

When a few bouts of uncomfortable straining are combined with the understanding that lifestyle changes can all but eliminate most constipation, preventive measures such as the following find their way into the self-treatment plans of most people: increased water intake to at least 8–10 glasses a day; increased fruits and vegetables; increased whole grains and fiber; decreased animal fats, such as cheese; decreased alcohol and caffeine; and increased physical activity. It's strongly suggested, even in a busy schedule, not to ignore the urge to have a BM.

Another simple technique used in other cultures but not found commonly in the U.S. is keeping a small footstool (at a height of about 6 inches) directly in front of the toilet on which to place both feet while defecating. This position flexes the hips and puts the pelvis in more of a squatting position, which is ideal for bowel evacuation.

Enemas should be taken only with a physician's approval and direction.

For medication-related constipation, treatment may include discontinuing or changing a medication or at least decreasing the dose. This is no easy decision if the medication relieves pain, stops seizures, or relieves severe depression, in which case the person might take a more aggressive approach to dietary and lifestyle changes, rather than discontinue the medication.

Common Medications

- Bulk-forming laxatives, such as methylcellulose (Citrucel) and psyllium (Fiberall, Metamucil, Serutan)
- Stimulant laxatives, such as bisacodyl (Correctol, Dulcolax, Fleet, Feen-a-Mint)
- Emollient laxatives, such as docusate sodium (Colace)
- Saline laxatives, such as magnesium citrate (Milk of Magnesia)

MASSAGE THERAPIST ASSESSMENT

Since evaluating bowel contents and peristalsis is well beyond the massage therapist's scope of practice, the assessment available to the therapist in attempting to treat functional constipation is based on the client's oral history. Taking into account the precautions outlined in this chapter regarding idiopathic constipation and the commonsense massage therapy cautions of not massaging a person who is experiencing abdominal pain, vomiting, and nausea, the decision to proceed with the step-by-step protocol is based on the client's accurate description of signs and symptoms.

THERAPEUTIC GOALS

The primary goal of massage therapy for treating constipation is for a BM to occur within 6–12 hours. Secondary goals include offering preventative education and self-massage techniques to help keep the BMs regular. Lastly, the massage therapist may be aware of troublesome symptoms warranting a physician's visit and can then appropriately counsel her client.

MASSAGE SESSION FREQUENCY

Constipation is not a chronic condition that should be regularly treated by a massage therapist; the bowels should move on their own, without manual prompting. Because it is inadvisable to routinely perform colon massage on a healthy client, listing massage frequency is not appropriate.

However, if the client is bedridden, temporarily immobile, suffers from postural abnormalities (such as hyperkyphosis) or other chronic medical conditions, and is taking constipating medications that he cannot discontinue, then helping evacuation of the bowel aided by regular massage is appropriate.

- Ideally: 60-minute sessions daily until evacuation is achieved
- Minimally: 60-minute sessions every other day, until evacuation is achieved

MASSAGE PROTOCOL

There are two theories about why massage of the colon produces results. One theory is that by applying direct, deep, rhythmic pressure to the colon, we are stimulating the body's natural peristaltic action. The other theory assumes that the same pressure and action gently force the movement of the fecal matter itself. Either way, it is reasonable to expect your client will experience a BM after you perform this work. The protocol is so effective that during a short internship at a nursing home where I performed multiple colon massages on elderly, bedridden residents every week, I gained the reputation as "The BM Queen"—not a title to be included on a resume, but one that brought no small relief nonetheless.

With this protocol, remember you are massaging and stimulating the colon and its contents. You must *work into and beyond* the multiple layers of very strong abdominal muscles in order to achieve results—and this means you are working very deeply into the abdominal cavity. It is a three-step process that includes starting very lightly to gain your client's trust and ending with your supported fingers 3 inches deep into the abdomen.

During colon massage, you will encounter various soft and hard, solid and bubbly substances beneath your fingers. The mobile, slightly fluttery, yet sometimes hard masses you feel are probably gas. Gas will break up with repeated strokes, and you may hear the colon "gurgle." You may encounter a solid, roundish mass that does not budge but does not feel like muscle; this is probably fecal matter. Trust yourself; you know what muscle feels like, and if you run into anything that does not feel like muscle, it's a good sign you are in the territory you hope to influence. Of course, your work on tender areas demands that you check in with your client and continue only as he directs.

This protocol has very limited efficacy if your client carries a large amount of excess adipose tissue (fat) around his abdomen.

Getting Started

Consistent with "slaying the dragon," it's best to initially position your client prone. You can place a small pillow in the abdominal region to create some pressure, if the

Thinking It Through

Most complaints of constipation encountered by the massage therapist do not have a serious medical component. However, even though functional constipation is fairly common, the therapist should use careful consideration before starting treatment. For example:

- If the client is constipated secondary to taking antidepressants, although he may be inclined to do so, I should counsel him *not to abruptly discontinue or alter the medication* because a very serious physical and psychiatric side effect could result.
- Many people insist they are constipated because their BM frequency does not match that of other family members. I should review the signs and symptoms of constipation with him, reassure him if he falls in the normal clinical range, but suggest that he see and consult his physician if he is still concerned.
- If constipation is secondary to narcotic medications, I must bring the relationship between narcotic intake and constipation to the client's attention, and let him decide his alternatives. Suggesting he reduce his pain medication or take an over-the-counter (OTC) replacement is outside my scope of practice.
- If the client regularly administers enemas or takes laxatives "to get cleaned out properly" and has few uninduced BMs, I should recommend that he see his physician.

client will allow it. Because the client has been straining, his gluteal muscles, piriformis, hip flexors, and lumbar spine region are hypertonic. There is an ulterior motive in starting on the gluteals: An effective colon massage is based on trust. Your client must allow you to work deeply into his entire abdomen, and by working carefully and thoroughly on another very personal region (the gluteals), you set the stage for trust when you begin working on his abdomen.

After placing your client supine, perform the remaining protocol with his legs bent, feet flat on the table. This position softens the abdominal muscles, allows you easier access, and is essential for optimal results.

All of your strokes, including the digital scooping techniques, will be smooth, *slow*, and rhythmic as you mimic peristalsis. You will always begin your protocol *at the point of the sigmoid colon* and work *counterclockwise—starting on the descending colon, then working the transverse colon, and then to the ascending colon—while your scooping fingers follow the clockwise direction of natural peristalsis* (Figure 12-2). You will perform three passes around the colon, each time working progressively deeper. By the time you perform your third pass, your fingers should be about 3–4 inches into the abdominal wall; superficial work will not be effective.

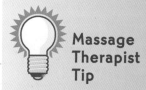

Massage Therapist Tip

Giving Permission to Pass Gas

In our culture, flatulence, the passing of gas, is considered impolite outside the confines of a highly private space. However, you will be stimulating your client's colon; it is to be expected—even welcomed—that he will pass gas. During the early stages of the protocol, be sure to casually mention that you expect he will pass gas, and that it's a welcome sign the massage is working. Assure him there is no need for embarrassment.

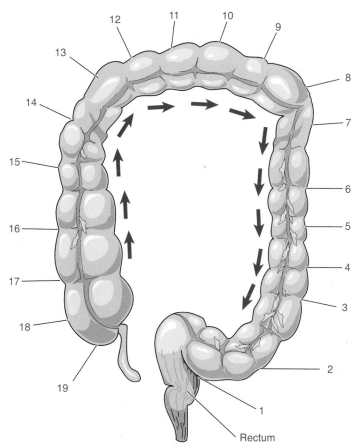

FIGURE 12-2 The direction of the colon massage. Starting at the sigmoid colon, begin scooping *toward the rectum* while working up the descending colon. When the bottom of the left rib cage is palpated, continue scooping *with little right-to-left scoops*, again following the route of the transverse colon. When the bottom of the right rib cage is palpated, continue scooping down the ascending colon; this time, *scooping in little down-up scoops*, following the path of the ascending colon. Numbers on the illustration serve as a guideline for direction, not the number points of treatment. Modified from LifeART image. Philadelphia: Lippincott Williams & Wilkins.

Contraindications and Cautions

- Active irritable bowel syndrome, Crohn's disease, or any intestinal inflammatory disease is a contraindication; however, because of the chronic constipation secondary to these conditions, the protocol could be performed with a physician's approval.
- A history of appendicitis-like symptoms and/or localized acute pain and fever are absolute contraindications.
- The complete absence of defecation after 3 days and/or the absence of defecation accompanied by fecal leakage are contraindications.
- Distention of the abdomen accompanied by nausea, pain, or vomiting is a contraindication.
- Pregnancy is a contraindication.
- A history of high blood pressure or cardiac compromise is a contraindication.
- Hydrotherapy should not be used unless the therapist has received specific training in the effects of heat and cold on the abdomen and bowel, and only if the client does not have any blood pressure or cardiac abnormalities.
- It's not wise to perform this protocol on a client who has just eaten a large meal.

Step-by-Step Protocol for **Constipation**

Technique	Duration
Position the client prone with a small pillow under his abdomen; support his ankles with a bolster. Ask permission to work on his gluteal muscles.	1 minute
Compression, medium pressure, evenly rhythmic, using your entire hand • Superior hamstring muscles • Lumbar spine region • Entire gluteal complex from the gluteal fold to the sacroiliac joint to the lateral head of the femur Work bilaterally.	4 minutes
Digital or heel of the hand kneading, deep pressure, evenly rhythmic • Along the border of the ischial tuberosity • Gluteus maximus, medius, and minimus • Piriformis muscle • Muscles in the lumbar spine region Work bilaterally.	10 minutes
Position the client supine, knees bent, feet flat on the table, head resting on a pillow. Drape appropriately: The area from the bottom of the rib cage to the top of the mons pubis should be exposed. Explain the colon massage protocol to your client when he is comfortably positioned. In a trusting, nonthreatening overture to a very aggressive protocol, place your hand on his abdomen and begin stroking with a flat, firm hand in a clockwise direction over the entire abdomen as you speak. Once he is relaxed and understands the protocol, you can begin the actual sequence.	3 minutes
Digital scooping, light pressure. Place all four fingertips of one hand directly over the region of the sigmoid colon; place the other hand on top of these fingers for both support and added pressure. Now begin a scooping motion, performing about five *stationary* scoops, in the direction of the rectum. (*This hand–finger placement is used for the entire protocol.*) • Directly over the sigmoid colon	2 minutes
Digital scooping, light pressure, moving up toward the left lower rib cage, about 2 inches at a time, using five *stationary scoops at each stop along the* way, pushing in the direction of the rectum • Entire descending colon	3 minutes
Digital scooping, light pressure, moving across the bottom of the rib cage, about 2 inches at a time, using five *stationary scoops each stop along the way,* moving your fingers in small right-to-left scoops. • Entire transverse colon	3 minutes

(continued)

Technique	Duration
Digital scooping, light pressure, moving up the ascending colon, about 2 inches at a time, using five *stationary scoops each stop along the way*, moving your fingers in down–up scoops in the direction of the bottom of the right rib cage. • Entire ascending colon	3 minutes
Stroke with a firm, flat hand, clockwise, while checking in with the client to make sure he is comfortable before you advance to the next, deeper step. • The entire route of the colon	1 minute
Digital scooping, medium pressure, at least five stationary strokes • Directly over the sigmoid colon	2 minutes
Digital scooping, medium pressure, at least five stationary scoops at each point along the route • Entire descending colon	3 minutes
Digital scooping, medium pressure, at least five stationary scoops at each point along the route • Entire transverse colon	3 minutes
Digital scooping, medium pressure, at least five stationary scoops at each point along the route • Entire ascending colon	3 minutes
Stroke with a firm, flat hand, clockwise, while checking in with the client to make sure he is comfortable with your moving to the next, deeper step. • The entire route of the colon	2 minutes
Digital scooping, deep pressure, at least five stationary strokes • Directly over the sigmoid colon	4 minutes
Digital scooping, deep pressure, at least five stationary scoops at each point along the route • Entire descending colon	4 minutes
Digital scooping, deep pressure, at least five stationary scoops at each point along the route • Entire transverse colon	4 minutes
Digital scooping, medium pressure, at least five stationary scoops at each point along the route • Entire ascending colon	4 minutes
Stroke with a firm, flat hand, clockwise, while thanking the client for cooperating with this protocol. • Entire abdominal region	1 minute
Cover the client's abdomen and ask him to rest for a while before getting off the table.	

HOMEWORK

Functional constipation caused by diet or lifestyle can be resolved by reversing the problems that created it. If your client is sedentary, suggest a walking regimen. If he is eating too much cheese or meat, suggest decreasing animal fats and increasing fruits and vegetables. In addition, although it is not possible for some clients limited by obesity or arthritis, you can teach your client to perform deep abdominal massage on himself.

Be careful not to go outside your scope of practice by offering a complete exercise or dietary regimen, or by suggesting that your client might find relief by taking OTC or prescription medications.

For Fast Results

If you have performed the colon massage protocol and expect the client to have results within 6–12 hours, you can offer the following assignments:

- When you get home, or as soon as possible, have a cup of hot water or hot lemon water. This will help stimulate a BM.
- If you don't have a BM by tomorrow, schedule another session.

Preventing Recurrences

- If your daily routine changes due to a vacation or new job, for example, be sure to continue to make time for your BM when you feel the urge. Don't ignore your body's signals.
- Increase your intake of fruits, vegetables, and fiber. There are healthy bran cereals on the market that help meet your daily fiber requirements.
- Drink 8–10 glasses of water every day. Keep a container filled and handy. Caffeine, soda, juice, and alcohol don't count.
- Buy a small footstool, about 6 inches high, and place it in front of your toilet. Put your feet on it each time you try to have BM; it will make passing the feces easier.

Performing a Colon Self-Massage

- Lay comfortably on your back in your bed, or in the bathtub filled with warm water.
- Raise your knees so your feet lay flat.
- Starting at the lower *left* side of your abdomen, just inside from your hip bone, place all of the fingertips of one hand into your abdomen and put your other hand on top of those fingertips to give you some support and strength.
- Now, start scooping into your abdomen as deeply as you can, moving your fingers clockwise in about 2-inch increments, working up to the *bottom of your ribs on the left side*. When you feel your rib cage, start scooping across your abdomen, from left to right, along the bottom of your rib cage, moving your fingers in little right-to-left movements. When you reach the bottom of your right rib cage (still scooping deeply into your abdomen), start moving *down the right side of your abdomen, working from the rib cage down to the area inside your right hip bone.*
- Try to relax and breathe during the entire procedure.
- *Remember your scooping is performed in a clockwise direction, but your hands are moving from the left side of your abdomen to the right.*

Review

1. What is the difference between functional and idiopathic constipation?
2. What is the range of "normal" BM frequency?

3. What are the signs and symptoms of functional constipation?
4. Name four contraindications for the colon massage protocol.
5. Explain, as you would to a willing client, how to perform a colon self-massage at home.
6. What is the first task you want your client to perform when he gets home after having your protocol?
7. During what timeframe is it reasonable to expect results from the protocol?

BIBLIOGRAPHY

National Institute of Diabetes and Digestive and Kidney Diseases. Constipation. Available at: http://digestive.niddk.nih.gov/ddiseases/pubs/constipation/. Accessed December 5, 2010.

Rattray F, Ludwig L. *Clinical Massage Therapy: Understanding, Assessing and Treating over 70 Conditions*, Toronto: Talus Incorporated, 2000:941–954.

WebMD. Digestive Disorders Health Center, Constipation, Age 12 and Older. Available at: http://www.webmd.com/digestive-disorders/tc/constipation-age-12-and-older-topic-overview. Accessed December 5, 2010.

Degenerative Disc Disease

Also known as:

DDD; Lumbago, if located in the lumbar region; Cervical Disc Disease, if in the neck; Thoracic Disc Disease, if located in the mid-back

Definition: A gradual deterioration of the intervertebral discs.

GENERAL INFORMATION

- Common causes: normal aging, prolonged sitting, spinal trauma
- Contributing lifestyle factors: repetitive, prolonged heavy lifting and twisting; abdominal obesity; smoking; poor nutrition
- Accelerated by trauma at any age
- Genetic predisposition
- Equal frequency among athletes and nonathletes
- Usually occurs during third, fourth, and fifth decades of life, with higher prevalence in women

Morbidity and Mortality

More accurately termed a "condition" than a "disease," DDD is often asymptomatic (manifesting no symptoms) because it results from the normal aging process. In fact, MRI studies indicate asymptomatic DDD is present in 25% of 40-year-olds and 60% of those older than 40 years of age. While the statistical prevalence of a sometimes symptomatic, ubiquitous condition is impossible to measure, low-back pain (LBP), the primary manifestation, is certainly measurable. From that standpoint, DDD statistically contributes to LBP prevalence, which is the leading cause of disability in the U.S. affecting those older than 45 years of age. In addition, 60–90% of the adult population annually suffers from LBP.

The prognosis, severity, and complications are directly related to the stage at which DDD is diagnosed and how promptly and effectively it is treated. The extent to which the disc can self-repair is unknown. Untreated, the degenerating discs can injure the nearby spinal cord or nerve roots, causing spinal stenosis (a narrowing of the canal through which the spinal cord passes), producing muscle weakness, and leading to damaged, nerve-related bowel and bladder dysfunction. Saddle anesthesia (perineal numbness) requires nerve-repairing surgery, which may relieve the pain but does not necessarily restore structure or function to the damaged disc itself. Intractable pain requiring surgical intervention is the most complicated and serious treatment of irreversible DDD.

PATHOPHYSIOLOGY

Understanding the healthy structure and function of the fibrocartilaginous spinal discs is essential before discussing pathophysiology. These lubricated, mini shock absorbers allow normal spinal movements of flexion, extension, hyperextension (leaning backward), rotation, and lateral bending (Figure 13-1). Spine stabilizers also include the longitudinal ligaments, deep musculature (erector complex), abdominal and hip muscles, flexors, extensors, and abductors.

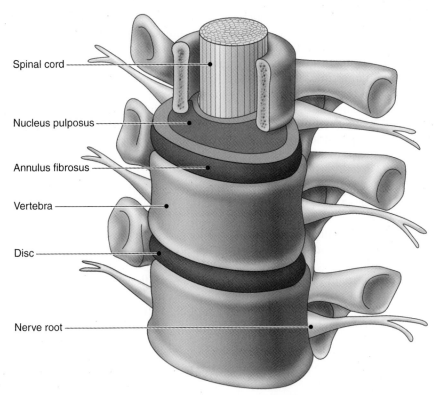

FIGURE 13-1 The fibrocartilaginous spinal disc. Tightly nestled in between each vertebra in the spine, a disc is composed of a jelly-like interior, the nucleus pulposus, and a series of tough, concentric outer rings, the annulus fibrosus.

The relationship between the abdomen and the spine is key to explaining the causes of DDD. If you think of the classic image of a pregnant woman in her third trimester, holding onto her back as she attempts to sit, you can easily understand the relationship between strain on the spine due to temporary or permanent anterior forces and DDD. Weak and stretched abdominal muscles (secondary to pregnancy or obesity), combined with tight hip flexors, can contribute directly to spinal instability and pain, thereby exacerbating the normal aging process of the spinal discs.

Just as increasing age leads to dry skin and brittle bones in even the healthiest of individuals, the intervertebral discs alter in structure and function after the second decade of life. The spinal disc's nucleus (center portion), normally consisting of 85% water, dries substantially with age, and the disc's annulus (concentric outer rings) turns from a relatively spongy consistency to that of old, tough, drying rubber. The height of the disc, usually about 0.25 inch, decreases, explaining in part why a person loses height with advancing years. Because of stiffness, and the lack of water, blood, and nutrients flowing into and out of the disc, the speed at which the disc can heal or repair itself is compromised.

Since it is not possible to function normally without sitting, twisting, and side-bending—all of which create insidious, accumulative tears in the discs—DDD occurs in stages that result in either serious dysfunction, mild back discomfort, or no symptoms at all.

Instability occurs first, as the usually tight-fitting discs start to slide around, bumping into nerve roots. The person may experience pain and discomfort. If treated at this stage, the condition can stabilize, and pain can be therapeutically controlled. During the second stage, osteophytes (new tiny bone growths [spurs]) begin to form from the constant, unusual wear and tear on the surrounding spinal joints. This further compromises nearby nerves and also causes stiffness. The damage from accumulated osteophytes is usually permanent. Finally, during the stabilization stage, the bony spurs have decreased spinal range of motion (ROM), stenosis may occur,

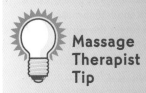

Massage Therapist Tip

Dermatomes

A dermatome is an area of skin where sensation is supplied by a single spinal nerve. For example, cervical spine impingement can manifest in numbness and tingling in the fingers. The nerves in the neck form an anatomic trail that feeds the motor and sensory function of the hand; thus, when the "electrical wire" in the neck is pinched in any way, the "circuit" does not work effectively, setting up signals "down the line." Another typical dermatomal signal used for massage assessment is "down the back of the leg pain," indicating a sciatic nerve compromise in the lumbar spine region.

Thinking It Through

Protective spasming, or protective hypertonicity, is a counter intuitive concept to most massage therapists. Let's think this through together, and give the muscles and bones a little personality in the process.

First, trauma or weakness to a joint sends a signal to the surrounding tissue that says, "Hey! The bones can't do their job in holding this joint stable just now; can we get some help from nearby tissue?!" Next, surrounding muscles "attempt" to take up a stabilizing role by "over reacting" to a nearby joint's weakness and establishing a protective hypervigilance, of sorts, in an effort to hold the bones in place. Physiologically, bone is stronger than muscle, so ultimately, the muscle "loses the battle," but not until a serious attempt has been made. This "serious attempt" causes hypertonicity and muscular spasms *that must remain untreated* until the joint can, once again, perform its normal stabilizing function.

Protective spasms typically occur after a motor vehicle accident when the patient has experienced whiplash, the neck joint is inflamed and unstable, and the surrounding muscles spasm and tighten to keep the neck erect. *It is an absolute contraindication to try to soften the muscles involved in protective hypertonicity.* If the therapist prematurely softens muscles before the joint has stabilized, the joint can actually seriously misalign, causing further damage.

bone may be grinding on bone, voluntary splinting causes secondary pain in adjoining tissues and joints, and the entire trunk now compensates to adjust to an irreversible and very painful condition.

Other age-related conditions that mimic the symptoms of DDD include osteoarthritis of the spinal joints, herniated disc, ligament sprain, spinal stenosis, and, most seriously, spinal tumor.

A medical diagnosis is essential both to determine the stage of this condition and to rule out other symptom-mimicking conditions. A DDD diagnosis is confirmed with the aid of a physical examination, an assessment of movements that reproduce pain, X-rays, CT scan, and/or MRI.

OVERALL SIGNS AND SYMPTOMS

- Intermittent pain, worsening with prolonged sitting, twisting, or lifting
- Episodic pain characterized by flare-ups alternating with periods of moderate discomfort
- Radiating pain and/or pins-and-needles sensation following a dermatome pattern (see online at http://thePoint.lww.com/Versagi)
- Muscle weakness in the area directly supplied by the affected (impinged) nerve
- Decreased spinal ROM

SIGNS AND SYMPTOMS MASSAGE THERAPY CAN ADDRESS

- The small, sturdy, stabilizing erector muscles that wrap around the spine become hypertonic as they attempt to hold the now unstable spine in place. The inevitable hypertrophy, muscle spasm, and pain-spasm-pain cycle can be relieved by massage therapy.
- The decreased ROM (and therefore secondary pain) resulting from prolonged immobility can be treated with massage techniques.
- The stress that accompanies living with chronic pain can be decreased with massage therapy.

TREATMENT OPTIONS

Treating symptomatic DDD ranges from conservative therapies to invasive surgery. Treatment goals include pain relief, increased ROM, and attempts to slow the normal degenerative process. If treated in the early stages, pain subsides within 1–4 weeks and a conservative treatment course follows.

During early treatment, the patient is encouraged to make symptom-reducing lifestyle changes. These include losing abdominal weight for the obese patient; quitting smoking for the cigarette smoker; avoiding high-impact, twisting sports for the athlete; and observing more efficient body mechanics and proper ergonomics, combined with regular stretches, for the desk jockey.

The application of heat for an aching back and cold for a severe flare-up is also considered conservative self-care during the early stages.

Physical therapy to improve lifelong poor postural habits and strengthen the abdominal core and surrounding back muscles, combined with retraining for safer bending and lifting, are additional effective conservative treatments. Traction can be effective if used judiciously. Exercise is considered essential, and a regimen of gentle, low-impact aerobic workouts, such as biking, swimming, and/or walking, is often combined with hamstring stretches and core strengthening.

Although, intuitively, bed rest seems appropriate for back pain, it is prescribed for very short-term periods of merely a day or two. Certainly, if the patient is experiencing intractable pain, bed rest will be called for. However, the secondary effects of immobility exacerbate DDD, and bed rest is not a common treatment. For the same reason, immobilizing back and neck braces is considered of limited, short-term value because the extended use of a brace, again, ultimately weakens surrounding muscles.

Chiropractic adjustments, application of TENS (transcutaneous electrical nerve stimulation performed by PTs), and epidural injections of anti-inflammatory steroids offer some relief. Long-term studies on the various treatment options show no single proven effective approach; the choices of modalities are usually based on an individual patient's preference and the physician's history of successfully treating DDD.

If unrelenting, severe pain and muscle spasm consistently interrupt the patient's activities of daily living and make normal functioning impossible, surgical intervention is the last viable treatment option. Surgery is considered only after 4–6 months of aggressive therapy, medication, PT, and lifestyle changes have garnered no relief. Surgical options include a spinal fusion or a disc replacement, each carrying a measure of risk and accompanied by side effects.

Medications are used to decrease the secondary symptoms caused by DDD, but no medication has yet been formulated that can stop or slow the ultimate degeneration of the disc.

Common Medications

- Nonsteroidal anti-inflammatory drugs (NSAIDs), such as ibuprofen (Motrin, Advil)
- Adrenocorticosteroids, such as prednisone (Deltasone, Orasone, Meticorten)
- Nonopioid pain relievers and fever reducers, such as acetaminophen (Tylenol, Feverall, Anacin, Panadol)
- Skeletal muscle relaxants, such as cyclobenzaprine hydrochloride (Flexeril)
- Opioid analgesics, such as oxycodone hydrochloride (OxyContin)
- Synthetic analgesics, such as tramadol hydrochloride (Ultram)
- Anti-inflammatory analgesic and fever reducers, such as celecoxib (Celebrex)

MASSAGE THERAPIST ASSESSMENT

Performing as an informed and responsible health care team member is the only arena in which a massage therapist will be treating and therefore assessing a patient who has DDD. The condition's symptomatic similarity to both serious and chronic disease, combined with the risk of doing great harm with a simple well-intentioned leg or hip stretch, makes working with a PT or orthopedic surgeon imperative. It is very helpful to have, and completely appropriate to ask for, a copy of the written X-ray, CT scan, or MRI report, which will clarify the exact location and extent of degeneration.

With that understanding, the following assessment techniques *are not intended for the therapist to assess the presence of DDD, but rather to assess the appropriate treatment for that day's session.* The assessment and the remaining focus of this chapter are for the treatment of DDD of the lumbar spine region:

- Palpation for paraspinal spasms
- Checking for trigger points and referred muscular tenderness, most commonly found (in lumbago) in the gluteal area and the hamstring complex
- Asking the patient if it is difficult to find a comfortable sitting or lying position
- Palpation of the hamstrings, gluteus maximus and minimus posteriorly, and the rectus femoris and the iliopsoas muscles anteriorly to determine hypertonicity

THERAPEUTIC GOALS

The chronic pain-spasm-pain cycle, trigger points, decreased ROM, and increased stress caused by DDD provide a clear-cut map for treating these patients. The therapist's job is to attempt to provide symptomatic relief of pain, spasm, and stress. Further, deep-breathing exercises are essential to help bring the patient into a parasympathetic state, help maintain vigorous breathing capability, and help prevent secondary pneumonia, so often brought on by age and debilitating conditions.

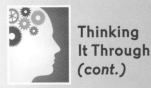

Thinking It Through (cont.)

During an acute flare-up phase of DDD, the paraspinal muscles often attempt to perform the job of the surrounding weakening, bony tissue. This creates extreme hypertonicity and muscle spasm that the therapist will be able to palpate. Here are some important questions for the therapist to think through—and perhaps ask her patient:

- Is the patient experiencing an unusual amount of pain? If the answer is yes, he may be having a flare-up, and massage of the back muscles is inappropriate. Relaxation techniques, not performed on the back, may be more helpful.
- Is the patient experiencing a typical "bad day" of pain? If the answer is yes, then the heat application and deep work to the back are appropriate.
- Is the patient experiencing the chronic pain and stiffness that usually accompany DDD? If so, the protocol in this chapter is appropriate.
- Is the patient holding his breath, wincing upon movement, and unable to find a comfortable sitting or lying position? These are sure signs of the presence of protective spasming, and the session should end with a call to the patient's physician.

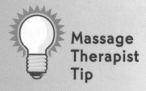

Massage Therapist Tip

Application of Heat and Cold

The use of a rice bag or other nonliquid medium for applying heat is *ineffective*. Although it might feel good, dry heat has no therapeutic value. A hot water bottle or a microwaveable gel pack (wrapped in a pillowcase) provides the needed weight and moisture for the heat to work into the muscle belly. The hot pack can be left in place—not placed directly on the skin—for as long as it's comfortable. Advise your patient not to fall asleep with a hot pack in place.

Cold application of ice requires more attention. The ice pack should be wrapped in a pillowcase or thin towel to prevent skin damage. To reduce spasm or inflammation, the ice pack must be left in place for about 5–10 minutes, *and then removed for about 30 minutes*. The cycle can be repeated a few times throughout the day. Ice packs left in place for a prolonged time ultimately *produce heat*, which is the exact opposite of the desired result.

MASSAGE SESSION FREQUENCY

- 60-minute sessions twice a week for 1 month, during active back discomfort, pain, and stiffness
- 60-minute sessions once a week until pain subsides and ROM increases
- 60-minute sessions at least monthly for maintenance

MASSAGE PROTOCOL

This therapy is hard work, as you knead and petrissage some of the strongest and largest muscles of the body. Focusing on the exact points of lumbar hypertonicity, muscle spasms, and radiating pain, you'll be working on the gluteal complex, hamstrings, rectus femoris, iliotibial (IT) band, iliopsoas, quadratus lumborum (QL), and the entire set of erector spinae muscles (Figure 13-2). (Check your anatomy text to review the origins and insertions of these muscles.) Also, remember you can (carefully) use your forearms and elbows to get into the deeper gluteal muscles as well as the QL. If you have not been taught how to find and release the QL or the iliopsoas, spending an hour with a more experienced colleague could be helpful.

Getting Started

Comfortable positioning is vital; your patient may not be able to tolerate a flat prone or supine position. Have plenty of pillows available.

You'll use hot packs to help soften hypertonic tissue and cold packs to quiet a flare-up or muscle spasm.

Although your therapeutic inclination will be to perform leg and spine stretches to address his limited spinal and hip joint ROM, these are best performed by the PT or orthopedic surgeon with whom you are consulting. For this reason, stretches are not included in the step-by-step protocol.

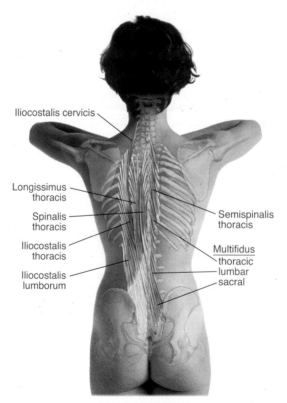

Iliocostalis cervicis

Longissimus thoracis

Spinalis thoracis

Iliocostalis thoracis

Iliocostalis lumborum

Semispinalis thoracis

Multifidus
thoracic
lumbar
sacral

FIGURE 13-2 The erector spinae muscles. This group is the deepest set of back-stabilizing muscles. From Clay JH, Pounds DM. *Basic Clinical Massage Therapy: Integrating Anatomy and Treatment*, 2nd ed. Philadelphia: Lippincott Williams & Wilkins, 2008.

Step-by-Step Protocol for Degenerative Disc Disease of the Lumbar Spine

Technique	Duration
Greet the patient's body with general warming compression. (The patient is lying comfortably prone.) Slaying-the-dragon techniques can include a scalp or foot massage.	3 minutes
Digital palpation, starting with medium pressure and working as deeply as the patient will allow. Feeling for trigger points, muscle spasms, and areas of tenderness. • Superior, middle, and lower trapezius • Rhomboids • Latissimus dorsi and into the thoracolumbar fascia • Gluteus maximus and medius • Serratus posterior • External obliques • Quadratus lumborum (QL) • Erector spinae	3 minutes
Apply a moist, heavy hot pack to the most compromised area based on the earlier mentioned palpation. During this time, simply lay your hand on the patient's back, perform further slaying-the-dragon techniques, sit in silence, or even leave the room to allow the patient to completely relax.	5 minutes
Remove the hot pack and place it on one upper leg on the superior hamstring region, as you prepare to work on the back. Effleurage, medium pressure, evenly rhythmic • The back from the base of the neck to the sacrum	3 minutes
Effleurage, deep pressure, evenly rhythmic • The back from the base of the neck to the sacrum	3 minutes
Focusing on areas of hypertonicity, spasm, and/or tenderness (assuming lumbar spine area involvement), digital or fist kneading, medium pressure, evenly rhythmic • Thoracolumbar fascia • Gluteus maximus and medius • Serratus posterior • External obliques • QLs	8 minutes
Digital or fist kneading, deep pressure, evenly rhythmic • Thoracolumbar fascia • Gluteus maximus and medius • Serratus posterior • External obliques • QLs	8 minutes
Stripping techniques, deep pressure, slow and evenly rhythmic, staying aware of your patient's possible flinching or wincing reactions • Erector spinae, thoracic and lumbar regions	8 minutes

(continued)

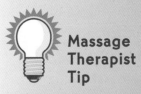

Massage Therapist Tip

Establishing a Long-Term Relationship

The physical duress of dealing with a condition that can easily alter the way your patient sits, stands, plays, and sleeps can be monumental. Add the emotional component of anticipatory fear, as he wonders if he'll have to take narcotics or undergo extensive spinal surgery. Try to develop a compassionate and diplomatic therapeutic relationship with this patient as you work together through his cycles of frustration, relief, and anxiety. Listen to him at the beginning of each session to determine his needs *for that session alone.* Show your professionalism by staying in touch with his PT and/or orthopedic surgeon. You have a real opportunity to establish a long-term professional association with this patient, who may continue experiencing symptoms for years.

Contraindications and Cautions

- Your patient's inability to find a comfortable lying position on the table or to lie still for any length of time is an indication that he needs to see his physician promptly.

- Suggesting or performing hip or spinal ROM exercises without knowing the exact status of the spinal disc involvement is contraindicated.

- Applying heat during a flare-up can lead to exacerbation of an inflammatory process and is therefore contraindicated.

- Performing manual traction to the spine, even simply involving myofascial releases, should not be performed without knowing the exact status of the spinal disc involvement.

- Knowing your patient's pain tolerance, combined with the knowledge of whether he's taking narcotics and/or muscle relaxants, will determine the depth of your work and the accuracy of your patient's response.

Technique	Duration
Stripping techniques, deep pressure, slow and evenly rhythmic • Piriformis	3 minutes
Effleurage, deep pressure, a little more swiftly than your initial effleurage technique • The back from the base of the neck to the sacrum	3 minutes
Standing at the side of the table, reach across the body, place one hand below the rib cage and above the iliac crest, and "rake" your fingers deeply toward the spine, using an alternating hand-over-hand technique. Use enough force to slightly tug the body off the table. • QLs • External obliques • Lateral latissimus dorsi Repeat on the other side.	2 minutes, each side 4 minutes total
Effleurage, deep pressure, a little more swiftly than your second effleurage technique • The back from the base of the neck to the sacrum	2 minutes
Place the hot pack on the other hamstring set. Effleurage, petrissage, digital kneading, effleurage • Hamstrings, focusing on the insertion up under the gluteus maximus	3 minutes
Remove the hot pack. Effleurage, petrissage, digital kneading, effleurage • Hamstrings on the other leg, focusing on the insertion up under the gluteus maximus	3 minutes
Turn your patient supine and place him in a comfortable position. Instruct him to take full breaths at least 3 times, inhaling deeply, holding the inhalation for a few seconds, exhaling slowly and thoroughly.	1 minute

HOMEWORK

If your patient is seeing a PT, he will already be performing daily exercises and stretches. Encourage him to demonstrate these exercises at the end of your session and to continue in his efforts at home. If he is obese, you can diplomatically suggest a weight-loss program and/or give him a registered dietitian's card. If he is a smoker, tactfully suggest a smoking-cessation program.

Without moving outside your scope of practice while simultaneously attending to the many lifestyle and preventive elements of your patient's long-term care, you can recommend the following homework assignments. Notice that each point includes instruction and encouragement; your patient will often be overwhelmed after months or years of doctor's appointments, and he may be taking narcotics. You want to make sure he understands *why* you are asking him to perform certain tasks.

- Take full, deep breaths throughout the day. Because you are in so much pain and your back is getting stiffer, it's easy to fall into the habit of holding your breath or not breathing deeply. This habit can lead to more problems and sometimes pneumonia, which, of course, you want to prevent. Several times throughout your day, take a really deep inhalation, hold it for a few seconds, and then force out all the air with a strong exhalation.

- Keep moving. Immobility will only worsen your DDD. Check with your physician and consider taking the stairs instead of an elevator, parking your car farther away from the store, and walking instead of driving to do a nearby errand. Create excuses to keep moving.
- Apply moist hot packs to your back when you're experiencing deep, aching pain. Apply ice packs when you're experiencing a flare-up or when you feel the pain is particularly bad.
- Try not to slump when you're sitting; sit upright. Good posture provides much better support for your spine and helps prevent the risk of further disc problems.

Review

1. What is DDD, and how common is it?
2. Is DDD always symptomatic?
3. List conservative, moderate, and aggressive treatment options.
4. Why should you treat DDD only while performing as part of a health care team?
5. Why is it important to ask whether a client is taking narcotic pain medication?

BIBLIOGRAPHY

About.com. Arthritis. What is Degenerative Disc Disease (DDD)? Available at: http://arthritis.about.com/od/spine/g/ddd.htm. Accessed May 6, 2010.

Benjamin B. Ligaments vs. Discs. *Massage Today.* July 2008:21.

Furman M. Cervical Disc Disease. EMedicine article, Topic 25. Available at: http://www.emedicine.com/pmr/topic25.htm. Accessed May 6, 2010.

Hendrickson T. *Massage for Orthopedic Conditions*, 2nd ed. Baltimore: Lippincott Williams & Wilkins, 2010.

Malange G. Degenerative Lumbar Disc Disease in the Mature Athlete. EMedicine article, Topic 68. Available at: http://www.emedicine.com/sports/topic68.htm. Accessed May 6, 2010.

MayoClinic.com. Degenerative Disk Disease: Common Back Pain Often Can Be Managed with Conservative Treatment. Available at: http://www.mayoclinic.org/news2007-mchi-4096.html. Accessed September 24, 2008.

Rattray F, Ludwig L. *Clinical Massage Therapy: Understanding, Assessing and Treating over 70 Conditions*, Toronto: Talus Incorporated, 2000: 617–636.

Rebuildyourback.com. Reversing Degenerative Disk Disease. Available at: http://www.rebuildyourback.com/herniated-disc/disease.php. Accessed May 6, 2010.

Spine-health.com. Pain Management Techniques for Degenerative Disc Disease; Deciding on Surgery for Degenerative Disc Disease; Lumbar Degenerative Disc Disease Treatment Options; What Is Degenerative Disc Disease? Available at: http://www.spine-health.com/conditions/degenerative-disc-disease. Accessed May 6, 2010.

WebMD.com. Back Pain Guide. Available at: http://www.webmd.com/back-pain/guide/understanding-spinal-disk-problems-basic-information. Accessed May 6, 2010.

WebMD.com. Back Pain Health Center: Degenerative Disc Disease—Topic Overview. Available at: http://www.webmd.com/back-pain/tc/degenerative-disc-disease-topic-overview. Accessed May 6, 2010.

Delayed Onset Muscle Soreness

Definition: A gradual increase in muscle soreness and pain a day or two after vigorous exercise, diminishing to complete recovery within 1 week.

GENERAL INFORMATION

- Caused by increasing an already established exercise regimen and/or initiating a new, overly aggressive workout program
- Occurs specifically in the overused muscle set, not the entire body
- Affects adult men and women at all levels of athletic prowess

PATHOPHYSIOLOGY

Since "muscle soreness" is ubiquitous in the medical literature, any discussion of pathophysiology begins with what DOMS is *not*. The normal muscle weakness or total body fatigue experienced during a vigorous workout is not DOMS. Further, DOMS is clearly distinguished from the acute, activity-halting pain indicative of a muscle strain or ligament sprain, accompanied by immediate, visible swelling and bruising.

Interestingly, the condition is an often sought-after source of pride by the weekend warrior who uses it as an indicator of the intensity of his new workout regimen.

During physical activity, microscopic tearing and subsequent swelling in the muscle fibers are the normal result of unusual force applied to a specific muscle and/or muscle complex. Muscles tear and rebuild, resulting in greater stamina and strength as the process is repeated and the exercise regimen continues. Examples of overexertion resulting in muscle tearing are a downhill skier taking an advanced hill too soon after mastering the bunny slopes, and a weight lifter adding both weight and repetitions before the muscles have adapted to the lower-weight workout.

Lactic acid buildup in muscles is the result of normal athletic activity, but this accumulation of an expected waste by-product does not cause the soreness that accompanies DOMS. Lactic acid washes out of the body after only a few hours of everyday movement.

The pain manifested during DOMS results from the following chain of events:

1. The muscle is pushed beyond its normal capacity.
2. Muscle fibers tear on a microscopic level, setting up a local inflammatory response.
3. Phagocytes (specialized white blood cells that respond to inflammation) rush to the area (a normal response to local trauma).
4. Swelling occurs, and then edema affects the surrounding tissues by *pushing fluid onto surrounding nerve endings.*
5. This phagocytic accumulation in a tightly enclosed area causes the pain associated with DOMS.

Many massage therapists incorrectly believe that postexertion muscle pain results from the accumulation of lactic acid. However, lactic acid is washed out of the body regularly, and its presence alone does not cause pain.

OVERALL SIGNS AND SYMPTOMS

- Localized pain, soreness, tenderness, and very mild swelling to a specific muscle or muscle set
- Sensitivity to touch and movement
- Decreased mobility secondary to pain
- Worsening pain within the first day or two after exertion, gradually decreasing to complete cessation after 1 week

SIGNS AND SYMPTOMS MASSAGE THERAPY CAN ADDRESS

- The removal of lactic acid buildup and the painful by-products of localized inflammation by increasing circulation to muscles constitute the baseline of most massage therapy techniques.
- The efficacy of massage therapy on DOMS is clinically well supported. One study reported a 30% decrease in DOMS in those who received a massage anywhere from 30 minutes to 14 days postexercise. Another study indicated massage could reduce myalgia (muscle pain) associated with DOMS by 25–50%, depending on the massage technique used.
- Other data support massage as moderately effective in facilitating recovery from repetitive exercise.

TREATMENT OPTIONS

The prevalence of DOMS in both professional and occasional athletes has contributed to the large body of sports rehabilitation research. Professional athletes' blood levels, diets, stretching methods, and pre- and post-event workout regimens are extensively studied, and weekend warriors search the lay literature for advice about pain relief. Passive recovery—doing nothing, letting the condition and the pain pass on their own—is one effective option. Many people, however, are not willing to withstand a week's worth of pain if the discomfort can be shortened or, better yet, prevented. Most treatment options include increasing blood flow to the affected muscle, decreasing the inflammatory process, or treating the muscle nutritionally.

Vibration of the muscle belly has been found to be an effective means of increasing blood flow. To decrease inflammation (which is *not* physiologically separate from increasing blood flow to the muscle), cold-water immersion and hot/cold water contrast baths have been found to be effective. (The image of the NFL linebacker still in uniform, submerging his entire lower torso postgame into a huge drum of ice water comes to mind.) In the nutritional approach, amino acid supplementation, a single protein meal during DOMS, and a postexercise protein mixture have been successful in muscle restoration and pain reduction.

People with DOMS are strongly urged to wait for an improvement in their condition before returning to the same causative exercise regimen.

Several preventive techniques are worth mentioning for two reasons: because exercise benefits lifelong health and because pain is not always a side effect of a dedicated exercise regimen.

1. Although stretching is not conclusively proven effective in preventing DOMS, a period of warm-up and cool-down stretches makes intuitive sense.
2. Experiments with increasing aerobic cardiac output before intense weight-lifting regimens have reduced DOMS.
3. Avoiding sudden increases in an existing exercise regimen, or gradually and slowly beginning a new workout program, can help reduce DOMS.
4. Limited evidence suggests that taking nonsteroidal anti-inflammatory drugs (NSAIDs) *a few hours before activity* may reduce DOMS.

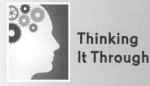

Thinking It Through

Most people have had the experience of seeing a physician who seems ill-suited to give advice in his field. An example would be an obese sports medicine specialist or a smoking pulmonologist. Since massage therapists are part of a health care team, it is essential that they represent a healthy lifestyle. Treating clients with DOMS provides a good opportunity to show that the therapist "talks the talk and walks the walk" when it comes to regular exercise. Questions a massage therapist might ask herself include the following:

- What do I do to keep myself on a regular exercise regimen?
- How do I treat DOMS when my muscles ache?
- What do I see as the most essential benefits of a long-term exercise regimen?
- When I stop exercising for any length of time, what effects do I notice?
- How does regular exercise affect my moods?
- How important is the fact that I may be serving as an example for those around me?

Common Medications

- NSAIDs, such as ibuprofen (Motrin, Advil) and naproxen (Aleve, Anaprox, Naprelan, Naprosyn)

MASSAGE THERAPIST ASSESSMENT

Of all conditions treated by massage therapists, DOMS may well be considered "home base." Much of the professional's work includes ridding the body of waste products, increasing circulation to muscles, and stretching joints to reduce stiffness. Assessing clients for the presence of DOMS will be second nature to most therapists.

A client will likely seek massage therapy for what she considers to be inexplicable stiffness and/or soreness after an extraordinary workout regimen. If her complaints indicate *postexercise* discomfort and local muscle involvement not accompanied by noticeable swelling or redness, the therapist can move ahead in treating DOMS with no assistance from another medical professional. The therapist can also, with caution, palpate the affected muscles and ask the client to demonstrate her limited range of motion (ROM). A painful client reaction that results from even slight palpation further confirms the presence of DOMS.

THERAPEUTIC GOALS

There are three primary therapeutic goals in the treatment of DOMS: increasing blood circulation to and removing waste products from the affected muscle set, increasing ROM at the proximal and distal joints, and breaking down adhesions that might have formed secondary to immobility.

There is one secondary therapeutic goal: resuming exercise. Exercise is proven to effectively limit the devastating effects of such conditions as Alzheimer's disease, cancer, and excessive, sustained stress. It is extraordinarily important for the therapist to encourage the client to continue her workout regimen and to praise her for her efforts. By reducing the client's pain, massage therapy can speed her return to regular exercise and sweating. The therapist should discourage the client from using the temporary pain caused by DOMS as an excuse to halt a potentially life-extending exercise program.

MASSAGE SESSION FREQUENCY

- Ideally: 60-minute sessions, twice during the week DOMS occurs
- Minimally: 60-minute sessions up to 1 month after DOMS diminishes

MASSAGE PROTOCOL

The session will combine careful assessment and vigorous therapy. Your client—whether a middle-aged housewife or a golf pro—is in pain, so your palpating assessment must be cautious.

You can easily use hot and cold packs as you "slay the dragon" elsewhere on the body. If you regularly employ a mechanical muscle vibrator, apply it directly to the appropriate muscle belly any time during the protocol. If you are using your hands for vibrating techniques, these following instructions, with the thigh as an example, may be helpful: Place your clenched fists on the lateral and medial surfaces of the thigh, and pump your fists up and down while maintaining tight contact with the thigh tissue. This will provide an effective vibration technique. Also, firmly planting your flat palm on any muscle belly and shaking your hand back and forth while applying firm downward pressure provide effective vibration.

Since your therapeutic goals include bringing blood to and removing waste from muscle tissue, you will frequently utilize deep, long (well-lubricated) effleurage techniques.

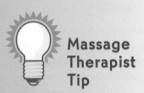

Massage Therapist Tip

Application of Topical Products

The labels on heat- or cold-producing, anti-inflammatory topical products promise increased circulation, increased warmth, decreased inflammation, and any combination of these. Available as lotions, creams, salves, sprays, and roll-ons, you can use these products and remain well within your scope of practice. Of course, no single product works for all clients, and the strong smell can be objectionable to both clients and therapists, regardless of effectiveness. Before planning to apply a product to your client's skin, call the manufacturer, and ask for the lab results and clinical studies indicating the exact effect you and your clients can expect. Also, ask about common allergic reactions. Reputable companies will be glad to send you literature and free samples. Always ask your client before applying any substance that has a potentially objectionable smell on her skin.

Step-by-Step Protocol for **Delayed Onset Muscle Soreness of Bilateral Lower Extremities**

Technique	Duration
With the client positioned comfortably supine, evaluate the extent of DOMS by palpating thighs and calves, noting the client's reaction. Assess bilateral knee and ankle range of motion (ROM).	2 minutes
Apply a heavy cold pack, wrapped in a pillowcase, to one thigh. Apply a heavy hot pack, wrapped in a pillowcase, to the contralateral (opposite) thigh. Ask your client to watch the clock and inform you after 5 minutes. Switch the cold and hot packs to the opposite thighs. This 5-minute rotation continues for the first 15 minutes of this extended (75-minute) protocol, during which you can allow the client to rest or slay the dragon by massaging shoulders, head, or feet.	(15 minutes of therapy applied before the usual 60-minute protocol begins.)
Remove hot/cold packs. Dry the skin. Effleurage, starting medium, working to deep pressure, slow and even rhythm, using your forearm or flat palm of your hand. • Lateral, anterior, and medial surfaces, right thigh	1 minute
Digital or knuckle kneading combined with muscle stripping, starting medium, working to deep pressure, slow and even rhythm • Lateral, anterior, and medial surfaces, right thigh	3 minutes
Digital kneading, deep pressure • Around the entire circumference of the patella and knee joint	2 minutes
Effleurage, deep pressure, slow then a little more quickly • Lateral, anterior, and medial surfaces, right thigh Repeat the entire sequence, working on the left thigh.	1 minute (7 minutes)
Position the client comfortably prone. Apply a heavy cold pack, wrapped in a pillowcase, to one calf. Apply a heavy hot pack, wrapped in a pillowcase, to the contralateral calf. Ask your client to watch the clock, and inform you after 5 minutes. At that point, switch the cold pack and hot pack to the opposite calves. This 5-minute calf-to-calf rotation of hot and cold packs continues as you work on your client's posterior thighs.	2 minutes
Effleurage, starting medium, working to deep pressure, slow and even rhythm, using your forearms • From just above the popliteal fossa until you feel the ischial tuberosity, right hamstrings	1 minute
Muscle stripping, starting medium, working to deep pressure • From just above the popliteal fossa until you feel the ischial tuberosity, right hamstrings	3 minutes
Effleurage, deep pressure • From just above the popliteal fossa until you feel the ischial tuberosity, right hamstrings Repeat the entire sequence, working on the left hamstrings.	3 minutes (7 minutes)

(continued)

Contraindications and Cautions

• If the client's muscle pain persists beyond 7 days and has not decreased in intensity, refer her to a sports medicine specialist or an orthopedic surgeon. Massage therapy is appropriate, but the session will focus on anxiety relief rather than pain reduction, and the importance of seeing a physician should be stressed.

• If the client presents with acute muscle pain, limited ROM, visible swelling and/or bruising indicative of a more serious soft tissue or ligament injury, local massage is contraindicated.

• Since transitory, multisite soreness and muscle pain may indicate a serious, systemic condition such as lupus, fibromyalgia, chronic fatigue syndrome, or multiple sclerosis, the client presenting with non–exercise-induced pain (or pain following very mild exercise) can receive a gentle Swedish massage; however, you should refer her to a physician.

Technique	Duration
Effleurage, starting medium, working to deep pressure, slow and even rhythm • Left gastrocnemius, soleus, plantaris, and popliteus muscles (the entire calf complex)	1 minute
Petrissage using a slow rolling motion, starting medium working to deep pressure • Left calf	2 minutes
Muscle stripping, starting medium, working to deep pressure • From the distal attachment at the Achilles tendon to just below the popliteal fossa	2 minutes
Effleurage, deep pressure • Left calf Repeat the entire sequence on the right calf.	1 minute (6 minutes)
Position the client comfortably supine. Perform hip, knee, and ankle passive ROM stretches (you do the work, the client surrenders the limb). Remember the stretch involves moving the joint to its "comfortable" point of resistance, asking the client to take a deep breath and then moving the joint slightly beyond the comfort zone. Do not create pain.	8 minutes
Vibration techniques, deep pressure • Entire left leg • Entire right leg	3 minutes 3 minutes
Effleurage, medium pressure at a brisk pace • The entire leg, from ankle to hip, bilaterally	2 minutes

Be sure that stretching techniques are performed only after warming the tissue with effleurage, petrissage, and kneading.

Getting Started

This step-by-step protocol utilizes hot and cold packs but will not incorporate the use of a mechanical vibrator or a topical product. Involve your client in her own therapy by asking her to time the 5-minute intervals for the hot/cold contrast therapy.

The techniques can be used on any affected muscle set. The protocol focuses on bilateral lower extremities affected by an overly exuberant new running regimen; it begins after your client informs you of her thigh and calf muscle pain, combined with knee and ankle stiffness.

Be sure to work the entire muscle set by including origins and insertions. Deep work into tendon insertion points will feel particularly soothing and will help prepare the limb for stretches.

HOMEWORK

Encourage your client to slowly return to her exercise regimen as soon as the pain decreases; there is no need to wait until she is completely asymptomatic. With an eye toward preventive measures, as well as treating the present DOMS, suggest the following homework assignments:

- Drink plenty of water before, during, and after your exercise sessions.
- Be sure to warm up before and cool down after working out.
- Work another part of your body, such as upper body weight lifting, while your legs, for example, are healing from DOMS. Consider cross-training in order to rotate muscle use, rather than repeatedly stressing the same muscle sets.
- Place alternating cold and hot packs on your potentially sore muscles following your next intense workout: 5 minutes of heat alternated with 5 minutes of cold for about 30 minutes.
- See your massage therapist the day of or the day after your next intense workout.

Review

1. What is the cause of the pain associated with DOMS?
2. List several standard treatments for DOMS.
3. If you intend to use topical preparations, what are your first steps?
4. Why is it important for a massage therapist to be fit?
5. Above and beyond the physical treatment of DOMS, why is it important to encourage a continued exercise regimen?

BIBLIOGRAPHY

Best TM, Hunter R, Wilcom A, et al. Effectiveness of sports massage for recovery of skeletal muscle from strenuous exercise. *Clinical Journal of Sports Medicine* 2008;18:446–460.

Broadbent S, Rousseau JJ, Thorp RM, et al. Vibration therapy reduces plasma IL-6 and muscle soreness after downhill running. *British Journal of Sports Medicine* 2008 Sep 23 (E-publication ahead of print copy.)

Davis WJ, Wood DT, Andrews RG, et al. Elimination of delayed-onset muscle soreness by pre-resistance cardioacceleration before each set. *Journal of Strength and Conditioning Resistance* 2008 Jan;22:212–225.

Dudley GA. Muscle pain prophylaxis. *Inflammopharmacology* 1999;7:249–253.

Etheridge T, Philp A, Watt PW. A single protein meal increases recovery muscle function following an acute eccentric exercise bout. *Applied Physiological Nutrition and Metabolism* 2008;33:483–488.

Frey Law LA, Evans S, Knudtson J, et al. Massage reduces pain perception and hyperalgesia in experimental muscle pain: a randomized, controlled trial. *Journal of Pain* 2008;9:714–721.

Herbert RD, deNoronha M. Stretching to prevent or reduce muscle soreness after exercise. *Cochrane Database Systematic Review* 2007:CD004577.

Kedlaya D. Postexercise Muscle Soreness. EMedicine article, Topic 117. Available at: http://www.emedicine.com/pmr/topic117.htm. Accessed May 6, 2010.

MayoClinic.com. Muscle Pain. Available at: http://www.mayoclinic.com/health/muscle-pain/MY00113/DSECTION=causes. Accessed May 6, 2010.

Nosaka K, Sacco P, Mawatari I. Effects of amino acid supplementation on muscle soreness and damage. *International Journal of Sports Nutrition and Exercise Metabolism* 2006;16:620–635.

Quinn E. Delayed Onset Muscle Soreness—DOMS—Muscle Pain and Soreness After Exercise. Sports Medicine. Available at: http://sportsmedicine.about.com/cs/injuries/a/doms.htm. Accessed May 6, 2010.

Rodenburg JB, Steenbeek D, Schiereck P, et al. Warm-up, stretching and massage diminish harmful effects of eccentric exercise. *International Journal of Sports Medicine* 1994;15:414–419.

Sports Medicine. Delayed Onset Muscle Soreness (DOMS). Available at: http://sportsmedicine.about.com/library/weekly/aa040401a.htm. Accessed May 6, 2010.

Vaile JM, Gill ND, Blazevich AJ. The effect of contrast water therapy on symptoms of delayed onset muscle soreness. *Journal of Strength and Conditioning Resistance* 2007;21:697–702.

Vaile JM, Halson S, Gill N, et al. Effect of hydrotherapy on the sign and symptoms of delayed onset muscle soreness. *European Journal of Applied Physiology* 2008;102:447–455. Erratum in: 2008 May;103:121–122.

Weil R. Muscle Soreness. MedicineNet.com. Available at: http://www.medicinenet.com/script/main/art.asp?articlekey=78966. Accessed May 6, 2010.

Fibromyalgia

Definition: A deep and superficial, soft tissue aching pain of at least 3 months' duration, characterized by specific tender points in 11 of 18 locations.

GENERAL INFORMATION

- Primary FMS: cause unclear; evidence suggesting neuroendocrine dysfunction
- Secondary FMS: caused by traumatic physical or psychological insult
- Duration measured in years; lifetime involvement not unusual
- Occurs in children and adults of all socioeconomics levels; strong prevalence in females aged 40–50
- More common with family history of depression and/or alcoholism and/or personal history of childhood physical and sexual abuse, drug abuse, or eating disorders
- Genetic predisposition

Morbidity and Mortality

About 3–6 million Americans (2–6% of the U.S. population) suffer from FMS. This condition often mimics similar diseases, and diseases occurring simultaneously with FMS can contribute to a confusing clinical picture. Associated conditions include menstrual difficulties, anxiety, depression, headaches, insomnia, temporomandibular joint (TMJ) dysfunction, bowel difficulties, chronic fatigue syndrome, noncardiac chest pain, myofascial pain syndrome, peripheral neurogenic pain, and some forms of arthritis.

Symptoms are exacerbated by overexertion, stress, long periods of immobility, depression, insufficient sleep, extreme weather changes, and the presence of simultaneous infectious illnesses.

There are no statistics to indicate prognosis. The severity of the chronic condition fluctuates, and complications often occur that affect the person's quality of life rather than the medical course of the syndrome. The pain is pervasive, and the condition can endure for decades. However, it is not progressive, does not deteriorate the joints or organs, and is not fatal.

PATHOPHYSIOLOGY

After years of labeling FMS as a psychological aberration or a nonexistent condition, clinicians have narrowed the pathophysiology to a probable central nervous system and/or endocrine disorder. A woman with FMS has hypersensitive pain-signaling activity in her brain and spinal fluid, and a dysfunction in the pain receptors in her muscles. The brain of a fibromyalgia patient reacts differently while reporting pain, and FMS patients show measurable abnormalities in nonpainful stimulus tests, in addition to sensitivity to light touch.

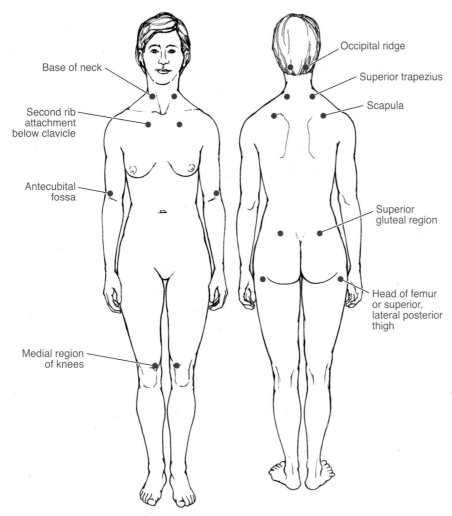

Base of neck

Second rib attachment below clavicle

Antecubital fossa

Medial region of knees

Occipital ridge

Superior trapezius

Scapula

Superior gluteal region

Head of femur or superior, lateral posterior thigh

FIGURE 15-1 Fibromyalgia. Locations of the tender points. Adapted from Werner R. *A Massage Therapist's Guide to Pathology*, 2nd ed. Philadelphia: Lippincott Williams & Wilkins, 2002.

Laboratory tests, MRIs, and muscle biopsies to determine the presence of FMS are usually nondiagnostic. According to criteria established by the American College of Rheumatology, the clinical diagnosis depends on confirmation of at least 11 of 18 tender points on the body, as shown in Figure 15-1.

OVERALL SIGNS AND SYMPTOMS

- Allodynia (a normally nonpainful stimulus perceived as painful)
- Pain lasting at least 3 months
- Pain and/or tenderness palpable in at least 11 of 18 points
- Generalized muscular aching
- Lack of restorative sleep, unrelated to the number of hours slept
- Pain and depression exacerbated by insomnia
- Pain exacerbated by exertion
- Moderate to profound fatigue
- Generalized stiffness, worse at the beginning and end of the day and after periods of immobility
- Distal paresthesia (numbness, tingling, burning, and stinging in the hands and feet)
- Cold intolerance

SIGNS AND SYMPTOMS MASSAGE THERAPY CAN ADDRESS

- Allodynia can be addressed with careful desensitization techniques.
- Decreasing the perception of pain is well within the massage therapist's scope of practice.
- Insomnia and its attendant anxiety and irritability can be addressed by placing the patient in a deep parasympathetic state.
- Generalized stiffness can be relieved with respectful and thorough range-of-motion (ROM) exercises, combined with gentle joint stretches.
- Breathing restrictions that typically accompany chronic pain and stress can be addressed during the massage therapy and homework sessions.

TREATMENT OPTIONS

There is no cure for fibromyalgia. Interdisciplinary and self-treatment regimens, which include exercise, physical therapy, talk therapy, medications, and lifestyle changes, can effectively manage the condition. Although the standard treatment is largely pharmaceutical, the wise patient does not rely on medication alone to relieve her symptoms, because all the suggested medications have long-term side effects.

Acupuncture, biofeedback, and chiropractic manipulations have met with some success. Physical therapies are reported as helpful; and aerobic exercise, combined with flexibility and strength training, is especially effective—when not undertaken too aggressively. Psychological approaches include cognitive behavioral therapy, hypnotherapy, and meditation. Alternative treatments include dietary supplementation, homeopathy, and a vegan diet.

Common Medications

Low doses of antidepressants help the person attain deep sleep, while increasing serotonin levels and decreasing pain. Research suggests that pregabalin (Lyrica), a medication traditionally classified as an antiepileptic, may help block nerve pain in patients with fibromyalgia, but the long-term side effects are yet to be determined. Lyrica is the first FDA-approved medication for the management of FMS.

The following medications are often given in combination, in an effort to control lifelong symptoms:

- Nonsteroidal anti-inflammatory drugs (NSAIDs), such as ibuprofen (Motrin, Advil) and naproxen (Aleve, Anaprox, Naprelan, Naprosyn)
- Tricyclic antidepressants, such as amitriptyline hydrochloride (Apo-Amitriptyline, Endep)
- Nonopioid pain relievers and fever reducers, such as acetaminophen (Tylenol, Feverall, Anacin, Panadol)
- Skeletal muscle relaxants, such as cyclobenzaprine hydrochloride (Flexeril)
- Synthetic analgesics, such as tramadol hydrochloride (Ultram)
- Tricyclic antidepressants, such as doxepin hydrochloride (Sinequan)
- Selective serotonin reuptake inhibitors (SSRIs), such as fluoxetine hydrochloride (Prozac), paroxetine hydrochloride (Paxil), and sertraline hydrochloride (Zoloft)
- Anticonvulsants, such as pregabalin (Lyrica)

MASSAGE THERAPIST ASSESSMENT

The initial assessment of an FMS patient is based on excellent history taking and not on the therapist's manual evaluation. The assessment could last at least half of the initial hour-long session. The patient will have had many medical misdiagnoses, and her frustration may need to be vented on the listening ear of a compassionate massage therapist. Trust must be built, and knowledge gained, before the tender patient is palpated.

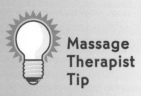

Massage Therapist Tip

Discovering Tissue Abnormality with Sensitive Hands

The tissue in and surrounding the typical FMS tender points may feel different. If you gently lay your hands or fingers on an identified tender point, you may feel what seems like thicker, leathery, fibrotic, mildly spasming, or "stuck" tissue with a significantly different texture than the healthy surrounding tissue. This is a confirming sign that your work in this area needs to be thorough yet gentle.

Because FMS is a common condition, the subject pervades the lay literature; therefore, the massage therapist must use caution when planning to treat a possibly self-diagnosed patient. Although it is outside the scope of massage practice to determine the 11 or more tender points, the therapist can ask whether the patient has been officially diagnosed with FMS and expect her to generally identify each area of pain.

The therapist should take detailed notes outlining each location of pain and its severity, using the 0–10 pain scale for each point. Exact initial intake is important, because this will serve as a map for future inquiries before each session.

The therapist should ask about the efficacy of other modalities that his patient is using to manage her FMS; this will help him plan the nature of the massage therapy session and guide future homework assignments. Of course, knowledge of pain-relieving and mood-altering medications is essential to help determine the patient's ability to respond to the depth of the massage treatment.

THERAPEUTIC GOALS

It is not reasonable to develop specific therapeutic goals when treating FMS. Pain that seems intolerable and diffuse during one session can disappear completely by the next session, when the patient's primary complaint might be profound fatigue secondary to nonrestful sleep. The only reasonable goal in treating FMS is to attempt to relieve one or two presenting complaints. Each therapy session, however, should address the patient's overall compromised physiologic state.

MASSAGE SESSION FREQUENCY

As mentioned, the first session includes a prolonged intake, so the actual hands-on session may last only 30 minutes. This is best, because a body in deep, chronic pain cannot usually tolerate a full-hour session initially.

- 30-minute sessions until the patient is comfortable and reports no side effects
- Increased session length to match the patient's tolerance
- Ideally: 60-minute sessions once a week for the duration of the condition

MASSAGE PROTOCOL

If you bring to mind your last bout of the flu, you will have some idea of the energy-sapping state your FMS patient daily inhabits. The pain, tenderness, and fatigue are unrelenting—and yet many of the suggested therapeutic modalities demand that she move her body when all she wants to do is lay on the couch. Your deep compassion must be combined with your responsibility to get her moving again. The pain-spasm-pain cycle must be stopped, circulation must be increased. Thorough charting is essential for mapping progressions and digressions.

Deep-breathing exercises are critical for maintaining thoracic capacity and preventing pneumonia and other infectious diseases. Pretreatment heat, or rotating the presence of a hot pack around the body during the session, can provide great comfort and prepare an area for treatment. (Cold is not applied to FMS patients.) Soothing, light-to-moderate pressure (you will rarely apply deep pressure) will help gain the patient's trust, while easing her into a parasympathetic state and increasing circulation.

The protocol below focuses on two bilateral points of tenderness, deep-breathing exercises, and almost full-body stretching and ROM techniques. Consider using the following technique in working on a tender point:

- Lay the tips of your fingers on a tender point; wait a moment, just rest.
- Slowly and carefully stretch the superficial skin out and away from the central point of pain, stretching the skin and tissues just below the skin, not engaging superficial muscle on this first move.

Thinking It Through

There is a clear clinical difference between a trigger point and a tender point, and the effective treatment of the FMS patient depends on the therapist's understanding of significantly different approaches. Trigger point work is rarely performed on a patient with fibromyalgia, because the deep insult could produce post-session pain. (Chapter 43 focuses on trigger points.) The therapist should keep the following in mind:

- FMS tender points are bilateral, are typically found in the areas indicated in Figure 15-1, manifest in localized pain or discomfort, and are transient.
- Trigger points can be bilateral but are often unilateral; they have a different character of pain in that they are deeply aching and constantly present. Trigger points also cause referred pain—pain that travels to another area of the body as a result of the myofascial compromise at the locus of the trigger point.
- FMS tender points are not deeply palpated directly and must be approached gingerly for effective, pain-free treatment.
- Trigger points are palpated, worked aggressively with an expected amount of discomfort, and can be treated with direct heat or cold and ROM exercises at the proximal or nearby joint.

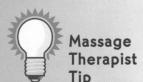

- Stop and rest. If the patient tolerated the first step, repeat the move, now engaging not only the skin but also the superficial muscle layer below the skin.
- Stop and rest. Repeat this technique until your hands engage the muscle belly below the tender point.
- Repeat this process, progressively moving deeper to the patient's tolerance.
- Finish the work with thorough, localized effleurage.

Getting Started

Clearly understand your patient's chief complaint before the session begins; have hot packs and plenty of pillows ready. Allow your patient to lead the way, yet remember that the most beneficial session includes addressing only one or two tender regions, increasing circulation, helping her breathe more efficiently, and stretching stiff limbs. This protocol addresses bilateral tender points above the scapula and in the lumbar region.

HOMEWORK

If a physical therapist and/or personal trainer are part of your patient's health care team, she is on the road to physically managing her condition. The following homework assignments, however, assume she is relying on you for motivation to get

Step-by-Step Protocol for **Fibromyalgia**

Technique	Duration
Starting with the patient supine, ask her to inhale deeply, hold it for a few seconds, and then forcibly exhale. Repeat 3 times.	1 minute
Compression, light pressure, using your whole hand • Entire anterior surface of the body, including the head and neck	2 minutes
Taking one of the patient's arms and cradling it securely with both of your hands, perform gentle stretching and ROM. Work slowly and rhythmically • At the shoulder joint • At the elbow joint • At the wrist joint Ask her to make a tight fist and to open her hand several times. Attempt to stimulate and to engage every muscle and joint of the upper extremity. Repeat on the contralateral arm.	4 minutes (8 minutes total)
Taking one of the patient's legs and cradling it securely with both of your arms, perform gentle stretching and ROM. Work slowly and rhythmically • At the hip joint • At the knee joint • At the ankle joint Ask her to tightly curl and uncurl her toes several times. Attempt to stimulate and to engage every muscle and joint of the lower extremity. Repeat on the contralateral leg.	5 minutes (10 minutes total)

(continued)

Technique	Duration
Ask your patient to inhale deeply again, hold it for a few seconds, and then forcibly exhale. Repeat 3 times.	1 minute
Turn the patient prone. Apply a moist hot pack to the bilateral suprascapular region.	1 minute
Compression, light pressure, using your whole hand • Entire posterior surface of the body, including the head and neck Move the hot pack to the lumbar region.	2 minutes
Using the technique described previously, place your fingers on the tender point above the spine of the left scapula. Compression, light-to-medium pressure, using your fingertips • Skin and superficial tissue only, no muscle involvement Stretch the superficial skin and some subcutaneous tissue • Away from the central area of the tender point Compression, medium pressure, using your fingertips • Superficial tissue and first layer of muscle Stretch the superficial tissue and first layer of muscle, using your flat hand. • Away from the central area of the tender point Compression, as deep as the patient can tolerate, using fingertips and hand • Working into the muscle as deeply as the patient will allow Stretch the deep tissue, using your hand • Away from the central area of the tender point Effleurage, slow, even, rhythmic strokes • Toward the ipsilateral axilla Repeat on the right side.	5 minutes (10 minutes total)
Remove the hot pack from the lumbar spine region after about 5 minutes. Repeat the previous procedure, starting first on the left side of the upper gluteal area, and then moving to the right side, and repeat the same procedure. (Final effleurage strokes will be directed toward the lateral area of the gluteal region.)	(10 minutes total)
Effleurage, slow, even strokes, medium pressure • Entire back from the lumbar region to the base of the neck	5 minutes
Position the patient supine. Compression, slow, even strokes, medium pressure • Entire anterior surface of the body	2 minutes
Stroking, using open fingers, slow, even, light pressure • Through the hair, from the top of the forehead out through the length of the hair	2 minutes
Allow the patient to rest, untouched, or ask if there is one more relaxation technique she might enjoy for the final few minutes.	

Contraindications and Cautions

• Deep work or aggressive overstretching is usually contraindicated.

• Modify pressure based on the patient's medication intake.

• Sleep may be induced as a result of the massage therapy session, so be sure driving arrangements have been made for the possible groggy patient post-session.

• Some research indicates a parallel between FMS and joint hypermobility. When performing stretching exercises, be aware if the patient moves too easily into hyperextension or hyperflexion, and adjust ROM and stretches accordingly.

moving. As with the focus of each massage session, self-care is for increasing circulation, stretching a stiff body, and maintaining efficient breathing. Emphasize that an element of each of these goals must be performed daily.

- One goal is to increase your ability to perform a gentle aerobic routine, with your final aim of a consistent 30-minute workout most days.
- You can choose dancing, walking, bike riding, swimming—any form of low-impact movement that you enjoy.
- If you can only start moving for 5 minutes, that's acceptable. The point is to move every day to the best of your endurance and ability.
- Keep an exercise journal to chart your progress.
- During your exercise, be sure to breathe deeply.
- While watching TV or driving, inhale deeply, hold your breath for a few seconds, and then exhale forcibly. Do this a few times every day. (Don't do this while driving if it makes you light-headed.)
- Before you get out of bed in the morning, stretch your whole body. Lay on your back and stretch your arms up over your head and out to the side; bring your knees up off the bed, roll your hips from side to side; tense and release your abdomen and gluteal muscles; roll your head from side to side; shrug your shoulders.
- In the shower, support yourself and try to stretch every joint and muscle; vigorously wash your hair and soap your body.
- If your budget and time allow, get a personal trainer or physical therapist who understands fibromyalgia, and ask him or her to help you create a progressive exercise routine.
- No matter how tired you are, try to move, breathe deeply, and stretch every single day.

Review

1. What is fibromyalgia?
2. Name the locations of several tender points.
3. What is the difference between a trigger point and a tender point?
4. List some lifelong interdisciplinary self-care techniques used by people with FMS.
5. Is there a diagnostic test to determine the presence of FMS?
6. What are your primary goals during each session?
7. Discuss a typical initial intake session with someone who has fibromyalgia.

BIBLIOGRAPHY

Ader D, Amour K, Matallana L, et al. National Institute of Arthritis and Musculoskeletal and Skin Diseases (NIAMS). Questions and Answers about Fibromyalgia. Available at: http://www.niams.nih.gov/Health_Info/Fibromyalgia/default.asp. Accessed May 6, 2010.

Chaitow L. Fibromyalgia: an evidence-based guide for working with FMS clients. *Massage Therapy Journal* Spring 2006:127–141.

Dalton E. Fibromyalgia: fact or fiction. *Massage and Bodywork* February/March 2006:60–68.

Ko G, Wine W. Chronic pain and cannabinoids: a survey of current fibromyalgia treatment approaches together with an overview and case studies of a new "old" treatment approach. *Practical Pain Management* 2005:28–36.

Rao SG, Gendreau FJ, Dranzler JD. Understanding the Fibromyalgia Syndrome. *Psychopharmacology Bulletin* 2008;40(4):24–56. Available at: http://www.medscape.com/viewarticle/569749. Accessed May 6, 2010.

Rattray F, Ludwig L. *Clinical Massage Therapy: Understanding, Assessing and Treating over 70 Conditions*, Toronto: Talus Incorporated, 2000.

Rooks DS. Fibromyalgia Treatment Update. Medscape. Cited from *Current Opinions in Rheumatology* 2007;19(2):111–117. Lippincott Williams & Wilkins, posted 02/16/2007. Available at: http://www.medscape.com/viewarticle/551891. Accessed May 6, 2010.

Shiel WC. Fibromyalgia. MedicineNet. Available at: http://www.medicinenet.com/fibromyalgia/article.htm. Accessed May 6, 2010.

16

Frozen Shoulder

Definition: An inflammatory thickening of shoulder synovial joint membranes characterized by functionally restricted and/or painful joint movement.

GENERAL INFORMATION

- Primary frozen shoulder: etiology unknown
- Secondary frozen shoulder: resulting from trauma, shoulder surgery, inflammatory disease, and/or previous shoulder conditions
- Onset between ages 40 and 70
- Duration depends on timing of diagnosis; usually resolves in 1–2 years
- Slight prevalence in females; rare in children

Morbidity and Mortality

Shoulder pain is the third most common musculoskeletal complaint in the workplace, followed by low-back pain (LBP) and neck pain. About 2% of the population suffers from frozen shoulder. It is more common in patients with diabetes, hyperthyroidism, and hypertriglyceridemia (increased triglyceride blood level), making these conditions possible risk factors for developing frozen shoulder. Researchers have been unable to determine whether these disorders are comorbidities or causative factors.

Although commonly unilateral, the condition occurs bilaterally in 16% of patients with a diagnosis of sequential frozen shoulder (one shoulder is affected, and then the other). In about 14% of these cases, the contralateral shoulder is affected before the first shoulder's symptoms resolve. Although 10% never recover full normal shoulder range of motion (ROM), relapse is unusual.

PATHOPHYSIOLOGY

X-rays rarely indicate previous joint abnormalities. The medical literature supports an inflammatory component, which may help explain the onset of subtle, gradual clinical symptoms, followed by remarkable pain and loss of function, and then, a waning of symptoms—all indicative of other inflammatory processes.

One common pathophysiologic explanation is as follows: An inflammatory process (of unknown origin) in the joint's synovial tissue creates a thicker synovial membrane, leading to tiny tears as the head of the humerus moves through normal ROM at articulating surfaces, where bone contacts bone (Figure 16-1). This low-level chronic inflammation leads to further local fibrosis (scar tissue), causing more inflammation upon movement as the cycle continues. Postoperative pathologic specimens support the preceding theory; however, similar reliable evidence is not available to indicate a strong inflammatory presence in the earlier stages of the condition.

Frozen shoulder occurs in three phases:

- *Phase 1 (acute stage), 2–9 months*: Pain of unknown origin usually originates at night, disturbing sleep; no significant functional loss, although pain can be felt at the far end of normal shoulder ROM.

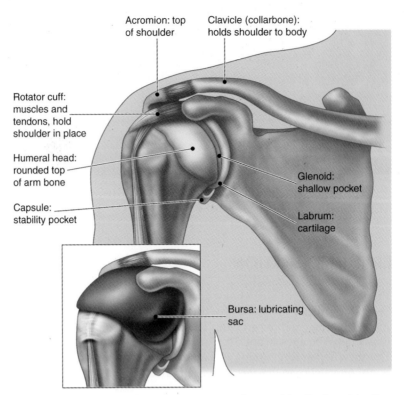

FIGURE 16-1 Anatomy of the shoulder joint. Synovial fluid is found at all articulating joints.

- *Phase 2 (subacute stage, stiffening phase), 3–9 months*: The shoulder feels frozen; ROM is functionally limited. Pain persists but is generally milder than in phase 1.
- *Phase 3 (chronic stage, thawing phase), 12–24 months*: Pain decreases significantly and ROM increases until the condition resolves.

Only a small percentage of patients complain of long-lasting ROM restrictions and pain.

Although it seems counterintuitive, frozen shoulder does not develop from disuse of the shoulder joint. No research supports increased diagnoses after stroke or paralysis in which functionality is dramatically decreased.

Diagnostic tests include bone thermography and Doppler. Arthroscopic findings indicate synovial tissue inflammation accompanied by intra-articular tendon thickening, scar tissue, and chronic inflammatory cells. However, physicians usually prefer a clinical (hands-on, noninvasive) diagnosis determined by the patient's oral history, pain level, and limited ROM.

OVERALL SIGNS AND SYMPTOMS

- Progressive unilateral shoulder pain, usually beginning at night, interrupting sleep
- Progressive shoulder functional restriction during normal ROM
- Pain while at rest and exacerbated with all shoulder activities
- Progressive worsening pain during vibration of the arm, psychological stress, and/or weather changes, especially exposure to cold

SIGNS AND SYMPTOMS MASSAGE THERAPY CAN ADDRESS

- The anxiety and breathing restrictions that accompany pain and loss of joint movement can be relieved with massage therapy techniques.
- Joint restrictions can be relaxed and low-level inflammatory debris can be cleansed from surrounding tissue with appropriate therapy.

TREATMENT OPTIONS

Although the etiology and pathophysiology of this condition remain unclear, treatment protocols supported by research relieve pain, increase ROM, and return the patient to normal or near-normal function.

Because no single approach has proven consistently effective, a combination is often prescribed. A progression from the least to the most invasive therapies includes the application of heat, oral pain medications, home exercise regimens, physical therapy (PT); PT combined with intra-articular corticosteroid injections, nerve blocks, arthroscopic release, including manipulation of the joint and scar removal, and, finally, open surgery. The medical literature indicates that early and aggressive treatment is most effective. Optimally, frozen shoulder can improve without surgery if diagnosed and treated during phase 1.

The best treatment is prevention, although preventing a condition of unknown etiology that presents with often subtle symptoms may be nearly impossible. Early mobilization and therapy during symptomatic onset may deter progression into later stages. Those performing repetitive or vibratory upper-extremity activities are counseled to attend to proper body mechanics, set up an ergonomically effective work environment, engage in preventive manual therapies, and rest frequently.

Common Medications

Typically, a patient will start a regimen of oral over-the-counter (OTC) analgesics and nonsteroidal anti-inflammatory drugs (NSAIDs) to control both pain and inflammation. If pain is not relieved, the patient will typically be prescribed with oral corticosteroids, then, steroidal injections directly into the joint. Narcotics are the medication of last resort.

- Nonopioid pain relievers and fever reducers such as acetaminophen (Tylenol, Feverall, Anacin, Panadol)
- Anti-inflammatory analgesics and fever reducers such as celecoxib (Celebrex)

MASSAGE THERAPIST ASSESSMENT

The massage therapist can *assess for treatment purposes only*. He does not assess for the existence of frozen shoulder, but rather to determine the therapy necessary for each specific session.

While sitting in a chair, the client is asked to demonstrate full shoulder joint movement, or active ROM (a standing position would alter the determination of true shoulder ROM). She should indicate the exact point at which the movement creates pain or "feels stuck." While the therapist keeps detailed notes, the client works through the shoulder's entire ROM capabilities including flexion, extension, abduction, adduction, circumduction, and internal and external rotation. The therapist should also record answers to questions about restrictions of daily activities. For example, difficulties with hair washing, bra fastening, reaching for the seatbelt, or lifting a gallon of milk can help determine the extent of the pain and lack of function. The therapist then performs the full shoulder ROM for the client (passive ROM) and makes any significant notes.

Finally, carefully probing the entire shoulder girdle and pectoralis complex, the therapist notes any point of tenderness, as well as hypertonicity and/or trigger points in the shoulder, upper chest, and arm.

THERAPEUTIC GOALS

Reducing the perception of pain, helping to improve ROM, decreasing breathing restrictions, reducing anxiety, and providing comfort are worthy goals in the treatment

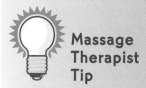

Massage Therapist Tip

Becoming Part of the Health Care Team

Although massage therapy alone cannot alter the course of frozen shoulder, your soft tissue work can directly influence your client's path toward wellness, as she works with her PT and physician. Ideally, a massage therapy appointment immediately preceding your client's PT appointment can prepare the tissue for a very effective (and less painful) PT session. To become a part of this health care team, you can call, with your client's permission, either the treating physician and/or the PT to diplomatically inform them that you, too, are treating their patient. You might say something like this: "I'm also treating your patient, Mrs. Smith, and would like to know how I can help your efforts to reduce her pain and increase her range of motion." A diplomatic massage therapist can often be rewarded with return phone calls from a PT or physician who understands that you share common goals and, in no way, are attempting to treat independently of medical counsel.

Thinking It Through

Treating frozen shoulder is an excellent time for a therapist to realize that his personal expectations and attitude while treating a client can profoundly affect treatment outcome. Since most frozen shoulders do resolve (often as mysteriously as they appear), therapy can be an exercise in diplomatic, cautious optimism that can be remarkably infectious to the hopeful client. The therapist can perform a "mental check" while treating not only frozen shoulder but also many chronic conditions.

- Am I expecting this client's symptoms to resolve?
- Are my verbal instructions during treatment and homework assignments presented optimistically?
- Am I seeing the client as "ill or handicapped" rather than on a progressive journey toward wellness?
- Am I asking the client to take full responsibility for her progress, or am I treating in such a way as to keep her dependent upon my therapy?
- Do I diplomatically remind the client, when she is feeling particularly defeated, that there is relief in sight and that research supports her full recovery?

of this complicated condition. The therapist must remember that he may encounter the client/patient at any stage, along her possibly long struggle with frozen shoulder, and functional restrictions fluctuate.

MASSAGE SESSION FREQUENCY

- Ideally: 60-minute sessions once a week
- Minimally: 60-minute sessions every other week
- Infrequent, inconsistent therapy will produce limited results

MASSAGE PROTOCOL

The following protocol is based on massage therapy for unilateral frozen shoulder at any phase of the condition. Since pain, limited ROM, breathing restrictions, and anxiety are always present with frozen shoulder, and given the assumption that you are working in conjunction with a PT or primary health care practitioner, you can modify the protocol according to the severity of your client's symptoms.

Your work will be very local and detailed to address extreme hypertonicity, deep in the client's shoulder joint. Contralateral attention to the uninvolved shoulder provides balance to the body. Positioning for contralateral therapy should not require the client to lie on the painful, involved shoulder; comfortable prone or supine positioning should be possible. Since you will require movement of the entire upper extremity through most of its functional capabilities, be sure to carefully and securely support the arm so the client can relax. Fear of an arm being accidentally dropped—and producing pain—will prevent her from reaching deep relaxation.

Your therapy will focus on bony prominences, muscle origin and insertion points, and especially at articulating surfaces in the shoulder joint where synovial fluid is created.

Although you will attempt to reduce breathing restrictions, it is not necessarily the anatomic diaphragmatic restriction that you are addressing but, rather, the psychological component of breath holding that accompanies chronic pain and anxiety. Therefore, your breath work will involve asking your client to breathe deeply throughout the session.

Maintain detailed intake, treatment, and progress notes that you can periodically share with the client's physician or PT.

Getting Started

Positioning is always dictated by the client's comfort level; in this case, your work is performed with the client side-lying on the unaffected shoulder. Contralateral work is performed with the client lying supine or prone. You will need moist hot packs and a "teddy bear" pillow (placed as if the side-lying client is holding a large, favorite teddy bear) that will provide support for the painful shoulder.

HOMEWORK

Although studies indicate that early, aggressive, and consistent stretching and strengthening programs at home can profoundly hasten a client's return to normal shoulder function, it is outside your scope of practice to assign any regimen beyond modest and noninvasive homework. You can assign the following with the knowledge that you are working within your scope, while simultaneously helping your client reach wellness:

- Apply heat to your shoulder regularly, except on days when you receive a shoulder injection or when the pain is acute.
- Roll your shoulders both forward and backward at least a dozen times throughout the day.
- Take deep breaths throughout the day by inhaling deeply, holding your breath for a few seconds, and exhaling with vigor. Do this at least 10 times a day.

Step-by-Step Protocol for **Frozen Shoulder**

Technique	Duration
Position the client side-lying with the unaffected side on the table. Place a small pillow under her neck and a larger pillow between her arms so the cervical spine is aligned and the affected shoulder rests in a correct anatomical position. Place a moist hot pack at the location of the head of the humerus so it drapes across the anterior and posterior portion of the shoulder girdle. Leave the pack in place; ask the client where she would like you to perform a few minutes of simple relaxation techniques.	5 minutes
Remove the hot pack. Effleurage, medium pressure, evenly rhythmic. • Pectoralis major, pectoralis minor, below the clavicular ridge all the way from the manubrium to the acromion process.	5 minutes
Effleurage, medium pressure, evenly rhythmic. • All muscles, tendons, bony prominences, and articulating joints of the shoulder girdle, especially focusing around the head of the humerus.	5 minutes
Effleurage, palmar and digital kneading, deep pressure, evenly rhythmic. • All muscles, tendons, bony prominences, and articulating joints of the shoulder girdle, especially focusing around the head of the humerus.	5 minutes
Ask the client to pinpoint where her shoulder feels "stuck" as you passively move her arm through its arc of ROM. Return the arm to its comfortable position. Follow these steps: • Warm the region using deep effleurage. • Move the arm to its painful or stuck point. • Stop movement and securely hold the arm. • Perform deep, slow, focused cross-fiber friction and kneading as near to the restricted area as the client's anatomy will allow. • Return the arm to a comfortable position and allow it to rest a moment. • Return the arm to the stuck or painful point following your client's input. • Ask the client to take a deep breath. • Move the arm to at least 1 inch beyond its previous point of pain or immobility; hold this position for a few seconds. • Return the arm to a relaxed position. • Effleurage, medium-to-deep pressure, to this entire area.	10 minutes
Effleurage, slow, medium pressure. • Anterior and posterior shoulder girdle area.	3 minutes
Find another area of shoulder restriction or pain and repeat the enumerated steps.	10 minutes

(continued)

Contraindications and Cautions

The presence of scar tissue, the client's desire to increase ROM, and her frustration with a "stuck" shoulder may tempt you to use more aggressive measures than are justified. It is not your job to "break up adhesions" or perform excessive scar work.

Pain relief and increased ROM will occur slowly in response to a combination of techniques. Neither you nor the client should expect immediate results.

Shoulder problems mimicking frozen shoulder symptoms include fracture, dislocation, rotator cuff tear, tumor, and infection. Do not treat self-diagnosed frozen shoulder until a physician has ruled out other more serious conditions.

An impingement is indicated if the client reports pain in the midrange of flexion or abduction accompanied by no pain at the beginning or end of the movement arc. Refer her to a physical medicine specialist.

Recent shoulder intra-articular corticosteroid injections are a contraindication for local massage therapy.

Technique	Duration
Position the client supine, maintain the pillow under her neck, remove the "teddy bear" pillow, reapply the hot pack to the anterior surface of the head of the humerus/shoulder girdle region (do not allow the client to lie on the hot pack). Ask the client to perform three rounds of deep breathing as she inhales deeply, holds the breath for a few seconds, and then forcibly exhales.	3 minutes
Effleurage, petrissage, effleurage, knead, effleurage. • The entire shoulder girdle and pectoralis major and minor complex of the unaffected shoulder.	10 minutes
Perform a few minutes of relaxation techniques before the client leaves the table.	4 minutes

- Self-massage your shoulder. Cup your palm around your shoulder, and then, as deeply as you can tolerate without creating pain, dig your fingers into your shoulder joint and massage it for a few minutes. You can do this while reading or watching TV.
- Move your arm to the point of pain or stiffness, and perform the above self-massage directly over the affected area.

Review Questions

1. What is frozen shoulder also called?
2. What causes frozen shoulder?
3. What are the symptoms of frozen shoulder?
4. What other conditions often coexist with frozen shoulder?
5. How many phases are there, what are they called, and what are their characteristics?
6. How is frozen shoulder usually clinically diagnosed?
7. What is the typical treatment regimen, from least to most invasive?
8. Does frozen shoulder typically resolve?

BIBLIOGRAPHY

Kane JW, Jackins S, Sidles JA, et al. Simple Home Program for Frozen Shoulder to Improve Patient's Assessment of Shoulder Function and Health Status. Medscape. Available at: http//www.medscape.com/viewarticle/417861. Accessed May 29, 2008.

Liebenson C. Shoulder disorders—Part 2: Examination. *Journal of Bodywork and Movement Therapies* 2005;9:283–292.

Liebenson C. Self-management of shoulder disorders—Part 3: Treatment. *Journal of Bodywork and Movement Therapies* 2006;10:65–70.

Mense S, Simons DG, Russell, IJ. *Muscle Pain: Understanding Its Nature, Diagnosis, and Treatment*. Philadelphia: Lippincott Williams & Wilkins, 2001.

Pearsall AW, Adhesive Capsulitis. EMedicine. Available at: http://www.emedicine.com/orthoped/topic372.htm. Accessed May 6, 2010.

Phillips G. Five massage therapists explain the most common injuries they see in a variety of sports, and how they treat them. *Massage Therapy Journal* 2008:33–44.

Rattray F, Ludwig L. *Clinical Massage Therapy: Understanding, Assessing, and Treating over 70 Conditions*, Toronto: Talus Incorporated, 2000.

Roy A, Adhesive Capsulitis. Emedicine. Available at: http://emedicine.medscape.com/article/326828-overview. Accessed May 6, 2010.

Werner R. *A Massage Therapist's Guide to Pathology*, 4th ed. Philadelphia: Lippincott Williams & Wilkins, 2009.

17

Headache—Migraine

Definition: Periodic, unexpected, debilitating, pulsating headache.

GENERAL INFORMATION

- Etiology unknown
- Triggered by stress; physical exertion; sleep deprivation; hot weather; certain foods, such as chocolate, citrus fruits, onions, coffee, MSG (monosodium glutamate); any form of alcohol; hormonal fluctuations; head trauma
- Early childhood onset with increased frequency during puberty, continued occurrence in 30s and 40s; rare after age 50
- Duration from hours to several days
- Strong genetic predisposition
- Prevalence in females
- Two types: migraine with aura (classic migraine) and migraine without aura (common migraine, 80% of migraine diagnoses)

Morbidity and Mortality

About 28 million people, or 10–20% of the U.S. population, suffer from migraine headaches, of which 17% are females and 6% are males. Before puberty, the incidence is higher in males; with the onset of puberty, the incidence and prevalence increase in both genders. After age 40, the incidence for both males and females declines dramatically. Persistent symptoms after the age of 50 often indicate other (more serious) etiologies. Some 70–80% of migraine sufferers report a first-degree relative (parent or sibling) who also has these debilitating headaches.

If migraines occur before the age of 50, they are *not usually* indicative of serious medical conditions. However, migraines at any age have been associated with an increased risk of stroke and seizure, Tourette syndrome, depression, anxiety, asthma, and brain lesions.

PATHOPHYSIOLOGY

Several theories attempt to explain the pathophysiology of this puzzling condition. A vascular theory proposes that the migraine "trigger" (a substance or event that initiates the headache) creates cerebral vasoconstriction (constricted blood vessels in the brain), followed by dramatically responsive cerebral vasodilation. The rush of intracranial pressure from the vasodilation causes profound pain. Interestingly, prodromal euphoria, irritability, yawning, depression, and/or excitability are also thought to be related to this change in intracranial pressure. (Prodromal refers to the earliest stage, before usual symptoms manifest.)

Another theory follows the trail of cerebral vascularity but maintains that a series of cascading neurotransmitters set up an inflammatory response in the brain. Finally, one study found postural dysfunctions such as the head-forward posture and extreme

137

low-back curvature as possible causative factors. No single theory explains the two types of migraines, the variety of triggers, onsets, and durations, or the inexplicable differences in intense migraine experiences.

Most migraines are appropriately diagnosed and treated by a primary care physician who approaches the patient clinically, taking into account her family history and personal symptoms. A physician may choose to perform a neurologic workup, but a CT scan or lumbar puncture is usually reserved for patients presenting with symptomatic complications beyond the normal migraine pattern. The great majority of migraine sufferers seen in an emergency center are referred to a primary care physician, not a neurologist.

OVERALL SIGNS AND SYMPTOMS

Any combination of the following signs and symptoms can occur in the migraineur, depending on her history, the trigger, the headache's severity, and whether she experiences auras:

- Unilateral cerebral disturbance or pain
- Blurred vision
- Dizziness or lightheadedness
- Peripheral visual auras, zigzagging lines in front of the eyes, ringing in the ears
- Extremely painful pulsating and throbbing in one or both sides of the head
- Hypersensitivity to light, and/or sound, and/or smells
- Nausea and vomiting
- Malaise

SIGNS AND SYMPTOMS MASSAGE THERAPY CAN ADDRESS

Massage therapy can do little to ease the signs and symptoms of a full-blown migraine while it is occurring; in fact, the migraineur would find bodywork unbearable, as any stimulus or approach to the body exacerbates symptoms. The following signs and symptoms that occur before and after the attack may be addressed by massage therapy:

- Scalp, face, neck, and shoulder hypertonicity are effectively treated with massage therapy techniques.
- The anxiety that accompanies the unpredictable nature of this condition can be addressed with soothing modalities.
- Self-help techniques can be taught to the migraineur, who is often eager for any nonpharmaceutical preventive measures.

TREATMENT OPTIONS

Often, a migraine sufferer's first response is to retreat; she will find a dark, quiet space in an attempt to ease the pain. Cool compresses to the neck and head, placed directly on the painful areas, can help. Strong anecdotal evidence indicates that complementary and alternative medicine (CAM) techniques, such as massage therapy, chiropractic adjustments, acupuncture, and acupressure, provide symptomatic relief, although these approaches have not been thoroughly studied. Two preventive herbs, butterbur and feverfew, have been found to be effective.

Prescription medications dominate the treatment for migraine headaches. Vasoconstrictors address constricted cerebral blood vessels, analgesics can reduce the pain that accompanies all migraines, tranquilizers calm anxiety, antiemetic medications help prevent nausea from dizziness, and some medications affect serotonin and dopamine levels in the brain. Migraineurs often take a combination

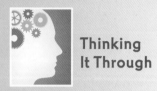

Thinking It Through

Because massage therapists are found more frequently in hospitals, clinics, and hospices, it becomes tempting, in a zealous effort to gain professional credibility, to overstate the physiologic effects of massage. Two effects have, in fact, been proven: Massage therapy techniques reduce anxiety and reduce the perception of pain. Multiple other studies are currently under way to further prove the profound effects of this work. Keeping in mind that understatement is the safer road, the therapist should think through how she might explain the following to a physician or health care professional who has entrusted a patient or client to the care of a massage therapist.

- What is the difference between "pain" and "the perception of pain"?
- How could a client be helped by anxiety relief?
- How can the power of touch affect most clients who are stressed?
- Why should a physician grant a massage therapist access to and the care of any seriously ill patient?
- Although massage therapists are gaining a foothold in medical environments, what might be some *disadvantages* of becoming one more member of a hospital team?

of medications, and, unfortunately, the duration of this powerful chemical cocktail can lead to a "rebound migraine"—a migraine that occurs as a side effect of the combinations and accumulation of medications used to treat the migraine itself. The long list of medications taken by most migraineurs—and the possible side effects—should be regularly monitored by the attending physician.

Common Medications

- Nonsteroidal anti-inflammatory drugs (NSAIDs), such as ibuprofen (Motrin, Advil); naproxen (Aleve, Anaprox, Naprelan, Naprosyn); ketoprofen (Oruvail, Orudis); and ketorolac tromethamine (Toradol)
- Nonopioid pain relievers and fever reducers, such as acetaminophen (Tylenol, Feverall, Anacin, Panadol)
- Antipsychotic, antiemetic anxiolytics, such as prochlorperazine (Compazine)
- Antiemetic, antivertigo, antihistamine sedatives, such as promethazine hydrochloride (Phenergan)
- Antiemetic gastrointestinal stimulants, such as metoclopramide hydrochloride (Reglan)
- Antimigraines, such as sumatriptan succinate (Imitrex), zolmitriptan (Zomig), eletriptan hydrobromide (Relpax), and rizatriptan benzoate (Maxalt)
- Narcotics, such as acetaminophen and codeine (Tylenol #3)
- Cranial vasoconstrictors, such as ergotamine tartrate and caffeine (Cafergot suppositories) and dihydroergotamine mesylate (Migranal spray)

MASSAGE THERAPIST ASSESSMENT

If a person is experiencing a migraine headache, she will probably not be found on a massage table. Driving to the appointment would have been impossible and unsafe. Being touched during a migraine attack is usually unpleasant at best. Therefore, this assessment assumes the client is in either the prodromal, post-headache stage, or the mildly symptomatic phase.

The therapist can perform a full intake outlining the client's history before palpating the head, neck, face, and shoulders to determine hypertonicity. The client can help by relating past occurrences, as well as self-help and medical treatments. Reasonable expectations regarding the outcome of a massage therapy session, as well as the techniques used, should be discussed in detail. The client's high hopes for relief and the fear of triggering stimuli need to be fairly addressed before the session begins.

THERAPEUTIC GOALS

Anxiety relief; reduced perception of pain; decreased hypertonicity in the head, neck, and shoulders; and providing a safe, quiet, noninvasive hour of peace are reasonable therapeutic goals.

MASSAGE SESSION FREQUENCY

- Before or after a migraine headache, 60-minute sessions may be exhausting; modify length to the client's tolerance.

MASSAGE PROTOCOL

Head, neck, face, and shoulder hypertonicity are the focal points of an effective treatment aimed at reducing the muscular side effects of excruciating pain. Application of cold packs to the side of the neck (but not on the carotid artery region), the back

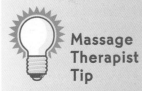

Massage Therapist Tip

An Assault on All Senses

If you have never experienced a migraine headache and want to empathize with a client who does have them, imagine what it would be like if each of your senses were simultaneously assaulted. Imagine a very low light feeling like a high-beam headlight being directed at your eyes; think about the subtlest of smells causing you to feel sick; determine what it might be like if your normal vision were compromised by sharp, wavy, moving lines that make it difficult to focus; add a sense of nausea combined with a fear of vomiting at any moment. Finally, accompany this sense-assault with a pain in your head so severe, it feels as if someone has taken an ice pick to your skull. You now have some idea of the horrible, unrelenting, unpredictable, and debilitating nature of the type of headache your client is enduring.

Contraindications and Cautions

- Do not apply heat to any portion of the client's body, but especially the head, neck, or shoulders. Increased vasodilation from the application of heat can exacerbate symptoms.

The following signs and symptoms are not merely contraindications and cautions for massage therapy, but are indications that your client should be referred to a physician promptly:

- A statement such as "This is the worst headache I've ever experienced; it's never been this bad"
- A migraine that has a more rapid onset than usual
- A change in frequency, duration, or severity of the migraine headache
- Headache onset by coughing, sneezing, or bearing down during a bowel movement
- Headache accompanied by fever, and/or a feeling of malaise, and/or neck stiffness
- Unexplained weight loss
- Fainting, difficulty speaking, or balance problems

Step-by-Step Protocol for Migraine Headache

Technique	Duration
With the client positioned supine, well-supported by pillows, place a cold pack on her neck or head, as she directs. Leave it in place for this opening technique. Greet the body with general warming compression. Do not touch the face, head, or neck at this point. Work slowly, *not* rhythmically; *vary your rhythm*, trying not to rock the body. • Start at the feet • Work up the legs • Include the abdominal region • Work the arms and hands • Include the pectoral region	5 minutes
Remove the cold pack. Stroking, even, long, careful, rhythmic strokes • Through the entire length of the hair from the scalp to the ends of the hair, over the entire head region	5 minutes
Cleanse your hands Digital kneading, medium pressure, evenly rhythmic • Bony prominences of the frontal, ethmoid, maxilla, and sphenoid (sinus configuration) bones • Work along the temporomandibular joint (TMJ)	5 minutes
Effleurage, using flattened fingers, medium pressure, evenly rhythmic • The entire face, working from the midline of the face, down toward the ears and the table	3 minutes
Digital kneading, medium pressure, evenly rhythmic • All muscles of the forehead, cheeks, and jaw	5 minutes
Effleurage, using flattened fingers, medium pressure, evenly rhythmic • The entire face	3 minutes
Digital kneading, medium pressure, *not rhythmic* • Occipital ridge	5 minutes
Digital kneading, medium pressure, *not rhythmic* • Posterior bony prominences of the cervical spine and posterior and lateral neck muscles • Include the insertions and origins of the sternocleidomastoid (SCM) on the mastoid and the sternum	5 minutes
Effleurage, medium pressure, rhythmic • All neck muscles	3 minutes
Effleurage, petrissage, effleurage, medium pressure, rhythmic • Bilateral superior trapezius muscles • Work away from the midline, out from the middle of the body to the lateral portion of the body	5 minutes

(continued)

Technique	Duration
Cleanse your hands.	
Effleurage, medium pressure, *vary your rhythm* • The face • The neck • The superior trapezius	5 minutes
Stroke, evenly rhythmic • Through the hair, from the scalp to the tips of the hair	5 minutes
Whole-body compression, evenly rhythmic • Starting at the feet • Working up the legs • Including the abdominal region • Working the arms and hands	6 minutes

of the neck, or the head can bring significant relief. Relaxation techniques to any part of the body, as requested by the client, will help reduce anxiety and pain perception.

Perform all techniques slowly and carefully, using light-to-medium pressure. Pressure that is too light can stimulate and irritate; too deep pressure might feel invasive. Be careful *not to use consistently rhythmic strokes*. This client is on the border of vertigo, and constant rhythmic techniques can trigger dizziness. Subtly vary the pace of the techniques, being careful not to initiate any rocking movements of the body.

Perform all neck and shoulder strokes *away from the head* to reduce the chance of increasing intracranial pressure.

Getting Started

Have a cold pack ready. Lights should be lowered, lotions should be scent-free, and the music set at a low volume. Silence might be best. Monitor your vocal tones and rate at which you speak to match your client's tolerance to stimuli. Make sure she has someone to drive her home, or that her session is timed so she can be left to sleep afterward.

The client will probably prefer a well-pillowed supine or side-lying position because lying prone may increase sinus, and therefore intracranial, pressure.

HOMEWORK

Write out any specific homework assignments for your migraine client. She may be so relaxed after her therapy session, or unable to concentrate because of her symptoms, or unable to focus because of her medications, that verbally assigning homework may be counterproductive. Keep your voice modulated and quiet, and don't overwhelm her with instructions.

- When you feel the next migraine headache coming on, begin massaging your face, scalp, and neck immediately. Use your fingertips, move slowly, but go in deeply enough to touch the bone under the muscle. Work in slow circles; try to work directly over any painful points.
- When you feel the migraine is coming on, get a cold pack, even just a bag of frozen fruit or vegetables. Put the pack in a pillowcase and place it directly on your neck or any painful spot on your head.

- Keep a journal of possible foods or activities that might have triggered your migraine; these triggers can help you and your physician to determine future preventive measures.
- If you feel you're getting headaches from your prescribed medications, return to your physician and ask her to reformulate your prescriptions.
- Continue to experiment with other CAM therapies; consider seeing a chiropractor or an acupuncturist.

Review

1. What are the two types of migraine headaches?
2. List several possible migraine headache triggers.
3. Why would a migraineur probably not seek massage therapy during a migraine attack?
4. List various classifications of medications commonly prescribed for migraine sufferers.
5. Describe some CAM therapies that might help migraineurs.
6. Based on one of the pathophysiologic theories, explain why cold packs might provide some relief.

BIBLIOGRAPHY

Blanda M. Migraine Headache. EMedicine article. Available at: http://emedicine.medscape .com/article/792267-overview. Accessed June 7, 2010.

Rattray F, Ludwig L. *Clinical Massage Therapy: Understanding, Assessing and Treating over 70 Conditions*, Toronto: Talus Incorporated, 2000.

Sahai S. Pathophysiology and Treatment of Migraine and Related Headache. EMedicine article. Available at: http://emedicine.medscape.com/article/1144656-overview. Accessed June 7, 2010.

Werner R. *A Massage Therapist's Guide to Pathology*, 4th ed. Philadelphia: Lippincott Williams & Wilkins, 2009.

18

Headache—Tension

Definition: A dull or vice-like pain of mild-to-moderate intensity experienced in the scalp, forehead, temples, jaw, and/or base of the skull.

GENERAL INFORMATION

- Causes: tightening of the head, jaw, neck, and upper shoulder muscles; depression
- Physical triggers: forward-head position, prolonged lateral head tilt, slouching, poor neck support while sleeping, poor workstation ergonomics
- Psychosomatic triggers: emotional stress, worry, and anxiety leading to shoulder elevation, holding the breath, jaw clenching.
- Aggravating factors: caffeine withdrawal, hypoglycemia (low blood sugar), fear, dehydration
- Onset: any age, but most common in young adults
- Duration from 30 minutes to several days
- Prevalence in females

PATHOPHYSIOLOGY

Although the research on headache etiology is ongoing, the current thinking is that the condition results from changes in the levels of the neurotransmitter serotonin in the brain. These fluctuations, combined with a possible inflammatory response that flushes the already tightly compacted cranial cavity with more fluid, cause increased intracranial pressure, resulting in the feeling of head pain. The person's response is to tighten the surrounding muscles (Figure 18-1), which then become hypertonic. This reaction produces a vice-like feeling in the head, as the cycle of head pain and hypertonicity continues.

Headache is the ninth most common reason for which Americans consult a physician. However, only a small percentage have a serious underlying pathology. Headaches are ubiquitous yet so varied that medical experts have identified primary and secondary headaches, as well as several classifications. A diagnosis of primary headache is simply the headache itself, with no accompanying pathology. A secondary headache results from, or coexists with, trauma (physical or emotional), or another incident or pathology. Classifications include cluster, migraine, chronic daily headache (CDH), rebound, vascular, mixed, and the most common, tension-type headache (TTH). Tension headaches, the focus of this chapter, are usually not debilitating, even if chronic, and the person can perform daily activities, and function at work and play.

OVERALL SIGNS AND SYMPTOMS

- Muscle tenderness and hypertonicity in the scalp, temples, forehead, neck, and upper shoulders
- Tightening sensation in the head muscles
- Mild-to-moderate steady, bilateral head pain

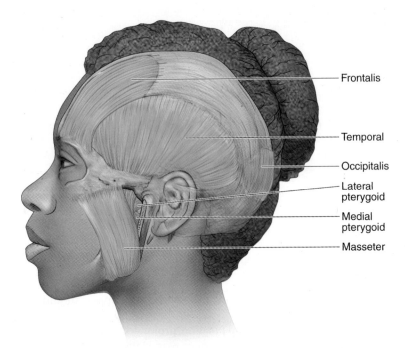

FIGURE 18-1 **Tension headache. Lateral and posterior views of the head muscles.**

SIGNS AND SYMPTOMS MASSAGE THERAPY CAN ADDRESS

- Helping a client achieve a parasympathetic state and addressing muscular hypertonicity are basic skills in every massage therapist's toolkit.
- Treating the client holistically—identifying muscular hypertonicity while simultaneously listening to the emotional and psychological components of the headache—is also well within the massage therapist's scope of practice.

TREATMENT OPTIONS

Physical therapy (PT) for headache sufferers with postural abnormalities can be effective in both relieving pain and preventing future occurrences. PT modalities may include the application of hot and cold packs, ultrasound, and electrical stimulation. Regular exercise, stretching, adequate sleep, stress-relief measures, and finding one's joy in life can also help prevent or reduce recurring headaches. Unrelenting headache pain is sometimes treated with cervical traction, local anesthesia injected into trigger points, and occipital nerve blocks.

The long-term use of even the mildest over-the-counter (OTC) pain medications can cause rebound headaches. A rebound headache results from the accumulation of the medications taken to treat the original headache.

Common Medications

- Salicylate nonopioid pain relievers, such as aspirin (Ecotrin, Empirin, Astrin)
- Nonopioid pain reliever and fever reducers, such as acetaminophen (Tylenol, Feverall, Anacin, Panadol)
- Nonsteroidal anti-inflammatory drugs (NSAIDs), such as ketorolac tromethamine (Toradol)
- Antipsychotic, antiemetic anxiolytics, such as prochlorperazine (Compazine)
- Antiemetic, antivertigo, antihistamine sedatives, such as promethazine hydrochloride (Reglan)

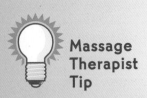

Massage Therapist Tip

It's Not Just "In the Head"

Trigger points often accompany the common tension headache. A trigger point is a localized, palpable area of extreme hypertonicity that causes radiating pain in regional—although not always directly localized—areas of the body. (Refer to Chapter 43 for more on trigger points.) The levels of aggressiveness and stretching that should accompany trigger point treatments are controversial, and a full explanation is outside the scope of this book. However, if you have been trained in identifying and treating trigger points, this work on the head, face, neck, and shoulders is appropriate for clients with tension headaches, as long as you use caution.

MASSAGE THERAPIST ASSESSMENT

Although she might not know exactly what set off the headache, the client will know the location, duration, and severity of her pain. Since a headache is one of the few conditions that can be pinpointed, the therapist's palpating assessment, combined with the client's detailed input, can provide an accurate treatment map. It's best to assess the client before she undresses, while she is sitting in a chair, and while the therapist is standing behind her. In this position, the therapist can palpate the client's face, jaw, temporomandibular joint (TMJ), neck, upper shoulders, and base of her skull to determine the exact points of pain and accompanying hypertonicity.

To determine the deficits in range of motion (ROM) and the extent of muscular hypertonicity, the therapist can ask the client to perform active (unassisted) head and neck ROM movements.

These movements include flexion, extension, and rotation from side to side, and they should be performed with only minimal discomfort.

Questioning the client about her medications, other complementary and alternative medicine (CAM) modalities she is using for pain relief, and whether she is seeing a physician will provide other essential information that can contribute to an effective session.

Headaches often accompany many conditions treated by massage therapists. It is important to know if the client has fibromyalgia, chronic fatigue syndrome, or TMJ syndrome, for example, in order to determine a treatment plan that addresses more than a localized headache.

THERAPEUTIC GOALS

Reducing muscular hypertonicity, restoring normal head and neck ROM, reinforcing a normal and relaxed breathing pattern, and helping the client reach a parasympathetic state are reasonable goals.

MASSAGE SESSION FREQUENCY

- 60-minute sessions twice a week during headache occurrence
- At least monthly preventive or maintenance sessions after the headache passes
- Underlying postural abnormalities, breath-holding patterns, and secondary effects of head tilt or forward-head posture will need to be addressed in subsequent, at least monthly, sessions.

MASSAGE PROTOCOL

Anatomic knowledge of the head and face muscles, joints, and bony prominences, combined with your sensitive hands that will seek out subtle areas of hypertonic tissue, perhaps buried under the hair or evident along the masseter, will serve both you and your client as you approach the highly personal treatment area. Your work will be performed slowly, deliberately, and only moderately deep as you focus on the head, neck, face, and shoulders. Working too deeply, quickly, or aggressively can lead to a recurring "kick-back" headache. This frustrating return of a headache, either hours or sometimes days after treatment, is in direct physiologic response to manual techniques that return blood flow too quickly to a constricted area.

Fascial release techniques are essential during this protocol because the scalp muscles are buried under a taut layer of tendon (galea aponeurotica), and the facial muscles can be surprisingly resistant to release. Placing your two thumbs on any facial muscle, and pushing them toward each other to create an S-shape in the underlying skin, is one effective fascial release technique that can be used, to varying depth, anywhere on the face. Gentle cross-fiber friction at muscle origins and insertions also provides fascial softening.

Thinking It Through

People who have tension headaches are often thought of as hypochondriacs, and their regular physicians, or other health care practitioners, might not take their discomfort seriously. A massage therapist, however, although not a diagnostician, has the luxury of spending an entire hour with the client and can sometimes unearth underlying pathologies that signal a visit to a neurologist, specialist, or talk therapist. Although pathologies are of concern, the compassionate therapist may be the first and only health care practitioner to look at the client's postural abnormalities and lifestyle stressors—themselves often the cause of headaches—and suggest a therapeutic path for pain relief. As the client offers her history, the therapist may ask himself the following questions:

- Is this client enduring recurring headaches, or worsening, noticeable changes in duration or severity, because she does not believe they are severe, when in fact these symptoms warrant another medical consultation?
- Who is attending to her underlying stressors? Should I tactfully suggest she seek psychological counseling and talk therapy because of her recent divorce?
- Did she experience a head trauma in the last 6–12 months that might have caused these headaches, and for which she never sought medical attention?

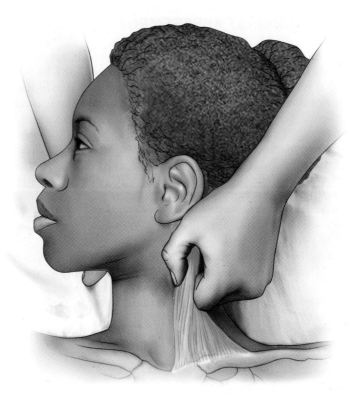

FIGURE 18-2 **SCM release. Grasping the SCM between the thumb and middle finger and alternating pressure between the two is an effective method of releasing hypertonicity in this muscle, which is often involved in clients with tension headaches.**

Hair tugging, when performed properly, can release the tough scalp tendon between the occipitalis and frontalis muscles. By spreading your open fingers and sliding them into your client's hair, make a gentle fist so your knuckles rest on the scalp itself, and then tug the hair forward and backward several times. This technique prepares the galea aponeurotica for successive kneading.

A sternocleidomastoid (SCM) release can be highly effective in treating a headache and is suggested during the step-by-step protocol. Although not customarily taught in massage therapy school, this release is relatively simple to perform. With your client lying supine on the table and her head turned to one side, you will be able to easily palpate the SCM. With your thumb and middle finger, gently grasp the muscle anywhere you can and push the alternating thumb and middle finger in opposite directions, effectively putting this muscle into a stretch (Figure 18-2). Following this gentle stretch with cross-fiber friction at both the SCM origin and insertion produces a very effective softening of one of the primary points of hypertonicity that typically accompanies a tension headache.

Precede all of your work with general effleurage to warm the tissue. Follow all work with gentle joint stretching and tissue lengthening. It is appropriate to ask your client, after about 20 minutes of massage therapy work, if her symptoms have decreased or subsided.

Shorten as many muscles as you can before working on a muscle set to allow greater accessibility to muscle origins and insertions. This is especially true of the posterior cervical muscles as you cross-fiber friction along the spinous and transverse processes. Cervical muscles are easily shortened when the client is lying supine and is asked to point her chin toward the ceiling, or when she is side-lying and asked to tilt her head backward.

Getting Started

Cool packs (not cold) on the closed eyes or forehead might comfort the client. Warm packs placed on the shoulders may also prepare the muscles for further work.

Step-by-Step Protocol for   Tension Headache

Technique	Duration
Position the client supine; no pillow under the head. Place a cool pack on the eyes or forehead; leave it in place for a few minutes as you work on her shoulders.	
Effleurage, medium pressure, evenly rhythmic, stroking *away* from the head and neck • From the occiput to the top of the deltoids. Perform bilaterally, alternating hands.	2 minutes
Place one hand at the top of the client's shoulder, the heel of that hand resting on the table; cup the occipital ridge in the other hand and hold her head stable. Gently but firmly push the shoulder. • Down toward the toes until you feel resistance. Hold for a few seconds and release. Repeat 3 times. Alternate hands. Perform bilaterally.	3 minutes
Effleurage, medium pressure, evenly rhythmic, stroking *away* from the head and neck. • From the occiput to the top of the deltoids. Perform bilaterally, alternating hands. Cleanse your hands.	2 minutes
After asking permission to do so, lay your hands on either side of your client's face. Effleurage, medium pressure, evenly rhythmic. • From the midline of the face, down toward the table, several times	2 minutes
Slide seamlessly to the TMJ. Perform cross-fiber friction, *working on one side of the face at a time, while bracing the face on the opposite side*. Perform digital kneading and effleurage, medium pressure. • From the TMJ to the base of the nose and back to the TMJ. Perform bilaterally.	5 minutes
Slide seamlessly to the forehead. Perform fascial release techniques, medium pressure. • From the center of the forehead, down to the temples, and back. You can work with both hands, bilaterally, simultaneously.	5 minutes
Slide seamlessly to the masseter muscle. Perform cross-fiber friction, medium pressure, *working on one side of the face at a time, while bracing the face on the opposite side*. • Start at the superior insertion point, work on both anterior and posterior ridges of the muscle, as well as the tiny belly, ending at the inferior insertion point.	5 minutes
Effleurage, medium pressure, slightly brisk pace • The entire face, lateral and posterior neck	1 minute
Cleanse your hands of all lubricant. Lay your client's head to one side. Perform nonaggressive, deliberate, thorough hair tugging. • Along the midline of the scalp from the forehead hairline to the occipital ridge. Give several brisk tugs at each position before moving on to the next position.	2 minutes

Contraindications and Cautions:

- During the physical assessment, you can expect the client to report tenderness, but a sudden withdrawal or wincing is not a normal response during palpation of client with TTH. Suspect an underlying pathology, and refer the client to her physician.

- If upon palpation the client feels warm to the touch, ask about fever or infection, both of which are contraindications for continuing a massage therapy session.

- Increased, uncomfortable pressure felt anywhere around the head by the client during assessment or palpation is unusual, and you should refer her to her physician.

- Nausea, vomiting, unusual eye pain, extreme agitation, or seeing spots before the eyes may indicate a serious medical condition, and you should refer her to her physician.

(continued)

Contraindications and Cautions: (cont.)

- Recent head trauma can cause a headache; even a seemingly innocuous knock on the head can create intracranial swelling sufficient to cause a headache. However, a motor vehicle accident, fall, sports injury, or blow to the head, although accompanied by an expected headache, often coexists with more serious conditions. Until a physician has ruled out accompanying complications, do not proceed if a client has experienced head trauma.
- New headaches in people older than 50 years of age, or in young children, require a referral to a physician before proceeding.
- Vertigo, or increased pain during the gentle assessment or when performing normal ROM of the head and neck, is a red flag to stop the treatment and refer the client to her physician.

Technique	Duration
Before proceeding, ask your client to take several slow, long, full, deep breaths.	2 minutes
Ask your client to roll her head slowly from side to side, stretching as far as she can comfortably move.	1 minute
Shorten the cervical spine muscles by positioning the client's chin toward the ceiling, as far as she can stretch. Do this by placing your fingertips along the occipital ridge and sliding up under the ridge until the entire weight of the head rests in your hands, and then point your fingertips toward the ceiling. The head will naturally fall into your hands. Hold her head this way for several seconds. Once you feel the head relax, roll it to one side, hold the head in one hand and digitally knead, with evenly rhythmic, medium pressure. • The entire occipital ridge, posterior surface of the scalp, into the spinous and transverse processes of the cervical spine Turn the head to the other side and repeat.	6 minutes
Effleurage, medium pressure, *stroking away from the head* • Both sides of the neck, along the entire course of the SCM	1 minute
Roll the client's head to one side to clearly identify the path of the SCM. Knead and lightly petrissage, several times, *down* the path of the SCM from the mastoid process to the manubrium. (You are "priming" the SCM for some relatively aggressive and unusual work and gaining the client's trust.) Grasp the SCM at any comfortable point, and alternate pressure between the thumb and middle finger for several seconds. Release and perform the same technique on the other side.	4 minutes
Stroke and effleurage, medium pressure, working *down* the neck from the occipital ridge • Bilateral sides of the neck	1 minute
Ask your client to take several full, deep breaths while rolling her head from side to side and working through several relaxed, active ROM positions.	4 minutes
With the client positioned side-lying, effleurage, petrissage, digital kneading, and repeat effleurage • The entire superior trapezius, cervical and thoracic muscles, working around the spinous and transverse processes from C-2 to T-12. Turn the client to the other side and repeat.	14 minutes
Stroking and compression, slow, even, deliberate • Through the hair, down the neck, down to the middle of the back	1 minute

Use adequate lubrication while working on the neck because stretching this delicate tissue without sufficient lubrication can irritate the skin. Slight lubrication helps with facial work, but be sure to ask for the client's permission to lubricate and/or touch her face before proceeding.

HOMEWORK

Although some people might expect to endure chronic headaches, the following preventive measures can reduce the incidence and severity. These homework assignments can easily be performed throughout the day.

- Get up from your desk every hour on the hour; roll your shoulders, turn your head from side to side, look up and down, and make funny faces to move your face muscles.
- Drink water throughout the day.
- Breathe deeply throughout the day, especially when you feel yourself getting tense.
- Ask family, friends, or colleagues to gently remind you when you are "wearing shoulder earrings," and bring your shoulders down to rest in their normal position.
- Get a phone headset instead of crimping your neck to the side.
- Ask your partner to notice if you are grinding your teeth at night; if you are, consider seeing a chiropractor or dentist.
- Look into seeing a chiropractor to relieve your neck and shoulder tenseness.
- Find ways to relax and enjoy yourself.
- Apply heat to your shoulders (*not to your neck*) when you are watching TV or reading at night after a particularly stressful day.
- Try not to sleep on your stomach, but if you must, support your head with pillows to maintain proper cervical alignment.
- If you continue to experience headaches while taking your medication, consider the possibility of a rebound headache, and check back with your physician.

Review

1. What distinguishes a diagnosis of a primary headache from that of a secondary headache?
2. List other classifications of headache.
3. Name the most common type of headache.
4. List several contraindications for the treatment of a client who has tension headaches.
5. Explain an efficient method of physical assessment during the intake process.
6. What is a "kick-back" headache, and what causes it?
7. How is a rebound headache caused?

BIBLIOGRAPHY

Benjamin PJ. Loosening the grip: how massage can soothe chronic tension headaches. *Massage Therapy Journal.* Summer 2006:49–59.

Kent D. Head, Neck and Shoulder Pain: How Trapezius Plays a Roll. Available at: http://www.kenthealth.com/articles/head-neck-and-shoulder-pain-how-trapezius-plays-a-roll.html. Accessed December 30, 2010.

Martin SA, Oswald BD, Mellick LB. Treating Headaches with Cervical Injections. *ADVANCE for Physicians Assistants* July–August 2008:31–35.

Mundo J. Handling Headaches: A Specialist's Self-Care Program. *Massage & Bodywork* June–July 2004:66–74.

Rattray F, Ludwig L. *Clinical Massage Therapy: Understanding, Assessing and Treating over 70 Conditions*, Toronto: Talus Incorporated, 2000.

Sargeant LK. Headache, Tension. EMedicine article, Topic 231. Available at: http://emedicine.medscape.com/article/792384-overview. Accessed May 29, 2008.

Sella GE. A muscular approach to headache. *Practical Pain Management* April 2006:28–33.

19

Human Immunodeficiency Virus and Acquired Immunodeficiency Syndrome

Definition: HIV refers to both the virus itself and the associated viral infection that attacks the human immune system; AIDS is a chronic, life-threatening disease resulting from a long struggle against HIV.

GENERAL INFORMATION

- Caused by HIV, a retrovirus (a virus that reverses normal cellular function)
- Transmission via infected blood, semen, and vaginal fluids through unprotected vaginal, anal, or oral sex, and the sharing of drug needles
- Transmission also possible during pregnancy, delivery, and breastfeeding
- Transmission through donated blood or blood products rare
- Transmission not possible through casual touching, hugging, coughing, shared eating utensils, mosquito bites, and tears
- Lifelong duration
- Prevalence in developing countries
- Pandemic disease (an epidemic occurring simultaneously globally)
- No cure

Morbidity and Mortality

Although misconstrued as a disease affecting those choosing same-sex partners, the HIV/AIDS global statistics indicate that 85% of HIV transmission occurs among heterosexuals. In the U.S., about one-third of all new diagnoses are related to heterosexual activities, one-half are related to male-to-male sexual contact, and IV drug users account for the remaining cases.

Worldwide, 42% of reported HIV cases are female; in the U.S., about 25% of new diagnoses are female. African American women are almost 23 times more likely to be diagnosed than Caucasian women. HIV infections in American children are now rare due to early screening and treatment of possibly infected mothers. Although most of those affected by HIV/AIDS live in developing countries, it is estimated that approximately 1.2 million U.S. citizens are currently infected, and that the virus and the syndrome have taken approximately 550,000 American lives. In the U.S., HIV/AIDS is the fifth leading cause of death among people aged 35–44, and AIDS is the leading cause of death among African Americans aged 35–44.

With a pandemic incidence rate nearing 40 million and the total measured death toll near 25 million, the cost of treatment is inestimable.

Not everyone infected with HIV develops AIDS, although that is the normal course of the disease. Not everyone suffering from AIDS will die from the disease, although survival is rare. The quality of the patient's nutrition, his socioeconomic status, the availability and intake of the appropriate medications, the control of opportunistic infections, and the person's ability to support his immune system affect progression and mortality. (An opportunistic infection is one that takes advantage of a weakened immune system.) It is possible to live asymptomatically for years and yet still carry HIV; during this time, a person can transmit the virus to unsuspecting sexual partners.

Risky sexual behaviors include unprotected sex (heterosexual, bisexual, and/or homosexual), multiple sexual partners, and having sex with someone who is HIV-positive. Higher HIV/AIDS incidence occurs among those already infected with a sexually transmitted disease (such as genital herpes or gonorrhea) and those sharing needles during IV drug use.

Transmission in the U.S. rarely occurs through the blood supply, because strict screening techniques were initiated in 1985 to detect the presence of HIV in all donated blood and blood products.

PATHOPHYSIOLOGY

A person's ability to fight disease—any disease, from the common cold to cancer—depends on a highly functioning immune system. The human immune system includes various white blood cells, some of which fight specific invaders. Certain ones oversee the entire immune process, including the powerful CD4 or T4 cells. The strength of the body's immune response is directly reflected by the CD4 cell count. When a persistent infection, a serious disease, or an opportunistic invader ravages the body, the CD4 rate reflects whether the immune system is winning or losing the battle.

Once infected with HIV, the body's immune system is forever compromised. Although a latent (symptom-free) period may occur immediately after infection and may even last a dozen or more years, ultimately, the toll of fighting this pernicious invader manifests as symptomatic HIV and/or HIV/AIDS. Rarely does an HIV-infected person live a normal, uncompromised life span.

Two tracking systems classify adults infected with HIV, monitor the progression toward HIV/AIDS, and help determine treatment. One system tracks the CD4 cell count; the second system, used concurrently with the first, monitors the patient's clinical symptoms.

Diagnostic tests, approved by the U.S. Food and Drug Administration (FDA), can detect the presence of HIV in the urine, saliva, or blood. Anonymous HIV testing is available in physicians' offices, public health clinics, hospitals, and some Planned Parenthood clinics. A home HIV test kit is also available through drugstores or by mail order. Testing is essential for anyone who has practiced risky behaviors, not only to ensure prompt personal care, but also to stop the spread to future unsuspecting sexual partners.

OVERALL SIGNS AND SYMPTOMS

Signs and symptoms are measured according to the stage of the disease. Since HIV/AIDS affects multiple body systems, common accompanying medical conditions are listed along with typical signs and symptoms.

Following an initial HIV infection, the symptoms mimic those of a cold or flu and might develop either immediately or weeks after exposure. Although a person may remain completely asymptomatic for years, the following temporary symptoms usually occur and last for 2–3 weeks:

- Fever
- Headache
- Fatigue
- Sore throat
- Muscular aches and pains
- Enlarged neck lymph nodes
- Mild skin rash

Throughout the initial, sometimes innocuous stage, the virus continues to multiply; it infects and weakens the now-compromised immune system. The CD4 count significantly declines, and symptoms progress in severity. Category A is the first clinical stage indicating symptomatic HIV. Symptoms and indicators include:

- Severe fatigue
- Weight loss
- Night sweats
- Fever
- Enlarged lymph nodes in the neck, armpit, or groin
- Persistent rashes
- Short-term memory loss
- History of HIV infection

Category B patients have a profoundly compromised immune system, and they are seeking medical treatment for both related and unrelated conditions but have not yet advanced toward a final diagnosis of HIV/AIDS. Symptoms and conditions include:

- Persistent mouth or vaginal yeast infection
- Cervical dysplasia (abnormal cells growing in the cervix)
- Persistent fever of 101.4°F or higher
- Diarrhea persisting longer than 1 month
- Sores on the sides of the tongue
- Shingles
- Pelvic inflammatory disease
- Numbness, tingling, and/or pain in the fingers and toes

Category C patients have developed AIDS, along with severe opportunistic infections or cancers. The following is a list of only a few of the signs, symptoms, and medical conditions:

- Soaking night sweats
- Persistent chills and fever higher than 100°F
- Persistent dry cough
- Shortness of breath
- White spots in the mouth or on the tongue
- Severe headache accompanied by neck stiffness
- Blurred vision
- Confusion
- Peripheral neuropathies
- Weight loss
- Cancer of the lymphatic system
- Tuberculosis
- Cancer of the cervix
- Kaposi's sarcoma
- Wasting syndrome (diarrhea, weakness, fever, and loss of weight and muscle mass)
- Severe headaches accompanied by stiff neck

SIGNS AND SYMPTOMS MASSAGE THERAPY CAN ADDRESS

- An educated, open-minded, and compassionate massage therapist can offset the effects of social and health care stigmas that often accompany a diagnosis of HIV/AIDS.
- Research supports a significant increase in the body's natural killer cells and the function of the immune system resulting from massage therapy techniques. (Natural killer cells are immune system cells that act as a first defense against any foreign body.)

- Massage therapy reduces stress hormones.
- Hypertonicity from inactivity and stress is relieved through massage therapy.
- Numbness and tingling from either the medications or the condition's progress can be relieved by appropriate massage therapy techniques.

TREATMENT OPTIONS

From the early onset of an HIV infection to the final stages of AIDS or AIDS-related cancers, the patient should be under the care of a physician specializing in immune disorders. Although primarily pharmaceutical, effective HIV/AIDS treatment also addresses nutrition, stress, exercise, and lifestyle habits in an effort to holistically support the failing immune system.

A regimen of powerful drugs aimed at halting viral reproduction is usually prescribed in combination with prophylactic (preventive) medications to stop the spread of opportunistic infections. These highly active antiretroviral therapies (HAART) can slow the rate at which the virus multiplies. The medications include two or three different prescriptions that must be taken consistently, at the exact same time every day, for the rest of the person's life. The inconvenience and expense are offset by the fact that this "cocktail" can give HIV-positive patients many productive years of life, although it does not cure the disease. Without the medications, death is imminent.

Since there is no cure, prevention is paramount. These lifestyle behaviors can help prevent HIV: supporting a healthy immune system by eating plenty of fruits and vegetables, exercising, not smoking, and reducing stress; avoiding IV drug use; decreasing alcohol use; avoiding unprotected sex or having multiple sexual partners; using latex or polyurethane condoms during sex; not using oil-based lubricants while using latex condoms (the oil breaks down latex, rendering the condom ineffective); and avoiding the sharing of toothbrushes or razors.

Common Medications

- Antivirals, such as zidovudine (AZT, Retrovir), saquinavir mesylate (Invirase), and nevirapine (Viramune)
- Antiviral antiretrovirals, such as tenofovir disoproxil fumarate (Viread)
- Anti-HIV antivirals, such as enfuvirtide (Fuzeon)

MASSAGE THERAPIST ASSESSMENT

The first step of the assessment is to determine how the diagnosis was made. Was it done by a physician or by a home test? This will tell the therapist how well the patient is being taken care of, how the therapist might join the health care team, and what his resources are as the disease inevitably progresses.

A complete medical history will provide the therapist with knowledge about disease progression, the type and efficacy of medication, present and past symptoms, and the patient's massage therapy expectations. In order to develop a helpful and yet reasonable treatment plan, the therapist must gently probe to discover symptoms, which may range from mild aches and pains to insomnia, to severe immunosuppression and depression.

Once the patient is on the table, a visual and manual assessment will identify areas of extensive bruising, possible IV drug use, skin fragility, possible tumors, hypertonic muscles, and respiratory distress.

THERAPEUTIC GOALS

The mercurial nature of HIV/AIDS means that one day, the patient will feel strong and able, and the next, he may feel inconsolable and exhausted. Taking his presentation into account, the therapist can help support the immune system, allow the

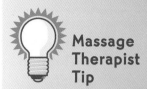

Massage Therapist Tip

Unbiased, Ungloved, and Unmasked

Whether the person sitting in your office has manifested HIV/AIDS because of a chosen lifestyle, a mother who had HIV, or a blood transfusion he received years ago is not your concern. Your concern is the simple, compassionate, glove-free, and mask-free manual and visual examination of a human being who needs your unbiased intent and massage therapy skills. It's not necessary to use gloves unless you have an open cut on your hand. A mask is not necessary unless you have a cold or the flu, or unless the patient has a contagious respiratory infection. This patient has probably endured overt and subtle judgments by health care practitioners and possibly friends and family. Any unnecessary barrier you erect may be misconstrued as yet another insult.

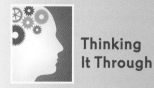

Thinking It Through

Because HIV/AIDS patients are susceptible to opportunistic infections and are taking large doses of strong medications, the toxic load on every organ and system in the body is profound. Even the mildest hour-long session could release toxins into the bloodstream, thus, causing very uncomfortable side effects. A massage therapist might ask herself the following questions before, during, and after a massage

Thinking It Through (cont.)

therapy session to ensure that her work does no harm:

- What are my patient's normal side effects from taking all his medications?
- Does he feel slightly warmer to my touch today; does he have a slight fever?
- How active is he? If he continues to exercise through his disease, how will this affect the depth and duration of his massage?
- How inactive is he? If he is very weak with not much muscle movement, what are our goals for this session?
- Is he dehydrated? Is he drinking enough fluids so his muscles and brain are sufficiently hydrated and his liver can process his medication? How can I encourage his hydration?
- Is his breathing labored or shallow? What can I do to help him breathe more deeply, not only on my table but also throughout the day?
- Is he bruising easily? How will this affect the depth and duration of his massage?
- Is he taking narcotics for his pain? Is he constipated? Can he offer reasonable feedback to my massage depth or pressure?
- How is he handling the normal, everyday exposure to toxins (on unwashed fruits and vegetables, in crowds of people)? Is my practice room as clean as it can be (doorknobs, sink hardware, linen)? Am I feeling my best today with no impending cold or flu?

patient to reach a parasympathetic state, help flush accumulated toxins from his bloodstream, increase lymphatic flow, and encourage deep breathing. All of these are reasonable therapeutic goals that can be accomplished in each session without placing too much duress on the patient, even when he is particularly tired.

MASSAGE SESSION FREQUENCY

Duration and frequency are determined by the patient's tolerance, by the strength of his immune system, and by the massage environment (hospital, home, hospice, massage therapy office). However, research indicates that increasing the frequency of massage sessions provides greater immune system support.

- Ideally: 60-minute sessions twice a week
- Helpful: 60-minute sessions once a week
- Supportive but not as physiologically effective: 60-minute sessions every other week
- Infrequent, inconsistent therapy can provide palliative support but little physiologic benefit

MASSAGE PROTOCOL

The following protocol is for a Category B HIV-positive male who continues to work and function despite his continual battle with opportunistic infections. He is taking his medications regularly and is fortunate enough to have the expense and care covered by insurance, but his stress level is very high.

Your mind-set when approaching a patient suffering from a profound systemic disease must be quite different from the mind-set for a person with a hypertonic muscle mass. Every stroke you choose must be weighed carefully as you focus on supporting the immune system. New research indicates that *slow, relatively deep massage strokes* are effective in helping generate natural killer cells and boosting overall immune function. This may seem counterintuitive as you approach your seemingly fragile patient. Certainly monitor your touch to the patient's tolerance, but err on the side of depth rather than performing a too light massage.

Since pneumonia constantly threatens to compromise or end this patient's life, deep-breathing exercises throughout the session—and in your homework assignments—are essential.

Providing passive range-of-motion (ROM) exercises after working on each limb will help flush toxins from the body by triggering lymphatic flow. Although your passive ROM is performed gently, it must bring the joint and limb to end-feel—the springy, slightly resisting point at the very end of the patient's normal ROM. To move short of end-feel is to perform ineffective ROM.

The numbness and tingling he may experience in his hands and feet can be addressed quite effectively with massage therapy. Chapter 25 includes massage instruction for neuropathies, and those skills can be used whenever the patient can tolerate focused, deep hand and footwork. The following protocol focuses on relaxation and immune support for a patient who remains relatively active and healthy. The neuropathy protocol, which takes 30–60 minutes, is one more skill to add to your toolkit but is not performed during this protocol.

Getting Started

Remember that this patient's aches and pains will vary from session to session, so be prepared to accommodate his immediate needs. Have plenty of pillows and blankets on hand for both comfortable positioning and warmth for a patient who may be cold on a hot August day. Again, beyond all clinical preparedness, listen with a compassionate, unbiased heart.

Step-by-Step Protocol for **HIV/AIDS**

Technique	Duration
With the patient lying prone, greet the body with general warming compression using medium-to-deep pressure. • Posterior calves, thighs, buttocks, back	2 minutes
Effleurage, petrissage, effleurage, compression, medium-to-deep pressure, evenly rhythmic • Gastrocnemius • Hamstrings • Buttocks Perform bilaterally.	4 minutes (8 minutes)
Passive ROM to end-feel, slow and rhythmic • Ankle joint (circumduction, plantar flexion, dorsiflexion) • Knee joint (extension, flexion) Finish with cephalic effleurage of the entire leg using deep pressure. Perform bilaterally.	2 minutes (4 minutes)
Effleurage, petrissage, compression, effleurage, medium-to-deep pressure, evenly rhythmic • All muscles of the back, from the lumbar spine region to the base of the occiput	5 minutes
Digital kneading, medium-to-deep pressure • Along each transverse process from T1 to L5 • Along and into the posterior costals, from the spine to the lateral side of the body	5 minutes
Gentle rocking, to and fro, evenly rhythmic, placing hands on • Posterior costal cage • Posterior, lateral gluteal region	2 minutes
Ask the patient to take one deep breath before positioning him supine.	1 minute
Passive ROM to end-feel, slow, evenly rhythmic • Knee joints • Hip joints • Shoulder joints Finish with deep compression and whole-body effleurage, working cephalically.	6 minutes 1 minute
Ask the patient to take three deep breaths while you gently place your hands on his anterior chest, offering slight resistance as he inhales and exhales. Do not come off the chest, but continue to apply gentle yet unyielding pressure on his chest as he breathes in and out deeply, 3 times.	3 minutes
Effleurage, petrissage, digital kneading, compression, effleurage, evenly rhythmic, medium-to-deep pressure • Foot, lower leg, thigh Perform bilaterally.	4 minutes (8 minutes)

Contraindications and Cautions

- Massaging over or near an open sore is a universal massage therapy contraindication and is especially important while working with an HIV/AIDS patient.
- Fever, particularly if low-grade and persistent, is a contraindication for bodywork, and the patient should see his physician immediately.
- Medication metaports, indwelling catheters, and feeding tubes require localized cautions.
- An open cut, even a minor hangnail or paper cut, on your hand dictates wearing gloves during the treatment.
- Keen awareness of the patient's fatigue, bruising, and possible narcotic intake will help determine session duration.
- If you have the slightest prodromal cold or flu symptoms, either cancel the session or wear a mask and wash your hands frequently.
- Short nails and the absence of rings will reduce the risk of breaking the patient's skin.

(continued)

Technique	Duration
Clockwise circles, performed with medium pressure, even and slow • Entire anterior surface of the abdomen, from the region of the diaphragm to above the mons pubis	2 minutes
Effleurage, petrissage, compression, effleurage, evenly rhythmic, medium-to-deep pressure • Hand, forearm, arm, shoulder region Perform bilaterally.	4 minutes (8 minutes)
With the patient's permission, perform a scalp massage, using slow, even digital kneading strokes. Focus on the occipital ridge. End with long, even strokes through his hair.	3 minutes
Compression, medium-to-deep pressure, very slow, rhythmic • Entire anterior surface of the body	1 minute
Ask the patient to take one more deep breath as you initiate very gentle rocking by placing one hand on either side of his pelvic region and rocking the body to and fro. At the point where the body takes over the rocking itself, move your hands away from the body and step away from the table.	1 minute

Although the patient's finances may be limited and his busy life may make scheduling a challenge, strongly suggest that he receives massage at least weekly. It's a good idea to call your patient the day after treatment, at least for the first few sessions, to see if there have been any negative side effects from your work.

HOMEWORK

Since HIV/AIDS infects the body for the patient's entire life, any suggestions you can make that will help support his immune system, keep him breathing deeply, and get or keep him moving can contribute to both the quality and the quantity of his years. Here are some homework assignments:

- Scrub all of your fruits and vegetables.
- Several times during the day, take a very deep inhalation, hold it for a few seconds, and forcibly exhale.
- Stretch while taking your daily shower; support yourself while rolling your shoulders, neck, hips, and ankles. Also, while in the shower, breathe deeply a few times.
- While watching TV or sitting or standing comfortably, move *every* joint in your body as far as it will go. Once you reach a comfortable point where the joint will move no farther, push a little beyond that point.
- Consider a gentle aerobic and strengthening program if you're not already active. Don't become sedentary.
- Drink plenty of water.
- Wash your hands frequently throughout the day, and especially after shopping or being out in crowds.
- Don't go into crowds if you're getting a cold or the flu.
- Suggest to friends who are not feeling well that they visit you after they are well.
- Find ways to relax, and make time for those techniques every day.
- Get plenty of sleep.

Review

1. Explain the difference between HIV and AIDS.
2. Which population is affected by HIV/AIDS?
3. What do the acronyms HIV and AIDS stand for?
4. Describe this disease's duration.
5. How is HIV/AIDS treated?
6. Is HIV always fatal?
7. Name behaviors that spread HIV/AIDS.
8. List behaviors that can prevent the spread of HIV/AIDS.
9. Is it common for a person to be infected with HIV/AIDS through the U.S. blood supply?

BIBLIOGRAPHY

Cutler N. Institute for Integrative Healthcare Studies. Massage Therapy and HIV/AIDS. Available at: http://www.integrative-healthcare.org/mt/archives/2006/12/massage _therapy_1.html. Accessed December 29, 2010.

Gnanakkan J. The Effects of Therapeutic Massage on HIV and AIDS Patients. *MassageToday.* October 2008, online version. Available at: http://www.massagetoday.cpom/mpacms/ mt/article.php?id+13288. Accessed December 29, 2010.

International AIDS Society-USA. Oral Manifestations of HIV Disease. Available at: http:// www.iasusa.org/pub/topics/2005/issue5/143. Accessed December 29, 2010.

MayoClinic.com. HIV/AIDS. Available at: http://www.mayoclinic.com/print/hiv-aids. Accessed December 29, 2010.

Medscape. Epidemiology of HIV/AIDS—United States, 1981–2005. Available at: http://www .medscape.com/viewarticle/534055_1. Accessed December 29, 2010.

Rattray F, Ludwig L. *Clinical Massage Therapy: Understanding, Assessing and Treating over 70 Conditions*, Toronto: Talus Incorporated, 2000.

San Francisco AIDS Foundation. Stages of HIV Infection. Available at: http://www.thebody .com/content/art2506. Accessed December 29, 2010.

Tran M, Nettleman M. HIV/AIDS. EMedicine article. Available at: http://www.emedicinehealth .com/script/main/art.asp?articlekey=58830. Accessed December 29, 2010.

WebMD. HIV and AIDS Guide. Available at: http://www.webmd.com/hiv-aids/guide/ default. Accessed December 29, 2010.

WebMD. HIV and AIDS Health Center: Human Immunodeficiency Virus (HIV) Infection – Medications. Available at: http://www.webmd.com/hiv-aids/human-immunodeficiency -virus-hiv-infection-symptoms. Accessed December 29, 2010.

20

Hyperkyphosis

Definition: An exaggerated, often progressive, increase in the normal posterior thoracic spinal curvature.

GENERAL INFORMATION

Hyperkyphosis is the correct term used for an exaggerated thoracic curve. (Lay, and often medical, literature mistakenly uses the terms interchangeably; the two terms are not synonymous.)

- Two forms: structural and postural
- Causes of structural hyperkyphosis: congenital factors, thoracic spine fracture, osteoporosis, arthritis, degenerative disc disease, ankylosing spondylitis, spinal cancers or tumors, paralytic conditions, spinal trauma
- Causes of postural hyperkyphosis: slouching, rounded-shoulder sleep posture (fetal position), persistent work-related postures
- Onset immediate or gradual, depending on etiology
- Duration: lifelong in structural form, short-term in postural form
- Prevalence of both structural and postural forms fairly evenly distributed among children, adolescents, and adults

PATHOPHYSIOLOGY

The term *kyphosis*, correctly used, refers to the *normal* posterior thoracic curvature that develops after an infant gains control of her head, begins crawling, and eventually stands upright. Normal spinal anatomy manifests a slight thoracic *kyphotic curve*.

The exaggerated forward rounding of the shoulders in both structural and postural hyperkyphosis compromises the musculature of the entire spinal column. The forward-head thrust position commonly assumed by people with hyperkyphosis leads to postural and structural problems, as well as head and jaw pain.

Scheuermann's kyphosis, a primary hyperkyphosis of unknown origin, develops in children (more often in males) between the ages of 10 and 15, and noticeably deforms the vertebrae. If untreated, Scheuermann's kyphosis results in lifelong deformity, muscular and joint pain, and/or organ compromise. Congenital hyperkyphosis, which occurs during fetal development, often worsens after the child is born; if untreated, it can lead to paralysis of the lower body.

Adolescent girls with poor posture, large-breasted women, anyone working at a computer or leaning over a desk, and those who frequently sleep in a fetal position have an increased risk of developing postural hyperkyphosis. This nonpathologic form of the condition usually disappears with normal physical development, changes in postural habits, physical therapy, weight loss, or breast reduction. Older adults with spinal arthritis or osteoporosis, or the long-term effects of an earlier trauma, are at greater risk for developing the less resilient, structural form of hyperkyphosis.

Untreated at any age, hyperkyphosis can lead to irreversible physical deformity, body image difficulties, ineffective breathing patterns, neurologic problems, and organ damage. Decreased lung capacity, which can develop regardless of the severity of the condition, is a continued medical concern because inefficient breathing patterns often result in bronchitis or pneumonia, both of which are more serious, and possibly life threatening, than the original hyperkyphosis.

The initial diagnosis is often made via a simple clinical intake and spinal palpation, followed by the patient assuming various spine-bending positions. X-rays reveal arthritic changes and identify spinal fusion, and they are essential if the patient manifests neurologic difficulties in the lower extremities. An MRI will indicate spinal tumors or soft tissue infection surrounding the bones or discs. Breathing tests determine the extent of thoracic compromise.

Hyperkyphosis does not usually directly shorten the person's life span. However, secondary conditions, such as recurring pneumonia, can affect the quality and quantity of years lived.

OVERALL SIGNS AND SYMPTOMS

Mild, transient, postural hyperkyphosis is often asymptomatic. Once muscles and bones compensate repeatedly over time, however, the following muscular signs occur:

- Shoulder protraction (drawing forward) and elevation (rising upward), combined with weaker middle and lower trapezius muscle, from shortened upper trapezius and levator scapula
- Rounded-shoulder effect from shortened and tightened pectoralis major and minor
- Noticeable "winging" of the scapula from weak serratus anterior

Signs and symptoms occurring as a result of the previous muscular signs include:

- Slouching posture
- Mild-to-moderate back pain
- Back pain upon movement
- Shoulder height imbalance
- Spinal stiffness and/or tenderness
- Forward-head posture
- Inefficient breathing patterns

SIGNS AND SYMPTOMS MASSAGE THERAPY CAN ADDRESS

A note of caution: Softening the surrounding musculature of a *structurally* hyperkyphotic spine that has been locked in hypertonicity for months or years can trigger extremely painful muscle spasms and result in an unstable spine. This chapter therefore presupposes that the massage therapist is addressing *postural* hyperkyphosis only. Unless she is working as part of a health care team, with the client's primary physician and/or physical therapist, or has advanced training, a massage therapist should not attempt to treat structural hyperkyphosis. (See Massage Therapist Assessment later in this chapter to determine the difference between structural and postural hyperkyphosis.)

- The back pain, shoulder height imbalance, and spinal stiffness and tenderness associated with postural hyperkyphosis can be effectively treated with massage therapy techniques.
- The secondary effects of the forward-head posture can be reduced or eliminated by massage therapy.
- Thoracic capacity can be increased and inefficient breathing patterns can be corrected with the intelligent use of specialized massage techniques.
- The temporarily immobile shoulder girdle will yield to massage therapy techniques.

TREATMENT OPTIONS

Noticeable deformity and chronic back discomfort or pain are often the triggers that prompt a visit to a sports or physical medicine physician, or an orthopedic specialist. Treatment is directly related to the condition's onset, severity, and symptoms. No matter how mild or severe the condition is, the treatment's effectiveness correlates to early intervention.

Postural hyperkyphosis often does not progress and can improve with focused, noninvasive treatment, such as massage therapy, physical therapy, chiropractic adjustments, exercise, joint mobilization, and stretching. In addition, improvements in workstation, posture, and sleeping habits can completely alleviate both the deformity and the pain associated with this milder form of hyperkyphosis. Over-the-counter (OTC) pain medication can relieve transient discomfort.

Depending on the age of onset and the progression, structural hyperkyphosis is generally treated more aggressively and invasively because of postural, breathing, neurologic, and organ complications, which are often accompanied by significant pain. In growing children and adolescents, wearing a back brace can prevent further curvature if the brace is applied early in the child's development. Full correction is sometimes possible using bracing alone. In adults where a slow, lifelong spinal compromise has caused a noticeable deformity, accompanied by only moderate pain, then pain medication, localized hot or cold packs, physical therapy, and breathing exercises may be helpful.

Spinal surgery is indicated in the case of tumor- or infection-related hyperkyphosis, intractable pain, severe progressive curvature, and neurologic problems. Vertebroplasty and kyphoplasty are recently developed, less risky, less invasive surgical procedures involving the injection of an inert cement into the vertebrae.

Common Medications

- Nonsteroidal anti-inflammatory drugs (NSAIDs), such as ibuprofen (Motrin, Advil)

MASSAGE THERAPIST ASSESSMENT

To ensure that the client has postural—and not structural—hyperkyphosis, the therapist should first ask whether she has seen a medical professional. If the client's response indicates that she experiences mild or moderate transient back pain and stiffness secondary to sleeping position, postural or work habits, or large breasts, the therapist can proceed.

Asking the client to bend forward, then observing her back for the absence of abnormal angles or curvatures, will further confirm postural hyperkyphosis. Finally, when lying supine on the massage table, the shoulders, after a few moments of relaxation and deep breathing, should naturally lie on the table with no abnormal, unmovable, or stiff shoulder forward rounding.

When the client is disrobed, under the sheets, and ready for treatment, palpation of the pectoralis major and minor; subclavius; sternocleidomastoid (SCM); levator scapulae; serratus anterior; suboccipitals; and anterior, lateral, and posterior intercostals and thoracic erector spinae will reveal hypertonicity, and the client may report tenderness. In addition, with the client in either the side-lying or the prone position, the hypertonic rhomboids, trapezius, and teres major and minor will render the scapula difficult, if not impossible, to move.

If the client has assumed the forward-head position in response to her rounded shoulders, the muscles surrounding her temporomandibular joint (TMJ) will be hypertonic, and she may complain of teeth clenching, which will result in tender anterior neck muscles and/or headache. The therapist should be aware of the client's further attempts at self-care via visits to a chiropractor or physical therapist.

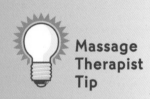

Massage Therapist Tip

Combining Assessment with a Gentle Stretch

The fact that your client is hyperkyphotic can be visually confirmed by asking her to lie supine on the table. Typically, her shoulders will be rounded and not lie flat. The rounding might be slight, perhaps no more than a hand's width, or you might be able to fit an entire fist between the posterior shoulder and the table. To help nudge the hypertonic pectoralis major and minor into a more natural, lengthened position, place your cupped hands over the top of your client's shoulders, and with a rocking, alternating motion, press her shoulders into the table, one after another. This should not cause pain but, in fact, often results in the client feeling as if she is "being opened up."

THERAPEUTIC GOALS

Easing the pain-spasm-pain cycle, flushing out local muscular waste products, stretching tight joints and shortened muscles, and improving thoracic capacity are all reasonable massage therapy goals for a client who has postural hyperkyphosis. Achieving these goals, however, is not possible without the client's adherence to daily self-care techniques.

MASSAGE SESSION FREQUENCY

- Ideally: twice a week for 2 weeks, then once a week for 6 weeks or until the postural abnormality is resolved
- Minimally: once a week for 2 months
- Infrequent, inconsistent sessions will be ineffective

MASSAGE PROTOCOL

Because of the extent of musculature involvement, the care that must be taken not to release hypertonic muscles too quickly, the various symptomatic differences clients will have, and the length of time and commitment required for the client to relearn postural adaptations, a single 60-minute protocol cannot address this condition. Instead, the protocol that follows offers a series of techniques with a suggested range of durations you can use depending on your client's symptomatic presentation before each session. Durations are suggestions only. Of all the recommended techniques, be sure to include those that address thoracic capacity in every session.

Some of this work is very aggressive and must be performed deeply. Be sure to soften the superficial tissue before going into the body with any invasive techniques.

During intercostal and parasternal digital kneading, ensure the client's comfort and drape appropriately. This is most easily done by gripping the sheet with one hand to keep it close to the client's chin while sliding your working hand under the sheet.

Hot packs can be applied to areas before they are massaged. Cold packs are effective if the client is experiencing spasm or pain.

Getting Started

A posturally hyperkyphotic client will be uncomfortable lying completely flat. Place pillows under her knees and under her head in the supine position. While prone, she may require a small pillow under her abdomen, or might want to hug a pillow close to her chest. Side-lying is ideal for treating postural hyperkyphosis, but be sure to provide cervical, thoracic, and pelvic pillowing support.

Have hot and cold packs ready. With any deep work on delicate or thin tissue, such as the anterior neck, be sure to use plenty of lubrication to avoid irritating the skin.

HOMEWORK

In order to free the shoulder girdle from the grip of hyperkyphosis, long-held incorrect posture must be reversed. Although the client will be well served by seeing a physical therapist who can recommend muscle stretching and strengthening exercises, the soft tissue work that you, the skilled massage therapist, can perform, combined with the following self-care suggestions, can lead to complete recovery.

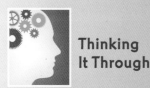

Thinking It Through

To fully understand the anatomic effect of the forward-head posture assumed by most clients with postural hyperkyphosis, the therapist can try going about her day for 30 minutes in this position. After about 15 minutes spent with her shoulders rolled forward, she can ask herself:

- What position does my jaw assume if I need to look forward?
- What happens to my forehead muscles as I try to look straight ahead?
- How does my breathing change in this position?
- What does my lower back feel like with my shoulders constantly pulled forward?
- How does this position affect how I feel about myself?
- Am I clenching my jaw?
- Are my abdominal muscles feeling strong and engaged or weak as a result of this position?

Step-by-Step Protocol for Hyperkyphosis

Technique	Duration
With the client supine, apply hot packs (over the sheet) on the left and right superior pectoralis major, below the clavicles. Leave in place as you greet the client's body with general warming compression, using medium-to-deep pressure applied evenly and rhythmically. • Use this time to evaluate the client's breathing pattern and scapular placement on the table. • Be sure to address the anterior thoracic and abdominal region in your compression techniques.	3 minutes
With the hot packs still in place, ask the client to take several very deep breaths as you perform effleurage, medium pressure, in a clockwise direction. • Over the entire abdominal region from the diaphragm to above the mons pubis	2 minutes
With the hot packs still in place, ask the client's permission to massage her head. Digital kneading, medium-to-deep pressure, evenly rhythmic • All the muscles of the head from the forehead hairline to the occipital ridge • Roll the head to one side, firmly holding it in one hand while you work deeply to the client's tolerance along the occipital ridge and into the laminar grooves of the cervical spine. Roll the head to the other side. Repeat.	5–10 minutes
Hold the entire weight of the head in your hands with your fingertips lodged just below the occipital ridge. Ask the client to inhale deeply as you apply pressure to the occipital ridge, which should allow the head to fall slowly backward into the palms of your hands, thrusting the client's chin toward the ceiling. Rest with her head in your hands until you feel a muscular release along the occipital ridge, and then return the head to its normal position.	2 minutes
Slide your hands down the anterior surface of the neck so each set of fingertips rests on the sides of the manubrium, at the top of the sternum. Begin digital kneading, medium-to-deep pressure, making small circles, evenly rhythmic. • From the sternum, addressing the attachment of the pectoralis major below the clavicle, out to the acromioclavicular joint	
Grip the sheet with one hand and keep it close to the client's chin. Ask permission to work along the sternum. With the other hand, digitally knead. • Attachment points of the intercostals and pectoralis major, and along the lateral border of one side of the sternum	
Avoiding breast tissue and nipple contact, effleurage • As much of the pectoralis major and minor as you can appropriately reach Switch the hand, maintaining modest draping, and repeat on the other side of the sternum and pectoralis major and minor.	3–6 minutes (6–12 minutes)

(continued)

Technique	Duration
Effleurage, medium pressure, in the direction of the axilla • As much of the pectoralis major as you can appropriately reach	1–2 minutes
Effleurage, muscle stripping, digital kneading, effleurage, medium-to-deep pressure • Pectoralis minor, bilaterally	3–5 minutes each side
With the client's permission, reveal the abdomen, using appropriate draping techniques. Effleurage in a clockwise direction, medium pressure, evenly rhythmic • The entire abdominal region from just below the rib cage to above the mons pubis	3 minutes
Ask the client to bend her knees. Digital kneading, medium pressure, evenly rhythmic • Along the border at the bottom of the rib cage, searching with your fingers to feel as if you are pushing up *under* the rib cage and engaging the diaphragm. If performed slowly and carefully, the client will not resist this technique. If the work is performed deeply enough, there will be no "tickle" response. Finish with slow, even deep effleurage, working clockwise • In the entire abdominal region	5–8 minutes 1 minute
Place the client in the side-lying position; pillow appropriately. Perform fascial stretching techniques, and skin rolling, as deeply as you can grip the skin • Along the border of the cervical spine, out to the lateral neck, down to the region of about C-7, along the superior border of the scapula, out to the lateral tip of the shoulder, down to approximately T-10. Finish with effleurage to the entire area.	8 minutes 1 minute
Position the client's arm (the one closest and not lying on the table) so you can access the entire scapula. Digitally knead, effleurage, petrissage, effleurage • Lateral, superior, and medial scapular borders, working the bony prominences, rotator cuff muscles, latissimus dorsi, teres major and minor, rhomboid major and minor. Attempt to *slightly move* the scapula as you work around the bone.	10 minutes
Effleurage, medium-to-deep pressure • From the occipital ridge, down the cervical spine, all along the scapula out to the tip of the shoulder and down to T-10	2 minutes
Ask the client, while still side-lying, to stretch out as far as she can and straighten her position on the table. In this position, undrape the quadratus lumborum (QL); working alternative hands using scooping motions, muscle stripping, digital kneading, effleurage, and petrissage, work deeply to the client's tolerance. • The QL working from the superior ridge of the pelvis to the lower edge of the posterior/lateral rib cage. Ask the client to take a deep breath and slightly soften and round her position. Repeat the previous technique, going in as deeply as you can.	5 minutes 3 minutes

(continued)

Technique	Duration
Turn the client to the other side and repeat all previous side-lying steps.	
Place the client in the prone position. Pillow for comfort. Apply a hot pack to the bilateral trapezius while you perform general relaxation techniques on her head, legs, or feet. Remove the hot pack. Effleurage, petrissage, effleurage, deep pressure • All posterior muscle sets, bilaterally, from the occipital ridge to, and including, the lumbar region	5 minutes 5 minutes
While applying gentle effleurage to the entire back, inform the client that you will be performing deep work that may feel a bit unusual. Ask her to give feedback if she is uncomfortable.	1 minute
Skin rolling, skin plucking, hacking (over the sheet), soft-fist beating, and fascial stretching techniques over the entire back from the superior trapezius down to the level of T-10. *Use no percussive techniques over the kidneys.* Work as deeply and aggressively as the client will allow, and then effleurage the area.	10 minutes
Effleurage, digital kneading, petrissage, effleurage, deep pressure, not necessarily rhythmic • Erector spinae in the cervical, thoracic, and lumbar region • Rhomboid major and minor • Teres major and minor	10 minutes
Shoulder mobilization—performed with the client prone. Gently place the client's arm so her hand lies in the small of her back, palm up. With one of your hands, brace her elbow; with the other hand, deeply palpate the medial border of her scapula. When you have a firm hold on the scapula, rest for a moment—and without warning the client—firmly pull the medial scapular border up, trying to move it so your fingers can reach "underneath." The client may initially resist this sensation, but firmly hold the scapula for as long as you comfortably can. Ask her to take a deep breath and tug on the scapula for one more inch, then slowly release. Follow with effleurage to the entire region. Repeat on the other side.	5–10 minutes
Shoulder mobilization—performed with the client side-lying. Position the client's arm to rest on her side. Digitally knead around the scapula and soften the superior trapezius. Place the client's arm behind her so her hand rests on the table (or as far behind her as it can comfortably rest), palm up. Gently rock the client's shoulder to and fro as you palpate the medial border of the scapula. When you feel as if you can grip the medial border of the scapula, with one firm, relatively quick grasp, tug the scapula toward you by a few inches, as far as it will move. Hold it. Ask the client to take a deep breath and pull the scapula 1 inch farther. Then slowly release the scapula and effleurage the surrounding area. Repeat on the other side.	5–10 minutes

(continued)

Technique	Duration
Position the client supine. Remove the pillow from the head region, and position yourself above the client. With a slow, methodical, and firm rocking motion, alternate pushing the client's shoulders down into the table. The final push is performed with equal pressure on both shoulders, holding this position for a moment. *If this technique creates any discomfort for the client, stop immediately.* The client might take a deep breath after this technique is performed, as the body resettles into its normal thoracic kyphotic curve.	5 minutes
Resisted breathing technique, client supine. Place your hands along the lateral and slightly distal borders of the client's rib cage. Apply gentle but firm pressure. As she inhales deeply, maintain your pressure on her thoracic cavity; she should feel substantial pressure and resistance as she inhales. Stay on the chest as she exhales, maintaining your pressure. Repeat 3 times. *Do not perform this technique on older adults or anyone with osteoporosis.*	5 minutes
Finish the session with any form of relaxing Swedish techniques preferred by the client.	

Massage therapy alone—without self-care—will yield no improvement. Here are some homework assignments:

- Frequently throughout the day, perform the doorway stretch (see Figure 6-1). Give yourself a reminder, such as every time you go to the bathroom or before and after meals.
- Fold your hands in front of your chest in a praying position; take a very deep breath as you raise your arms and stretch them as far behind your head as you can. Take another deep breath with your arms in the air, and slowly return them to the starting position. Do this six times throughout the day.
- Interlace your fingers together behind you at the level of your lower back. Take a deep breath as you raise your arms as high as you can push them. Press your shoulder blades together. Repeat three times a day.
- Lie on the floor or on your bed with your arms stretched completely out to the side, as far as you can reach. Take several deep breaths as you feel the full length of your spine settle into the bed or floor. Try to feel your shoulder blades pressing against the floor or bed.
- Lie on your side and curl into a tight fetal position. Tense every muscle in your body. Take a deep breath and slowly uncurl; roll onto your back and spread your arms out wide to either side.
- When you feel yourself slouching, immediately stand up, alternating raising, lowering, and rolling your shoulder blades backward. Take a deep breath and assume your previous position in a straighter posture.
- Ask friends, family, and coworkers to gently remind you when they notice you are slouching.

Review

1. Explain the difference between kyphosis and hyperkyphosis.
2. Name the two forms of hyperkyphosis.
3. List some of the causes of both forms of hyperkyphosis.

4. Why should a massage therapist not attempt to treat structural hyperkyphosis?
5. List as many muscles as you can that can be affected by both forms of hyperkyphosis.
6. Explain why a forward-head posture often occurs secondary to hyperkyphosis, and describe some of the effects of this position.
7. Why are breathing exercises and thoracic cavity mobilization important in the treatment of this condition?

BIBLIOGRAPHY

An HS. Kyphosis: Description and Diagnosis. Spine Universe. Available at: http://www
.spineuniverse.com/conditions/kyphosis/kyphosis-description-diagnosis. Accessed
June 13, 2010.

Joseph TN. Medical Encyclopedia: Kyphosis. MedlinePlus. Available at: http://www.nlm.nih
.gov/medlineplus/ency/article/001240.htm. Accessed June 13, 2010.

MayoClinic.com. Kyphosis. Available at: http://www.mayoclinic.com/health/kyphosis/
DS00681. Accessed June 13, 2010.

Rattray F, Ludwig L. *Clinical Massage Therapy: Understanding, Assessing and Treating over 70
Conditions*, Toronto: Talus Incorporated, 2000.

Vaughn JJ. Patient Education: Hyperkyphosis. The Kentucky Spine Institute. Available at:
http://www.kyspine.net/HTML/hyperkyphosis.html. Accessed June 13, 2010.

21

Iliotibial Band Syndrome

Also known as:

ITBS; Iliotibial Band Friction Syndrome

Definition: An inflammatory condition resulting from repeated distal iliotibial band friction over the lateral femoral condyle of the knee.

GENERAL INFORMATION

- Primary cause: knee overuse during running or cycling
- Secondary causes: prolonged lower extremity immobility and/or prolonged sitting; habitual unilateral, lower extremity weight-bearing stance
- Contributing factors: running on hard or banked surfaces, inefficient or improper running techniques, worn-out or improperly fitting shoes, foot pronation, cycling long distances with improperly adjusted bicycle seat
- Gradual onset
- Prevalent in active and casual athletes, ages 15–50
- Presentation usually unilateral
- Second most common running-related sports injury

PATHOPHYSIOLOGY

The iliotibial (IT) band is located in almost a straight line from the anterior superior iliac spine (ASIS) to the lateral aspect of the tibial condyle. Originating at the tensor fascia lata and ending in a ligament-like structure, this dense fascial band crosses and helps stabilize the knee joint (Figure 21-1). This stringy, strong, mobile band also assists the lower extremity during inward and outward hip rotation, and extension and flexion of the knee. The only firm bony attachments exist at the proximal ASIS and the distal tibial condyle. The two, very distant, bony attachments allow this long structure to move freely, while continuously adjusting anteriorly and posteriorly during normal gait.

ITBS develops when irregular knee movement causes repeated unusual friction over the embedded bursa lateral to the knee joint. As mild inflammation develops, pain ensues, subtle abnormal gait or leg use follows, and the entire IT band becomes shortened and hypertonic, producing a cycle of pain and stiffness. Although ITBS is clinically an inflammatory condition, the classic symptoms of heat, redness, and swelling are usually absent, and only localized pain is used as a diagnostic indicator.

Diagnosis is confirmed based on clinical symptoms, the patient's complaints and history, palpation indicating a hypertonic IT band, reproducible localized pain, and occasionally the presence of an abnormal, stiffened gait. The patient can clearly identify point tenderness at the lateral knee and often complains of radiating pain up the lateral thigh. Leg and hip strength testing may indicate weakness in knee flexors and extensors and/or hip abductors. Knee pain experienced at rest, with no history of repetitive use or trauma, is *not* indicative of ITBS.

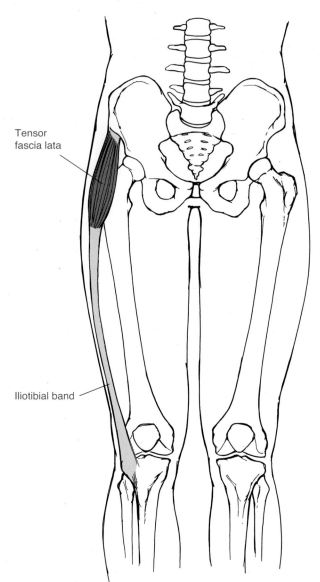

FIGURE 21-1 **Tensor fascia lata and iliotibial band of the lateral thigh. From Hendrickson T.** *Massage for Orthopedic Conditions*, **Philadelphia: Lippincott Williams & Wilkins, 2003.**

OVERALL SIGNS AND SYMPTOMS

Develops early in syndrome:

- Local aching or burning at the lateral aspect of the knee *during activity*; resolves, but sometimes worsens, with activity
- Radiating pain up the lateral aspect of the thigh *during activity*; resolves, but sometimes worsens, with activity
- Pain when ascending or descending the stairs or running downhill
- IT band hypertonicity

Develops later in syndrome:

- Feeling a "snap" or hearing a "pop" while walking, running, or cycling
- Pain during non training walking
- IT band hypertonicity and thickening
- Anterior pelvic tilt; hyperlordosis

Develops if untreated:

- Pain at rest
- Stiff-legged gait
- Extreme IT band hypertonicity
- Adhesions along the IT band

SIGNS AND SYMPTOMS MASSAGE THERAPY CAN ADDRESS

Since the IT band is an easily accessible soft tissue structure with clearly defined bony origins and insertions, ITBS is effectively addressed with massage therapy techniques.

- Hypertonicity is addressed with deep, aggressive manual techniques combined with heat applications.
- The shortened IT band is stretched using both on-the-table and homework exercises.
- The low-level knee joint inflammation is addressed with tissue flushing techniques.

TREATMENT OPTIONS

ITBS usually disappears if the person reduces, stops, or corrects the offending activity. If symptoms persist, treatment is conservative. Manual therapies, including massage, heat application, and stretching are effective. Physical therapy techniques help strengthen the patient's lower extremities if he wants to maintain and continue his exercise regimen. Non-weight-bearing cross-training techniques, such as swimming using only the upper body and arms, are suggested for the dedicated athlete who wishes to maintain his cardiovascular routine while his lower extremities heal. Although conservative, treatment must be continuous—even after activity correction and pain relief—if the patient wants to remain symptom-free.

Inflammation is easily controlled with the use of ice, rest, and nonsteroidal anti-inflammatory drugs (NSAIDs). Heat is used for chronic, dull, aching discomfort. Ice is applied for local flare-ups and more intensive pain. Local corticosteroid injections are used only when the ITBS does not respond to more conservative techniques. Surgery is rarely necessary.

Common Medications

- NSAIDs, such as ibuprofen (Motrin, Advil)

MASSAGE THERAPIST ASSESSMENT

A "weekend warrior" or consistent runner or cyclist may or may not have visited a physician's office before seeking massage therapy for ITBS. Assessment, not diagnosis, is fairly straightforward based on the client's history and simple palpation techniques.

The therapist should ask the client about his athletic habits, including questions about the condition of his running shoes, whether the track he runs on is slanted, and in which direction he consistently runs. He can describe the duration of his bicycle rides and whether his bicycle seat has been professionally fitted for his cycling habits and leg length. The therapist should also have him remove his shoes and observe whether the inside edges are more worn than the outside edges (indicating overpronation).

With the client standing in front of the therapist, she asks permission to palpate the *bilateral* IT bands from the ASIS all the way down to the lateral sides of

**Thinking
It Through**

Regular exercise is essential to prevent chronic disease, help ensure a smooth aging process, and reduce symptoms in myriad medical conditions. Although ITBS most often results from improper or excessive exercising and the short-term treatment may involve exercise reduction or cessation, it is wise for the therapist to advise the client to maintain some form of activity. She might encourage him to continue his exercise regimen by considering the following:

- If ill-fitting shoes are the cause of my client's ITBS, together we can find a running store whose staff includes experienced runners. I can recommend his going there to get properly fitted, and buying a new pair of running shoes for motivation when he returns to his exercise program.
- If foot pronation has contributed to my client's pain, I can refer him to an expert foot physician who can examine his feet and prescribe orthotics or special shoes in anticipation of his returning to his exercise regimen.
- If my client is a cyclist and has not benefited from a professional evaluation of his riding position and bike equipment, we can search online and find proper cyclist alignment techniques and/or a bike shop that will properly adjust his bike seat.
- If my client is hesitant to return to weight-bearing exercises for fear of ITBS

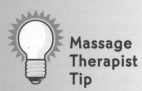

the knees. She notes hypertonicity and tenderness on the affected side. Reproducible lateral knee pain should be evident upon deep palpation and when the client is asked to walk swiftly or run across the office. (A normal walking gait may not reproduce the pain.) The therapist can ask if he has heard a popping or snapping sound while running or cycling. The therapist observes the client from a sideways position and looks for hyperlordosis (swayback).

Finally, the therapist inquires about self-care measures, other health care professionals the client has visited, and medication intake.

THERAPEUTIC GOALS

There are two primary massage therapy goals for clients with ITBS: decreasing hypertonicity and increasing IT band flexibility. In addition, teaching home stretching exercises and encouraging clients to return to a regular exercise regimen as soon as possible are essential.

MASSAGE SESSION FREQUENCY

- 60-minute sessions once a week, until pain and hypertonicity completely resolve
- 60-minute sessions once a month, for maintenance

MASSAGE PROTOCOL

Helping a client who has ITBS is a classic work for the massage therapist. You can use many of the simplest, highly effective techniques you learned in massage school to achieve significant results.

The approach must be aggressive and deep in order to be effective. However, "no pain, no gain" is *not* a massage therapist's mantra. Effective, deep techniques are best accomplished this way:

1. Begin with warming techniques (jostling, vibrating, and shaking the tissue).
2. Stay keenly aware of the client's response.
3. Follow the tissue with hands intelligently aware of anatomy.
4. Work sufficiently deeply that you feel as if you have the entire IT band at your disposal.

Before beginning the session, your communication with the client should clarify that he *may experience some discomfort, but that you will never work to the point of causing pain.* Light, superficial massage for ITBS is ineffective.

Getting Started

If the client has a dull, aching pain, use hot packs. If he complains of a sharp, nagging pain, use ice packs. Review the table and homework stretches you will perform and assign for ITBS, so that you're comfortable and confident before you begin. Have adequate pillows to provide for a prolonged, comfortable side-lying position. Regardless of his level of athleticism, remember to praise your client for his efforts and encourage him to continue exercising.

HOMEWORK

Massage therapy must be accompanied by consistent, daily self-care if your client is to remain pain-free and return to his exercise program or athletic regimen. Applying

Step-by-Step Protocol for Iliotibial Band Syndrome

Technique	Duration
Position the client comfortably prone. Apply and secure a moist hot pack along the affected iliotibial band as you proceed with the following warm-up techniques.	1 minute
Compression, deep pressure, evenly rhythmic, brisk pace, using your whole hand • Achilles' tendon, to the gastrocnemius, to the hamstrings, to the ischial tuberosity • Move over onto the lateral aspect of the thigh, lateral aspect of the pelvic crest, and then (after asking the client's permission) deep into the entire gluteal complex. Start on the unaffected leg, and then move to the affected side, leaving the hot pack in place until you must move it to work on the affected lateral thigh.	5 minutes
Effleurage, petrissage, effleurage, deep pressure, not necessarily rhythmic, *starting proximal and working distal*, massaging the affected leg only • Gluteal complex • Hamstrings • Gastrocnemius • Achilles' tendon	5 minutes
Position the client comfortably side-lying, pillow between his knees, with his unaffected IT band lying on the table. Remove the hot pack. Position yourself in front of the client, facing his head while standing at the level of his knees. Make two fists, and apply your softly clenched fists on the anterior and posterior surface of his thigh. Very vigorously and deeply simultaneously jostle, shake, or vibrate: • Hamstring complex • Quadriceps complex	3 minutes
Skin rolling, skin plucking, wringing and/or flat-hand tissue broadening techniques (using no lubrication), working deeply but to the client's tolerance • Down the entire length of the IT band from the ASIS to the lateral aspect of the knee	5 minutes
Digital kneading and muscle stripping, using very precise, exact fingertip techniques as if trying to pry loose the entire IT band, working deeply. • The entire route of the IT band	5 minutes
Using your thumbs (use a small but sufficient amount of lubricant) deeply, rhythmically cross-fiber friction the entire IT band, working from • The ASIS • Down the front of the pelvic crest • To the femoral head • Deeply into the tensor fascia lata • Down the entire length of the IT band • To the insertion on the lateral tibial condyle	5 minutes

Contraindications and Cautions

• A client who presents with lateral knee pain but has no history of athletic endeavor or knee trauma may be suffering from either a neoplasm or an infection of unknown origin. Do not perform therapy on the affected leg. However, a general Swedish relaxation massage is fine, followed by a referral to a physician.

(continued)

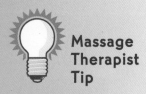

Technique	Duration
Effleurage, petrissage, effleurage, deep pressure, brisk pace • From the ASIS • Down into the hamstrings and quadriceps • Into the gastrocnemius and the tibialis anterior • Deep into the Achilles' tendon	5 minutes
With the client still on the table, securely braced, perform the following table stretches: • Ask the client to flex his ankle as hard as he can so his toes are stretched toward his knee (not pointing his toes), while positioning himself in a fetal position. Ask him to tense his leg muscles for as long as he can possibly hold this position, and then release. • Ask the client to immediately open his position so he is completely stretched out on the table, still side-lying, and stretch to "become long" and hold that position as long as he can, and then release. • Stand behind the client; ask him to position himself close to the edge of the table where you are standing. Ask him to hold onto the opposite edge of the table. While securing him so he feels safe, ask him to slowly drop his top (affected) leg behind him and slightly off the table until he feels a significant stretch. (Stop this stretch if he experiences even mild back pain.) Ask him to hold it as long as he can, then return to a stable position. • Position the client supine, stand at his side. Ask him to place the heel of the affected leg on the knee of the unaffected leg. Place your hand on the affected knee. Gently push the bent knee across the client's body, moving it as close to the opposite side of the table as you can get it without causing pain. *Be sure the hips lie flat on the table and that the client's gluteals do not come off the table during this stretch; he should remain lying flat to achieve an effective stretch.* Ask him to take a deep breath if this is uncomfortable. *Stop if this stretch hurts his back.* Release the stretch and return to a comfortable supine position. Repeat 3 times. • Standing at the client's side, ask him to place the flat of the foot of the affected leg against the inside of the unaffected knee. His knee should now be bent outward, slightly off the table. Place your hands on his affected knee and thigh and begin pushing his bent leg up toward his head, keeping it lying as flat on the table as you can. Keep going until you meet sufficient resistance; ask the client to take a deep breath, and then move an inch farther. Release the stretch and return to a comfortable supine position. Repeat 3 times.	10 minutes
Digital kneading and muscle stripping, using very precise, exact fingertip techniques as if trying to pry loose the entire IT band, working deeply • The entire route of the IT band	5 minutes
Jostle, shake, vibrate, using your fists or the flat of your hands, deeply, vigorously • Quadriceps complex • IT band	5 minutes

(continued)

Technique	Duration
Effleurage, petrissage, effleurage, stroking • Quadriceps • IT band • Around the knee • Tibialis anterior	6 minutes

moist hot packs when he experiences a deep, dull pain and ice when he experiences sharper pain are two active measures he can take toward self-care. Although you cannot suggest taking medication, you can counsel your client to call his family physician for over-the-counter (OTC) pain medication suggestions. Most important, however, are the following daily exercises, which will stretch his IT band and surrounding muscles.

Talk through and *demonstrate*—yes, lie on the floor in your doorway—each exercise before your client leaves your office to make sure he understands these homework assignments:

- Standing IT band stretch (Figure 21-2): Cross your unaffected leg in front of your affected leg. Bend over and reach for your toes. Sweep your fingers along the floor (or as close as you can get) back and forth about 6 inches. Take a deep breath, and as you exhale, try to reach closer to the floor. Repeat three times.
- Side-leaning IT band stretch (Figure 21-3): Stand sideways, about a foot away from a wall, with your affected side nearest the wall. Reach out to the wall for support. Cross your unaffected leg in front of your affected leg, keeping the foot of your affected leg flat on the floor. Lean into the wall with your hip and hold for 15 seconds. Repeat three times.
- Lying-on-your-back hamstring stretch (Figure 21-4): Lie on your back, on the floor in a doorway, with your affected leg closest to the doorframe.

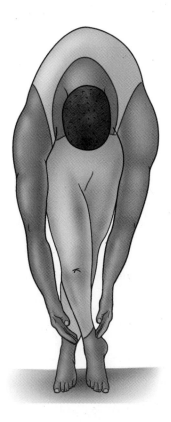

FIGURE 21-2 **The standing IT band stretch.**

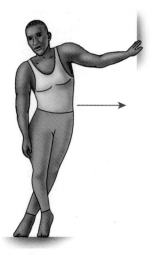

FIGURE 21-3 **The side-leaning IT band stretch.**

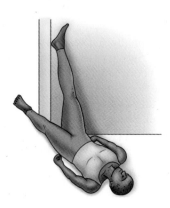

FIGURE 21-4 **The lying-on-your-back hamstring stretch.**

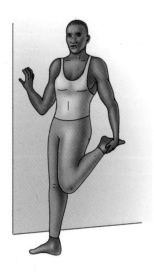

FIGURE 21-5 **The standing quadriceps stretch.**

Swing your leg up and lean it against the frame; allow your other leg to stay on the floor, lying through the doorway. Slightly shimmy your body through the doorway until you feel a stretch at the back of your leg (your hamstrings) as your affected leg remains up on the wall. Stay in this position while you feel the stretch for at least 30 seconds. Bring your leg down, rest. Repeat three times.

- Standing quadriceps stretch (Figure 21-5): Stand facing a wall about an arm's length away. Reach out and brace yourself with the arm of your unaffected side. With the arm of your affected side, reach down and grasp the ankle of your affected leg. Try to touch your heel to your buttocks. Stay stable and stand straight. Hold the stretch for about 30 seconds. Repeat three times.

Review

1. Name the causes of ITBS.
2. What are the symptoms of ITBS?
3. How would you describe the medical treatment for ITBS?
4. What are the effective yet mild massage therapy techniques for treating ITBS?
5. Explain the mechanics of effective stretching.
6. Describe the techniques for the safe application of ice.

BIBLIOGRAPHY

Cluett J. Orthopedics Iliotibial Band Syndrome: Information about this common sports injury. About.com. Available at: http://orthopedics.about.com/cs/sportsmedicine/a/itbs.htm. Accessed June 13, 2010.

Hendrickson T. *Massage for Orthopedic Conditions*, 2nd ed. Baltimore: Lippincott Williams & Williams, 2009.

Martinez JM. Physical Medicine and Rehabilitation for Iliotibial Band Syndrome. EMedicine article. Available at: http://emedicine.medscape.com/article/307850-overview. Accessed June 13, 2010.

National Institute of Arthritis and Musculoskeletal and Skin Diseases. Questions and Answers about Knee Problems. Available at: http://www.niams.nih.gov/Health_Info/Knee _Problems/default.asp. Accessed June 13, 2010.

Pinzon EA. Chronic overuse sports injuries. *Practical Pain Management*. May/June 2008:42–51.

Sportsinjuryclinic.net. Runners Knee: Iliotibial Band Syndrome. Available at: http://www .sportsinjuryclinic.net/cybertherapist/front/knee/irunnersknee.html. Accessed June 13, 2010.

Stirling JM. Iliotibial Band Syndrome. EMedicine article. Available at: http://emedicine .medscape.com/article/91129-overview. Accessed June 13, 2010.

Wanich T, Hodgkins C, Columbier JA, et al. Cycling injuries of the lower extremity. *Journal of the American Academy of Orthopedic Surgeons* 2007;15:748–756.

22

Insomnia

Definition: A sleep disturbance characterized by difficulty falling asleep or staying asleep, or awakening too early.

GENERAL INFORMATION

- Physiologic etiology poorly understood
- Caused by anxiety, mental ruminations secondary to real or imagined stress-inducing life events, medication side effects
- Common predisposing factors: over-the-counter (OTC) decongestants, pain medications, dietary supplements containing caffeine or stimulants, prescription thyroid hormones, antidepressants, corticosteroids, heart medications, caffeine, alcohol, or nicotine taken too close to bedtime
- Acute insomnia duration less than 1 month
- Chronic insomnia duration 1 month or longer
- Increased prevalence with age

Morbidity and Mortality

At least one-third of adults in the U.S. complain of difficulty sleeping, and 10–15% suffer from clinically diagnosed insomnia. Approximately 9–15% of the same population report insomnia serious enough to cause daytime impairments.

About 85–90% of insomnia cases result from a coexisting medical or psychiatric condition. In fact, insomnia coupled with a medical or psychiatric diagnosis annually doubles the incidence of hospital admissions and physician office visits.

Insomnia often occurs immediately prior to a diagnosis of depression. It is used as a diagnostic signal for recurring depression, is associated with increased suicide risk, and is a precipitating factor in manic episodes of bipolar disorder.

Insomnia is associated with a decreased life span. The mortality rate in older adults with heart disease, stroke, cancer, and attempted suicide doubles with accompanying insomnia.

PATHOPHYSIOLOGY

The number of hours of sleeplessness is not a good indicator of insomnia. Although 7.5 hours is the average amount of sleep most adults need, advanced age, illness, personal constitution, and subjective evaluations of overall health and mood indicate that the "normal" sleep cycle ranges from 4 or 5 to 10 hours. A distinction should be made between the sleep's quality and quantity, and whether inadequate sleep is merely secondary to an expected sleep disturbance. On-call hospital residents or mothers of newborns, for example, experience insufficient or nonrestorative sleep, but they do not necessarily have clinical insomnia. A sleep disturbance lasting more than a month, however, is considered a clinical condition and is a cause for medical intervention.

Insomnia is classified as primary or secondary. Primary insomnia can be pinpointed to life events, such as unusual or excessive stress, a job change, travel, financial worries, or a new pet in the home. (Some references identify primary insomnia as that which presents with no known physiologic basis.) Secondary (comorbid) insomnia is sleeplessness with or resulting from a coexisting medical or psychiatric condition.

The condition is associated with musculoskeletal pain, arthritis, cancer, menopause, dementia, Alzheimer's disease, Parkinson's disease, pain syndromes, gastrointestinal and metabolic disorders, chronic fatigue syndrome, and fibromyalgia.

Consequences of acute or chronic insomnia include impaired concentration, performance, memory, reaction time, and coordination. Further, increased workplace absenteeism, diminished social functioning, increased pain perception, and compromised quality-of-life issues result from even mild sleep disturbances.

A polysomnography, or sleep test, usually administered in an overnight sleep clinic, measures sleep-wake cycles. However, the results merely indicate the presence of a sleep disorder and rarely provide sufficient diagnostic information.

OVERALL SIGNS AND SYMPTOMS

- Difficulty falling asleep
- Early morning awakening
- Daytime sleepiness, fatigue, malaise
- Accidents or errors at work or while driving
- Impaired judgment

SIGNS AND SYMPTOMS MASSAGE THERAPY CAN ADDRESS

When techniques are used to specifically quiet the person's mind and body and the session is given in the appropriate environment, massage therapy can help reduce stress and anxiety and thereby induce sleep.

TREATMENT OPTIONS

Cognitive behavioral therapy (CBT) is a nonpharmaceutical, behavioral treatment option that is relatively effective. CBT consists of educational steps aimed at teaching the insomniac how, where, and when to sleep, and combines talk therapy with relaxation techniques.

Preventive measures include reading medication labels of cough, cold, and pain relievers to discover the presence of stimulants and caffeine; avoiding exercise before bedtime; avoiding caffeine, nicotine, or alcohol anytime after lunch; avoiding naps; keeping the bedroom as a place strictly for sleep (not for reading, eating, watching TV, etc.); creating a quiet, dark, slightly cool environment in which to sleep; and observing a consistent bedtime.

Medications are commonly used to induce or maintain sleep; approximately $2 billion are spent annually on sleep-promoting agents, and about 25% of adults with sleep difficulties resort to OTC sleep medications. The insomniac's goal is to find a nonaddictive, effective medication that does not cause morning drowsiness. Alcohol is sometimes used as a sleep aid, and although it can be effective, quality of sleep is usually poor. OTC sleep aids containing antihistamines can cause drowsiness and are often the medication of choice for the occasional insomniac, even given the usual side effect of a morning-after dry mouth.

Melatonin, a natural hormone produced in the brain and directly related to the sleep-wake cycle, is available in tablet form without prescription and is found in most health food stores. With few, if any, side effects, it can hasten the onset and deepen the quality of sleep.

Physicians usually do not recommend the long-term use of sleep aids, citing adverse side effects and the risk of dependency.

Thinking It Through

Even if sleep is induced as a result of an expert massage therapy session, the client must be roused after 60 minutes and returned to the real world. It is unlikely that the client can experience deep, restorative sleep in a mere 60 minutes. The question then becomes, "Does it serve the client to perform sleep-inducing techniques in the massage therapy treatment room?" The exercise for the massage therapist involves thinking through *where and for how long* the session takes place. She might ask herself the following questions:

- If I successfully put this client to sleep on the massage table in my treatment room, can I allow her to sleep until she awakens? Do I have two treatment rooms—one of which I can leave undisturbed, the other one in which I can treat my next client?
- If I know a client is coming to see me for insomnia, should I schedule her for the last appointment of the day?
- Should I allow a client who has fallen asleep on my table and is in a profound state of relaxation to drive home after her appointment? Should I ask her to be sure someone accompanies her to the session?
- Would it be best to go to my client's home in order to treat her insomnia?
- If my client requests that I massage her in her home and in her own bed so she can simply fall asleep and stay asleep after the massage, is this appropriate and ethical? Am I comfortable in the home environment?

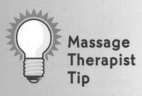

Common Medications

- Benzodiazepine hypnotics, such as estazolam (ProSom)
- Benzodiazepine hypnotic sedatives, such as temazepam (Restoril)
- Sedatives, such as triazolam (Halcion)
- Sedative hypnotics, such as zaleplon (Sonata), zolpidem tartrate (Ambien), and eszopiclone (Lunesta)
- Melatonin receptor agonists, such as ramelteon (Rozerem)

MASSAGE THERAPIST ASSESSMENT

Since only about 50% of adults who experience insomnia tell their primary physicians about this condition and most health care practitioners fail to ask about sleep habits, the massage therapist is in a unique position to ask about sleep with every new client intake, as well as at the beginning of every session. If the client complains of malaise, difficulty concentrating, or drowsiness—especially in the absence of any obvious medical condition—a question about her recent sleep habits is in order. The therapist should also be aware of common medication side effects and any possible comorbid symptoms from a client's current medical diagnosis. If a client informs the therapist of an impending wedding, divorce, house sale, job loss or promotion, or any stress-inducing life event (both positive and negative events can produce physiologic stress), the therapist should expect that the client has at least a temporary sleep disorder.

THERAPEUTIC GOALS

Helping a client achieve a deep parasympathetic state—whether or not sleep is induced—is a worthy therapeutic goal. The body is thus "reminded" what deep relaxation feels like and can begin its journey toward reversing the effects of stress.

MASSAGE SESSION FREQUENCY

Given that insomnia may last for weeks or months; that the therapist may be treating this condition in a home, practice room, or medical setting; and that the protocol can last from 15 minutes to 1 hour, massage session frequency should be individualized.

MASSAGE PROTOCOL

Two simple sleep-inducing techniques are used by many massage therapists working in hospitals, hospices, nursing homes, and private practices. These techniques are highly effective in treating the insomnia experienced by agitated psychiatric, pediatric, cancer, intensive care unit, or critical care unit patients, and those enduring intractable pain or unrelenting stress.

The following two protocols can be provided alone or in combination with other relaxing Swedish techniques. Duration is not indicated in the step-by-step parts because you may be offering these techniques in a hospital setting, in your treatment room, or in the client's home, and durations will vary according to the situation and the client. As soon as sleep is attained, however, the session should cease.

Slow-Stroke Back (or Front) Massage

This protocol assumes the client is positioned prone, but in many cases (as in a hospital or nursing home environment), the patient may be able to lie supine only.

- Stand at the side of the hospital bed or massage table, facing the client's head. Lay your *non-lubricated* hands (either directly on the client's skin or over clothes) at the base of the client's neck (Figure 22-1). Using only the weight of your hands (no lighter, because this will be stimulating to the body, and no

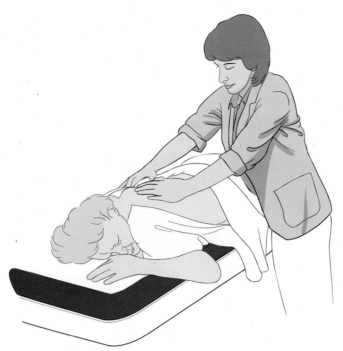

FIGURE 22-1 **Beginning the slow-stroke back massage.
LifeArt image. Philadelphia: Lippincott Williams & Wilkins.**

deeper, because your intent is not to massage muscle) and maintaining full hand (not fingertip) contact, slowly slide your hands down the client's back to her sacrum. It should take you about 1 minute to travel the length of her spine.
- When your hands reach the sacrum, slowly "brush off" your hands to either side of the body.
- Return to the base of the neck immediately and repeat. *This work is unidirectional—running down the spine only.*
- Duration: 15–20 minutes

Hold and Stroke

This technique can be performed with the client lying in any comfortable position.

- Facing the massage table, standing at about the location of the client's waist, gently place one of your hands on your client's shoulder and the other on her hand. Simply rest *for a full minute*. Focus, and determine your intent. Breathe slowly and evenly. Do nothing. Do not speak.
- Once you are focused, begin stroking *down* the arm with the *non-lubricated* hand that was holding your client's shoulder. Use the weight of your full, open hand; do not use your fingertips. Move slowly. This work is performed to the depth at which you would normally apply lubricant and goes no deeper than superficial fascia.
- Repeat three times on one arm.
- Move silently to the contralateral upper extremity and repeat.
- Use slow-stroke back (or front) techniques to the trunk of the body.
- Moving to the lower extremities, place one hand near the head of the femur and the other as far down the leg as you can comfortably reach. Again, center yourself and focus in silence.
- Repeat the slow stroking down the leg.
- Silently move to the other lower extremity and repeat.
- Finish with about 5 minutes of slow-stroke back (or front) massage.
- Duration: 15–30 minutes

Step-by-Step Protocol for	Insomnia	
Technique	**Duration**
Slow-stroke back massage	15–20 minutes
And/or a combination of any of the following Swedish relaxation techniques	30–45 minutes
With the client positioned prone or supine, general warming compression, medium pressure, evenly rhythmic, very slowly • Head to toe	
With the client positioned prone, effleurage, petrissage, effleurage, stroking, evenly rhythmic, medium pressure, very slowly • The entire back, from the base of the skull to the sacrum	
With the client positioned either prone or supine, gently rock the body • Applying alternating pressure on either side of the pelvis, hands on the gluteus medius	
Stroking through the hair, slowly raking your fingers through the length of the hair from the scalp to the tips. Alternate gentle, rhythmic scalp massage with long, slow strokes through the hair.	
Slow, large, clockwise circles, light pressure, rhythmic • On the abdomen, from below the ribs to just above the mons pubis	

Getting Started

As simple as these techniques are, they can cause back spasms in a massage therapist who is not used to performing slow, focused work. Be careful to bend your knees, work from your core, breathe deeply, and shift your weight rather than stretch from your shoulders as you perform these highly effective but surprisingly demanding massage therapy techniques.

Warm packs are often very soothing and can be applied anywhere on the client's body. A heated table pad is also comforting. Make sure the post-session environment has been considered before beginning the session.

Remember, as soon as the client achieves sleep (watch for deeply even, rhythmic breathing or a light snore), work for about another minute and then gently move away from the body and stop treatment.

If the client is comfortable with complete silence, consider foregoing the use of music.

HOMEWORK

As ubiquitous and seemingly innocuous as insomnia is, be aware that its long-term presence can profoundly affect mortality and quality of life, and that insomnia often coexists with serious medical or psychiatric disorders. Therefore, client homework assignments involve quality-of-life and self-awareness issues.

- Be aware of OTC decongestants, pain medications, dietary supplements containing caffeine or stimulants, prescription thyroid hormones, antidepressants,

corticosteroids, heart medications, caffeine, alcohol, or nicotine taken too close to bedtime.
- If your bedroom is the family's "Grand Central Station," find ways to restructure the room so it is a calmer place and more conducive to peaceful sleep.
- Notice if there are any long-term side effects of the sleep aids you've been using.
- Find a naturopath who can talk to you about alternative supplements.
- Keep a sleep journal, and write down sleep disturbances and habits to report to your physician.

Review

1. How would you explain the difference between primary and secondary insomnia?
2. What are some nonpharmaceutical treatment options for insomnia?
3. Name some practical considerations for a massage therapist who is treating a client experiencing insomnia.
4. Describe the slow-stroke back massage.
5. Describe the hold and stroke technique.

BIBLIOGRAPHY

Doghramji P, Moxin C. Treatment options for patients with insomnia. *ADVANCE for Physician Assistants* May/June 2008;29–34.

MayoClinic.com. Insomnia. Available at: http://www.mayoclinic.com/print/insomnia/DS00187. Accessed June 13, 2010.

Mok E, Woo CP. Massage benefits stroke patients. *Complementary Therapies in Nursing & Midwifery* 2004;10:209–216.

Neubauer D. Optimizing the Long-Term Treatment of Insomnia. Medscape.com. Available at: http://www.medscape.com/viewarticle549102. Accessed December 9, 2008.

Riley WT, Hunt CE. Manifestations and Management of Chronic Insomnia: NIH State-of-the-Science Conference Findings and Implications. Medscape.com. Available at: http://www.medscape.com/viewprogram/4784. Accessed June 13, 2010.

Versagi C. Hands of Peace: How to Touch the Dying. *Massage Magazine*. November/December 1999:68–77.

23

Multiple Sclerosis

Definition: An inflammatory disease of the central nervous system (CNS) in which the myelin sheath deteriorates, resulting in the destruction of nerve fibers.

GENERAL INFORMATION

- Exact etiology unknown
- Multiple triggers: genetic, environmental, and autoimmune factors; history of serious viral or bacterial infection
- Usual onset: age 20–40; occurrence as early as age 15 and as late as age 45
- Most common chronic CNS disease among young adults in the U.S.
- Lifelong duration
- Twice as prevalent in young women as in young men; after about age 30, both genders affected almost equally
- Higher prevalence in Caucasians living in temperate climates

Morbidity and Mortality

Approximately 300,000 Americans are currently affected by MS, with 25,000 new cases diagnosed annually. Once diagnosed, patients typically follow a clinical course of flares and remissions. Although complete asymptomatic remission does occur, it is rare. Debilitation directly relates to the form of MS, genetic history, environmental factors, and how aggressively and consistently the disease is treated. The average life expectancy after diagnosis is 25–30 years. There is no cure.

Complications include minor to severe decrease in quality of life, contractures, mild to complete debilitation, secondary infections, clinical depression, and altered self-image.

PATHOPHYSIOLOGY

Nerve signals travel at lightning speed within the CNS (brain and spinal cord) via fibers from the brain to the spinal cord and back again. These delicate nerve fibers are surrounded and protected by a fatty, slick coating called the myelin sheath (Figure 23-1). Innumerable signals—for vision, smell, gross and fine muscle movement, and so on—allow graceful and efficient function.

Demyelination is damage to the myelin sheath from disease or injury, after which signals do not travel smoothly. As the body attempts to repair the damaged sheath, scar tissue builds and hardens (sclerosis) in multiple spots along the myelin sheath—thus, the name multiple sclerosis. Hardened, scarred patches of myelin sheath cause halting or stuttering signals from and to the brain, leading to symptoms like muscle weakness, spasticity, and eye pain.

Here's an easy way to understand demyelination. Decades ago, household electrical cords were covered in a black, fuzzy, threadlike material. The flow of electricity from the wall socket to a lamp was sometimes inconsistent as it ran through these fibers. Troublesome grandchildren (myself included) found it a great source of entertainment (and irritation for the grandparents) to jump up and down on these cords,

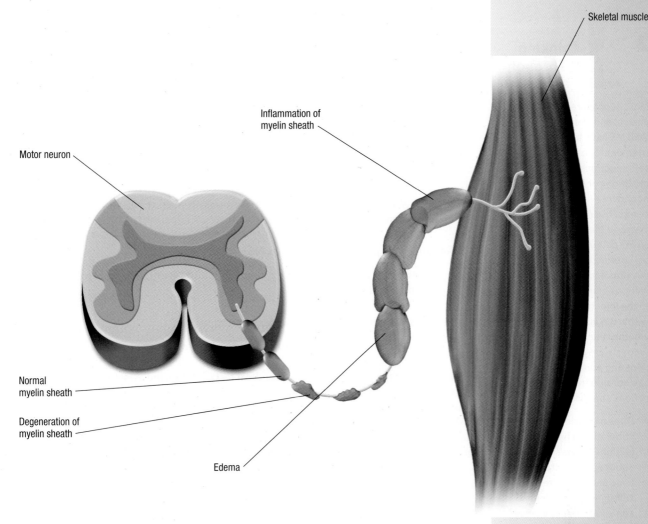

FIGURE 23-1 **A myelinated motor nerve. MS involves the destruction of the myelin sheath, thereby impairing nerve signals.**

causing a flickering—if not a total extinguishing—of the lamp's light. Demyelination is similar. The normally smooth electrical conduction from the brain (wall socket) to the body (lamp) "flickers" because the smooth flow of "electricity" (nerve signals) has been interrupted. Destruction of the smooth surface coating of nerve fibers in MS has the same effect as ill-mannered grandchildren stomping on electrical cords; it interrupts the smooth electrical flow, and thus functions, distally.

The CNS has both motor and sensory nerves. If you pick up a hot cup of coffee, the *motor* nerves in your hand provide the strength and coordination to grasp and hold the cup; the *sensory* nerves provide information to the brain, registering, "Aha—hot liquid." Therefore, nerve damage can result in *both* motor and sensory abnormalities.

There is no single clinical portrait of a typical MS patient; in fact, patients are often misdiagnosed because symptoms associated with such conditions as scleroderma, fibromyalgia, lupus, and even CNS tumors often mimic those of MS. In addition, the clinical course of the condition varies widely and highly depends on the initial form of MS. MS patients usually linger for years or decades in the stage at which they are diagnosed before gradually progressing to a more serious form. Rarely, MS is diagnosed as malignant, in which case the condition worsens rapidly and leads to an early death.

Patients with benign MS:

- Experience one or two early flares
- Can continue to live relatively symptom-free for decades

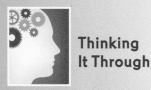

Thinking It Through

Most people are needle-averse, and many people with MS have to administer weekly or monthly self-injections into alternating thighs or belly fat, and/or endure IV infusions to control their symptoms. A massage therapist treating an MS patient must be aware of these important concerns: the sites and frequency of injections or infusions, whether the injection has occurred within the last 24 hours, and whether the injection site is tender. Here are some questions and points the therapist can consider regarding her patient's medications:

- Does my patient complain about giving herself injections? Does she know about auto-injectors?
- If my patient has recently self-injected, I should not apply local heat because I could increase the rate of drug absorption; conversely, I should not apply cold, which might impede drug absorption.
- Is she bruised locally from her injections? How close can I work around her injection site, and how should I adjust my pressure in this area?
- Since flu-like symptoms lasting 1–3 days are a common side effect of most MS self-administered medications, I should remind my patient to schedule our massage sessions either immediately before or a few days after her injection.

- Experience longer survival than in the other forms of MS
- Sometimes remain in the benign stage (15% of patients), but more typically progress to a more serious form of MS

Patients with relapsing/remitting MS (the most common form):

- Experience long periods of remission, during which recovery is almost complete, interspersed with definite flares
- Can remain in this form for life but more often develop the next, more serious form

Patients with secondary progressive MS:

- Follow a similar clinical pattern as relapsing/remitting MS, but healing during remission is less successful

Patients with primary progressive MS:

- Experience constant, low-grade flares that allow very little time to heal
- Often steadily decline

Patients with malignant MS (the rarest form):

- Experience severe flares that rapidly progress into severe disability or death

No single clinical examination or medical test confirms the existence of MS. The clinician depends on each patient's symptomatic and family history, combined with the results from spinal taps, MRIs, and nerve conduction tests, to make a near-final diagnosis. Even after clinical testing is completed, a firm diagnosis is not possible without these two factors: (1) The patient has experienced two flares at least 1 month apart, affecting different parts of the body; and (2) test results have ruled out similar conditions.

Prognosis is determined by the form of MS from the initial diagnosis, the severity and frequency of flares, and the efficiency with which the body heals during remissions.

OVERALL SIGNS AND SYMPTOMS

Symptoms manifest according to the form of MS, whether medication has been recently administered, the presence or absence of flares, and whether the patient is in remission. Overall, however, the following represents the most common symptomatic picture of the MS patient:

- Weakness, spasm, stiffness, and/or cramping in the extremity muscles
- Paresthesia (numbness, tingling, and burning) in the hands and feet
- Pain in the eye or eyes, with compromised vision
- Dysfunction in urinating and sexual performance
- Stumbling and/or loss of coordination
- Impaired cognition
- Depression
- Nausea, diarrhea, and indigestion
- Profound fatigue

SIGNS AND SYMPTOMS MASSAGE THERAPY CAN ADDRESS

- The careful administration of massage therapy techniques can help relieve muscle cramping, spasm, spasticity, and hand and foot paresthesias.
- The secondary limb and joint compensatory stiffness, contractures, and localized edema can be addressed with effective soft tissue and range-of-motion (ROM) techniques.

- Depression can be reduced, and an altered self-image can be improved, by compassionate bodywork.

TREATMENT OPTIONS

After the initial diagnosis is confirmed and a baseline MRI is taken, serial MRIs (multiple scans taken at consistent intervals to track disease progression or remission) are used to determine the treatment plan. Although a holistic approach to MS is important and incorporates gentle cardiovascular exercise, strength training, high-quality nutrition, stress reduction, and an increase in the quality and quantity of sleep, the treatment for the condition is largely pharmaceutical.

Although steroids can quiet flares, drugs that limit the immune system's response to inflammation and secondarily reduce flares, while prolonging periods of remission, are now the ones most commonly used to treat MS. Interferon betas allow many patients to live almost symptom-free. These drugs, which are immunomodulators, help manage relapsing MS and reduce the development of brain lesions (injury to nerves in the brain caused by demyelination). Chemotherapeutic agents, also called antineoplastics, quiet the immune system but are reserved to treat the most severe cases of MS. Drug cocktails (combinations of two or more medications) can address a variety of symptoms. All of these medications have serious long-term adverse side effects.

Common Medications

- Nonsteroidal anti-inflammatory drugs (NSAIDs), such as ibuprofen (Motrin, Advil)
- Antiviral immunoregulators, such as interferon beta-1b, recombinant (Betaseron)
- Antineoplastics, such as mitoxantrone hydrochloride (Novantrone)
- Antiviral, antiproliferative immunomodulators, such as interferon beta-1a (Avonex, Rebif)
- Immunomodulators, such as glatiramer acetate (Copaxone) and natalizumab (Tysabri)

MASSAGE THERAPIST ASSESSMENT

No two MS patients will present with the same complaints, and even the same patient will present with different symptoms before each session. The following questions will help the therapist assess the patient's immediate concerns and determine short- and long-term treatment goals:

- In which stage of MS has she been diagnosed?
- When was her last flare?
- Is she in pain today? Where?
- Is she experiencing bowel or bladder difficulty?
- When was her last injection? Which site? Is it tender?
- Which activities of daily living (ADLs) are the most challenging?
- How are her muscles compensating for her altered gait?
- Does she experience paresthesias? Where?
- What other health care specialists is she seeing?
- Which specific symptoms would she like to address today?

THERAPEUTIC GOALS

Because of the mercurial symptomatic picture presented by most MS patients, therapeutic goals will shift frequently. Given both the musculoskeletal involvement of MS and the understandable accompanying stress, the following three general goals

Thinking It Through (cont.)

- Is her physician suggesting over-the-counter (OTC) pain relievers, such as NSAIDs, which can be taken an hour before each injection and then about every 6 hours after the injection for the first 24 hours? If she is not aware of this avenue of pain relief, how can I suggest that she approach her physician without going outside my scope of practice?

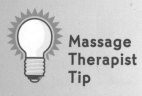

Massage Therapist Tip

Never Stretch the Limbs of a Multiple Sclerosis Patient

You've learned to instruct a client to "Stretch to the point of resistance, take a deep breath, and then stretch slightly beyond that point." *Exactly the opposite is true when working with MS patients.* Here's why: (1) These patients can't tolerate any form of sympathetic nerve firing, which might cause a spasm. (2) They might have an inadequate physiologic reporting mechanism to sense how far they can stretch. (3) If they have contractures, you can cause harm with even mildly overzealous passive ROM. When treating or assigning homework to an MS patient, remember that *stretching must be performed only to the point of slight resistance, and then stopped.* Any further stretching or strengthening exercises should be performed by a physical therapist.

can be combined with the patient's specific concerns: relieving musculoskeletal pain, stiffness, and spasm on the affected and compensating sides of the body; reducing stress; and helping maintain thoracic capacity and efficient breathing patterns.

MASSAGE SESSION FREQUENCY

- Ideally: 60-minute sessions once a week
- If patient tolerance is limited, two 30-minute sessions in the same week
- Mildly effective: 60-minute sessions every other week
- Inconsistent, infrequent therapy yields little improvement but can provide situational stress relief

MASSAGE PROTOCOL

MS is a complicated medical condition, and patients endure it for their entire lives. Therefore, you have an opportunity to maintain a long-term therapeutic relationship; you can make a significant difference in their quality of life and help them manage their level of pain. Remember, you will never accomplish all that needs to be done in one session, and patience and keen listening skills will help keep each session in perspective.

Deep-breathing exercises can be interjected at any point during your session. Passive ROM (remembering not to fully stretch) will help ease stiffness and prevent contractures. If you notice edema, gentle effleurage and stroking performed cephalically will help. If your patient experiences a spasm during your session, stay with the spasm—don't come off the body, but instead gently hold the limb, stop massaging for a moment, and continue to apply gentle pressure. The spasm will stop and you will be able to continue your work. In this way, you are training the body to "let you in," and the cumulative effects cause the muscles to more readily yield to your work.

Detailed, medium-pressure digital work into and around each joint is extremely important to maintain joint health, assist lymphatic flow, help reduce contractures, and soften hypertonic tissue. At each session, digitally explore each joint to familiarize yourself with the body so you can objectively track functional and anatomical progression or digression. The ill effects of contractures, spasticity, and spasm are bilateral, so remember to work both sides of the body.

Keeping copious and detailed SOAP notes will increase your effectiveness and help the patient realize that she is making progress, even if it's minimal. Your patient is seeing multiple medical specialists and dealing with an insurance company; your notes, or at least a treatment summary, may be requested by a physician or an insurer.

Getting Started

Before her first appointment, ask whether she uses a cane or a wheelchair. Arrange your reception and treatment rooms accordingly. Practice transferring a patient from a wheelchair to the massage table (with a colleague, for example) to ensure a confident, accident-free process. During inclement weather, have towels available at the door so you can wipe off the wheelchair wheels and not track snow, rain, or mud into your professional area.

Since each MS patient is unique, for protocol purposes, the following treatment is based on a 45-year-old Caucasian woman with relapsing/remitting MS. She is not currently in a flare, walks with a stumbling gait, and occasionally uses a cane. Both legs are primarily affected, and she injects Avonex into alternating thighs every other week. Her last injection was 1 week ago into her superior left thigh. Lying prone is uncomfortable; she prefers side-lying or supine. She is concerned about thigh and calf spasms, as well as mild, bilateral ankle edema.

Step-by-Step Protocol for **Multiple Sclerosis**	
Technique	**Duration**
Note: This protocol is slightly longer than 60 minutes due to the amount and detail of therapy involved; times can be altered according to patient tolerance. After positioning the patient comfortably supine, ask which massage technique she finds particularly relaxing (e.g., scalp massage, face massage, or total body stroking). Perform this technique to initiate deep relaxation.	2 minutes
Effleurage, medium pressure, slow, evenly rhythmic, working cephalically • Right lower extremity • Right foot	1 minute
Effleurage, petrissage, effleurage, medium pressure, slow, evenly rhythmic, *start proximally* • Right lower extremity	3 minutes
Digital kneading, medium pressure • Origins and insertions of the quadriceps • Around the patella • Origins and insertions of the IT band • Origins and insertions of the tibialis anterior • Around the malleolus	
Effleurage, medium pressure • Entire lower extremity	4 minutes
Stroking, using your fingertips only, brushing cephalically • Around the malleolus and up about 4 inches toward the knee	1 minute
Effleurage, medium pressure • The foot below the malleolus	1 minute
Digital kneading, medium pressure • Every toe, between the toes, between all metacarpals, plantar and dorsal surface of the foot, in between all bones and ligaments, around the malleolus	3 minutes
Effleurage, medium pressure • The foot and malleolus	1 minute
Passive ROM (watch the extent of your stretch, move only to mild resistance and stop) • At the hip • At the knee • At the ankle (attempt full circumduction and plantar and dorsal flexing and extending)	4 minutes
Effleurage, slightly more briskly, medium pressure, not necessarily rhythmic • Entire lower extremity	1 minute

Contraindications and Cautions

- Never work deeply or vigorously enough to overheat a muscle complex or to raise the patient's core temperature. MS patients react poorly to heat, and you could initiate a flare.

- Do not apply hot packs; even a table warmer could produce too much heat and cause a flare.

- Do not use mechanical muscle vibrators to quiet a spasm; use your hands only. A mechanical vibrator can stimulate the sympathetic nervous system.

- Be aware of the day, time, and location of the patient's last injection; avoid working around puncture sites within 24 hours of the injection.

- Since many MS patients experience vertigo, ask permission before using any rocking techniques.

- Watch for red, inflamed, hot, or swollen areas over bony prominences. The patient may not be able to feel these signs and symptoms of skin infection or breakdown. If symptoms exist, refer the patient to a physician immediately.

(continued)

Technique	Duration
Perform the previous protocol on the left leg, using caution around the injection site.	19 minutes
Position the patient side-lying. Effleurage, medium pressure, slow, evenly rhythmic • Hamstrings • Gastrocnemius • Heel	2 minutes
Effleurage, petrissage, effleurage, medium pressure, slow, evenly rhythmic • Hamstrings • Gastrocnemius • Heel	4 minutes
Digital kneading, medium pressure, slow, evenly rhythmic • Origin and insertions of the hamstrings (work up into the ischial tuberosity) • Origins and insertions of the gastrocnemius • Around and into the calcaneus	4 minutes
Effleurage, medium pressure, slow, evenly rhythmic • Lower extremity	1 minute
Stroking, using your fingertips only, brushing cephalically • Around the malleolus	1 minute
Reposition patient on the other side, and repeat the previous side-lying protocol.	12 minutes
End the session with a few minutes of a deep relaxation technique.	2 minutes

HOMEWORK

You can provide much-needed holistic support as your MS patient attempts to maintain her regular ADLs and bolster her wobbly self-image. While reminding her not to work to the point of heat exhaustion and to always be gentle with herself, you can offer the following homework assignments:

- Purchase a big exercise ball; blow it up until it's firm, not squishy. Place the ball next to a couch, a sturdy armchair, or the wall. Put one hand on a secure surface to steady yourself, and sit on the ball. Gently begin bouncing. Bounce as long as you can. Take frequent deep breaths. You'll start to feel this in your thighs. When you feel the slightest bit tired, stop and rest. Then continue bouncing. This simple exercise helps keep your thigh muscles strong and is extremely effective in maintaining your sense of balance.
- Find a gentle yoga or tai chi class; either one will help strengthen your balance and maintain your flexibility without overheating your central body core or major muscles.
- Consider swimming or a water aerobics class, but be sure that the water is not too warm. You should not sweat while in the water or when getting out of the pool.

- Take deep breaths several times throughout the day. Inhale deeply, hold it for a few seconds, and then forcibly exhale.
- Investigate personal deep relaxation techniques that work for you, and set aside time to practice one daily.
- Be sure to get enough hours of deep, restful sleep.

Review

1. Describe the various stages or forms of MS.
2. What is the medical treatment for MS?
3. List three cautions that you should observe when massaging an MS patient.
4. Why should your SOAP notes be particularly thorough when documenting sessions with MS patients?
5. How might you have to alter your massage treatment room to accommodate your patient?
6. Is there a cure for MS?

BIBLIOGRAPHY

Bar-Or A. The Immunology of Multiple Sclerosis. Available at: http://www.medscape.com/viewarticle/572284. Accessed May 31, 2008.

Cohen BJ. *Memmler's The Human Body in Health and Disease*, 11th ed. Baltimore: Lippincott Williams and Wilkins, 2008.

Jeffrey DR. Managing Clinically Definite Multiple Sclerosis. A CME Course. Available at: http://www.medscape.com/viewprogram/8268. Accessed June 29, 2010.

Jeffrey S. BEYOND and PRECISE Results Suggest Equivalence for Multiple Sclerosis Treatments. Available at: http://www.medscape.com/viewarticle/573185. Accessed June 29, 2010.

Jeffrey S. Multiple Sclerosis Gene Discovery First Major Genetic Advance in 30 Years. Medscape. Available at: http://www.medscape.com/viewarticle/560661. Accessed June 29, 2010.

May TS. Most Cases of "Benign" MS Progress After 20 Years, but Survival Is Longer. Medscape. Available at: http://www.medscape.com/viewarticle/564612. Accessed June 29, 2010.

Rattray F, Ludwig L. *Clinical Massage Therapy: Understanding, Assessing and Treating over 70 Conditions*, Toronto: Talus Incorporated, 2000.

Werner R. *A Massage Therapist's Guide to Pathology*, 4th ed. Philadelphia: Lippincott Williams & Wilkins, 2009.

24

Muscle Cramp; Charley Horse

Muscle Spasm

Definition: An involuntary contraction of a voluntary skeletal muscle.

GENERAL INFORMATION

- Caused by trauma, muscle overuse, emotional stress, chilled muscles, prolonged immobilization, ischemia (temporary lack of oxygen in localized tissue), dehydration, or insufficient calcium, sodium, magnesium, potassium, or vitamin D
- Muscles commonly affected: gastrocnemius, soleus, hamstrings, deep back muscles (especially the erector spinae complex), and sternocleidomastoid (SCM)

PATHOPHYSIOLOGY

A review of normal muscle anatomy and physiology will help clarify the pathophysiology of a muscle spasm. Muscle tissue is one of the most sanguineous (well-vascularized) tissues in the body. In order to function quickly and efficiently on both gross and fine motor levels, a muscle must receive a constant flow of fresh blood from and release metabolic waste into the bloodstream. As muscles move, Golgi tendon organs (GTOs; nerve receptors located in tendons) signal the brain about the extent a muscle can stretch before injury will occur. The vigilant GTOs constantly fire signals during normal muscle activity and will produce sudden and severe pain if an overly zealous exerciser, for example, stretches too far and thereby possibly risks snapping a tendon off a bone. When a tendon is injured or inflamed, the GTOs "register their objections" by firing continuous pain signals in order to prevent the person from continuing offending activity.

Conversely, immobilized muscle produces its own set of painful signals. Local ischemia, which accompanies immobilization, leads to metabolite buildup, causing pain and further muscle immobilizing, thereby continuing the pain-spasm-pain cycle (see Figure 3-1).

There is no diagnostic test for identifying a muscle spasm. The clinician palpates for the presence of tightened, painful muscles and will take an oral history of recent activity, lack of activity, or the presence of recent trauma or disease.

OVERALL SIGNS AND SYMPTOMS

- Temporary skeletal muscle pain, spasm, and/or cramping
- Temporary decreased range of motion (ROM) secondary to muscle shortening and pain
- Unusually firm, hard, and/or congested muscle tissue

SIGNS AND SYMPTOMS MASSAGE THERAPY CAN ADDRESS

- The pain-spasm-pain cycle is effectively broken with skilled therapeutic massage.
- ROM is increased with passive techniques applied to the post-spasm muscle and proximal joint.
- Accumulated toxins can be hastened out of the muscle and sent into circulation with the use of several massage modalities.

TREATMENT OPTIONS

Rest, *ice*, and nonsteroidal anti-inflammatory drugs (NSAIDs) or muscle relaxants are suggested during the first 3 days if muscle spasms occur secondary to trauma. Rest, *heat*, NSAIDs, and, more rarely, muscle relaxants are suggested for chronic or infrequent muscle spasms that result from minor injury, exercise, or immobilization.

When a spasm results from exercise dehydration, water and sports drinks are suggested before, during, and after activity. Spasms occurring secondary to metabolic imbalance or circulatory diseases often do not resolve until the primary condition is addressed.

Common Medications

- NSAIDs, such as ibuprofen (Motrin, Advil)
- Skeletal muscle relaxant, such as cyclobenzaprine hydrochloride (Flexeril)

MASSAGE THERAPIST ASSESSMENT

The client experiencing a muscle spasm may present after unusual or excessive physical activity, such as shoveling after the first snow storm of the year, or because of one sudden, unusual awkward movement, such as jerking to catch something. Before proceeding with the treatment of a seemingly innocuous muscle spasm, however, the therapist must be assured that no underlying metabolic pathology exists. In addition, a therapist should not treat muscle spasm secondary to recent injury or trauma. Before continuing in the safe treatment of a muscle spasm, the therapist can:

- Ask the client about the specific, suspected origin of the muscle spasm.
- Ask him to clearly identify the exact location of the spasm.
- Find out whether he experiences chronic spasms or if this is an unusual occurrence.
- Ask how he normally treats the spasm.
- Ask if he is diabetic, dehydrated, experiencing unusual stress, or is a smoker.
- Ask if he is seeing a physician, chiropractor, or physical therapist for his spasms or for any medical condition.
- Palpate the muscle belly to determine the character of the spasm. Is it accompanied by heat, coolness, or increased hypertonicity?
- Ask the client to demonstrate his ROM at the affected limb.

THERAPEUTIC GOALS

Reasonable goals for treating muscle spasm include softening hypertonic muscles, quieting the firing GTOs, removing accumulated metabolic waste, increasing circulation to the affected muscle, enhancing the healing process, and relieving the pain.

Massage Therapist Tip

Treating a Sudden, Painful Spasm of Unknown Cause

When a client, or even a colleague or an acquaintance, suddenly experiences an intolerable muscle spasm and requests that you "do something, anything," your first thought as a massage therapist is to dive right in and massage the muscle belly. But unless you know the cause of the cramp, you could easily make matters worse. You can safely contract and massage the antagonist muscles—those muscles that perform the opposite action of the spasming muscles. For example, if the hamstrings are in spasm, you could work on the quadriceps. This will quiet the muscle spasm without placing your client at risk. Once you determine the client's history, you can proceed with a full treatment protocol.

Thinking It Through

As uncomfortable as a muscle spasm may be, it should not be massaged if there is even a remote possibility that the spasm is a result of physical trauma. Post-traumatic muscles that go into spasm are compensating to protect an injured area; this is referred to as *splinting* or *guarding*. In the case of whiplash, for example, the cervical muscles, tendons, and ligaments that hold the head upright are so injured

Thinking It Through (cont.)

that they cannot support the 10-pound head. Therefore, surrounding muscles splint or guard the surrounding anatomy. These muscles work so hard at compensating that they painfully spasm, yet their job is to provide support for the head. *If the massage therapist loosens these muscles, the head will not have the much-needed support; the muscles will release, causing further, possibly serious, injury to the already injured area.*

The careful therapist must think through her treatment of a muscle spasm and consider the following before proceeding:

- Is the spasm the result of trauma?
- If I massage splinting muscles, what will be the effect?
- Should I perform relaxation massage on the surrounding tissue and not work on the splinting area?
- Would an application of ice packs for a few minutes provide temporary relief without loosening the muscles and creating functional instability?
- Should I consider not treating this client, and instead refer him to a physician until the splinting has passed?
- How can I best explain to this client that I should not work on his painful muscles?

MASSAGE SESSION FREQUENCY

- Ideally: 60-minute sessions once a day until the painful spasm is under control
- Preventive: 60-minute sessions once a week if the client is sedentary

MASSAGE PROTOCOL

Once you have determined that it is safe to proceed, your approach to a spasming muscle should be gentle but firm, and your protocol will have a definite beginning, middle, and end. Haphazard work will produce unnecessary pain and may injure the client.

Your first task is the application of ice for an acute spasm (if it occurred within the last 3 days) or heat (if the spasm is chronic or if it occurred longer than 3 days ago). You must attempt to break the pain-spasm-pain cycle and use the gate control theory of pain to your advantage (see Chapter 3). Use frequent deep-breathing techniques to help relax your client and bring oxygen to the blood-starved muscles. You'll "slay the dragon" while the ice or heat begins to work, and then gently perform techniques that will bring blood to the muscle belly and quiet the GTOs. Take your time and don't overwork the muscle set; start at the tendon sites, not on the muscle belly; be sure to work on surrounding and antagonist muscles and not solely on the painful muscle.

Passive ROM and deep vibratory techniques—both highly effective and necessary components of this protocol—should not be performed until well after you are sure the spasm has quieted. Even then, you may find that as you attempt to reposition the client, or as he gets off the table at the end of the session, the muscle may re-spasm. These repeated spasm cycles will quiet with rest, heat or ice, anti-inflammatories, and time.

The following protocol is based on the treatment of nontraumatic back muscle spasms resulting from snow shoveling.

Getting Started

Try to gather information from a telephone intake before your client arrives to ensure that you can safely treat him. Once you determine it is safe to proceed, have ice and hot packs ready.

This protocol focuses on treating the rhomboids, so the client will probably be positioned prone for an extended period. Allow him to move his head from side to side, and shift positions frequently so he does not lay prone for 60 minutes. This sustained position is usually not well-tolerated and can produce sinus congestion and headache. The side-lying position can be a helpful alternative.

HOMEWORK

Your client's healing is only possible if he continues to attend to his muscle spasm after he leaves your table. Appropriate homework assignments are determined by the client's acute or chronic symptoms.

Acute Muscle Spasm

- Place an ice pack or bag of frozen vegetables on your spasming muscle for 5–10 minutes every hour. Repeat frequently.
- Find the end of your muscle, the place where it attaches to your bone. Deeply massage into this area. Don't cause further pain and don't massage directly on the painful muscle.

Step-by-Step Protocol for Muscle Spasm of Bilateral Rhomboids

Technique	Duration
Position the client comfortably prone or side-lying. Apply a heavy, moist hot pack (over the sheet) directly on the spasming muscles.	
Use slaying-the-dragon techniques to the lower back or legs. Ask the client to inhale and exhale, slowly and deeply, several times.	3 minutes
Remove the hot packs. Place your hands directly on the spasming muscles. Just remain in contact with the spasming muscles. The client's body must know you intend no harm before you proceed.	1 minute
Effleurage, medium pressure, very slow, evenly rhythmic • In all directions, over the entire back, being sure to work over the rhomboids (Lighten your pressure if the client retracts when you work over the rhomboids but be sure to engage the rhomboids with some pressure.)	1 minute
Compression, light pressure, evenly pumping • The entire back beginning at the lumbar spine region, working laterally out to the sides of the body and then toward the spine; work up the entire spine and back until you reach the base of the skull	3 minutes
Compression, medium pressure, evenly pumping • The entire back beginning at the lumbar spine, working laterally out to the sides of the body and then toward the spine; work up the entire spine and back until you reach the base of the skull	4 minutes
Effleurage, medium pressure, slow, evenly rhythmic • The entire back, working in all directions	3 minutes
Place your hands on the rhomboids. Rest them on the tissue. Feel for the quieting of the spasm	1 minute
Digital kneading, medium pressure, very slow, evenly rhythmic • Superior and lateral border of the bilateral scapulae (Do not approach the rhomboids yet.)	5 minutes
Effleurage, medium-to-deep pressure • Around the thoracic vertebrae and bilateral scapulae	3 minutes
Digital kneading, medium pressure, very slow, evenly rhythmic. Combine this movement with deep effleurage periodically "cleaning" the area. • Lateral border of the bilateral scapulae and into the deep spinalis complex from T-1 through T-12	6 minutes
Place your hands on the rhomboids; be sure they have quieted and are no longer spasming before you proceed.	1 minute

(continued)

Contraindications and Cautions

- Gastrocnemius cramps are often associated with third-trimester pregnancy. The cause is thought to be either vitamin insufficiency or spinal disc involvement secondary to the baby's placement against the spine. Since pregnant women are also at risk for lower extremity blood pooling and blood clots, it is best to get a physician's clearance before treating muscle spasms in a pregnant client.

- A *unilateral* dull, aching, sometimes cramping sensation in the gastrocnemius (or any muscle) accompanied by heat, redness, slight swelling, pain, and localized tenderness are dangerous signs and symptoms of a potentially lethal deep vein thrombosis (DVT). Never massage a muscle that feels unilaterally warm, appears reddened, is even mildly swollen, and is uncomfortably tender to the touch. The client should see a physician before you proceed.

Contraindications and Cautions (cont.)

- Diabetic patients often suffer from chronic arteriosclerotic vascular disorders, which cause leg pain and cramping. Be sure to get a clearance from the client's physician before proceeding with deep work.
- Chronic smokers often have circulatory disorders that can inflame vessels. Be sure to get a physician's clearance before performing deep work on a chronic smoker.
- Women who take birth control pills are at increased risk for DVT.
- Never massage a set of muscles that are splinting or guarding after trauma or injury. Immediately refer the client to a physician.
- Do not stretch or work deeply into a spasming muscle until it has completely relaxed.
- Do not apply heat to a muscle spasm that occurred as a result of injury or trauma.

Technique	Duration
Gently but firmly grip all three edges of one scapula in your fingertips, and try to move it on the back of the thoracic cavity. If the adipose tissue or musculature prevents this move, ask the client to lay his arm onto his lower back, which will help the scapula "pop out" and move off the back. Gently but firmly continue to move the scapula, passively, as much as you can. Repeat on the contralateral scapula.	3 minutes 3 minutes
Immediately slowly effleurage, medium pressure - Rhomboids	2 minutes
Effleurage, petrissage, effleurage, digital kneading, medium-to-deep pressure, *not evenly rhythmic* - Along the transverse processes of the cervical spine, thoracic spine, around both scapulae, into the QLs (bilateral quadratus lumborum), down to the lumbar spine and sacrum	6 minutes
When you are certain that the spasming has completely stopped, digital vibration, deep to tolerance, rhythmic - Directly over the spasming muscles, on both lateral borders of the scapulae	5 minutes
Immediately change your pace and slowly but deeply effleurage - Over the entire posterior thoracic region, focusing on the scapulae	4 minutes
Ask the client to sit up on the side of the table, facing away from you. Position the sheet for modesty. Place his feet on a stool for support if necessary. Make sure the spasming has not recurred because of this repositioning. Ask him to take a couple deep breaths.	2 minutes
Effleurage, very slowly, medium pressure, using long soothing strokes - Over the entire back, up into the base of his skull, down to his lumbar spine region	4 minutes

- Slowly and carefully perform ROM exercises without placing the muscle into even the slightest stretch.
- Call your physician to determine if you should be taking NSAIDs, or if she wants to prescribe a short-term muscle relaxant. Don't drive if you're taking muscle relaxants.
- Return for another massage session as soon as your schedule allows.
- Rest.

Non-Acute Muscle Spasm

- Apply a moist hot pack directly onto the affected muscle; leave it on for as long as it's comfortable.
- Find the end of your muscle, the place where it attaches to your bone. Deeply massage this area, but don't cause further pain.
- Find the exact affected muscle. Massage into the muscle belly. Start superficially, working progressively deeper. Do not cause pain.

- Perform slow, careful ROM exercises, moving your joint until you can't move any farther; hold this stretch for about 20 seconds and then release. Don't bounce. Repeat several times.
- If you are exercising, be sure to drink plenty of water for adequate hydration.
- Stretch before and after your regular workout.
- Rest.

Review

1. List some causes for muscle spasms.
2. Explain muscle splinting or guarding.
3. When is it unsafe to massage a muscle spasm?
4. Describe the difference in the use of ice or heat in the treatment of either acute or chronic spasm.
5. List the signs and symptoms of a DVT. What should you do if you suspect a DVT?
6. What would cause painful leg cramps in a woman in third-trimester pregnancy?

BIBLIOGRAPHY

Joseph TN. Charley Horse. MedlinePlus. Available at: http://www.nlm.nih/gov/medlineplus/ency/article/002066. Accessed December 22, 2008.

Rattray F, Ludwig L. *Clinical Massage Therapy: Understanding, Assessing and Treating over 70 Conditions*, Toronto: Talus Incorporated, 2000.

Werner R. *A Massage Therapist's Guide to Pathology*, 4th ed. Philadelphia: Lippincott Williams & Wilkins, 2009.

Wible J. *Drug Handbook for Massage Therapists*, Philadelphia: Lippincott Williams & Wilkins, 2009.

25

Neuropathy: Diabetic Peripheral Neuropathy and Chemotherapy-Induced Peripheral Neuropathy

Definition: Diabetic peripheral neuropathy—damaged and painful distal sensory and motor nerves secondary to uncontrolled blood glucose.

Definition: Chemotherapy-induced peripheral neuropathy—damaged and painful distal sensory and motor nerves secondary to the administration of a neurotoxic chemotherapeutic agent.

GENERAL INFORMATION

Diabetic Peripheral Neuropathy

- Multifaceted causes under continuing study; strongest evidence pointing to uncontrolled (high) blood glucose, vascular insufficiency, degeneration of nerve fibers secondary to oxidative debt (lack of oxygen)
- Most common complication of diabetes mellitus (DM)
- Classification based on blood glucose levels; degree of sensory, motor, or autonomic nerve involvement
- Onset: mild discomfort, developing insidiously; acute pain occurring after years
- Duration of acute pain about 12 months
- Progression to open wounds, ulcers; amputation common
- Prevalence in people who smoke, drink alcohol heavily, are hypertensive, have uncontrolled DM, or a long history of DM

Chemotherapy-Induced Peripheral Neuropathy

- Causes: administration of neurotoxic (nerve-damaging) chemotherapeutic agents, such as Taxol, Taxotere, Abraxane, Oncovin, Navelbine, Platinol, Paraplatin, and Eloxatin
- Sensory nerves most often affected
- Onset gradual, mildly symptomatic; discomfort increasing with each additional chemotherapy dose; usually moving proximal as pain worsens
- Duration usually several months, peak discomfort at 3–5 months after the final chemotherapy dose
- Most symptoms diminishing within a year; rarely irreversible
- Prevalence in people who drink alcohol heavily, are severely malnourished, and have previously undergone chemotherapy for an earlier cancer

Morbidity and Mortality

Diabetic Peripheral Neuropathy

About 10–20% of newly diagnosed diabetic patients suffer from DPN. Half of all elderly diabetics manifest symptoms, and approximately 30–50% of all diabetic patients with either type 1 or type 2 DM will manifest symptoms of DPN.

The most serious comorbidities include foot ulceration and lower extremity amputation. Although not life threatening, unless uncontrolled infection occurs in an already medically compromised patient, these secondary effects of DPN severely limit the patient's quality of life and are the most common cause of hospitalization in the diabetic population.

Chemotherapy-Induced Peripheral Neuropathy

The most serious concern for medical oncologists treating CIPN patients is that the condition can quickly become "dose-limiting"—that is, the pain or discomfort is so disturbing to the cancer patient that she may choose to discontinue taking the life-saving chemotherapeutic agent. The conundrum is that the discomfort, unto itself, may be minimal; but added to a medical journey already fraught with "too many medications," this side effect may be the "straw that breaks the camel's back," and the patient will refuse chemotherapy. Medical oncologists obviously consider this an understandable but highly unwise decision and therefore take great measures to try to reduce the symptoms of CIPN.

PATHOPHYSIOLOGY

The two main divisions of the nervous system are the central nervous system (CNS; the brain and spinal cord) and the peripheral nervous system (PNS). The PNS has two branches: the somatic nervous system and the autonomic nervous system. The somatic system, which includes the peripheral nerves, is composed of fibers that transmit sensory information *to the CNS* ("this cup is hot," for example) and transmit motor signals *from the brain to the skeletal muscle* (the ability to quickly put the cup down). Compared to other nerves in the body, these fibers are extremely long, traveling from the brain to the periphery of the body—the hands, fingers, feet, and toes.

To function properly, these fragile nerves must regularly receive generous amounts of carefully regulated nutrients and oxygen, and the body's blood glucose level must remain stable. Clinical studies indicate that the efficient functioning of the nerves is also directly related to the level of oxygen they regularly receive. When the blood glucose level spikes or remains high, or when a chemotherapeutic agent severely reduces the ability of peripheral nerves to utilize oxygen, there is a greater risk of DPN and/or CIPN. In addition, fiber length makes the nerves vulnerable to injury from physical trauma anywhere along a nerve's winding path to and from the brain and the distal body regions.

Diagnostic methods for both DPN and CIPN include simple subjective, symptomatic reporting of the location, duration, and intensity of the sensory or motor disturbance; observance of heel-toe gait; and the administration of electrodiagnostic, muscle strength, pinprick, cranial nerve, and nerve conduction tests.

OVERALL SIGNS AND SYMPTOMS

DPN and CIPN share common symptoms.

- Initial, subtle discomfort in a bilateral "stocking-and-glove" distribution of sensory and/or motor nerves
- Progressive sensory symptoms: paresthesias, such as burning, tingling, numbness, and a pins-and-needles sensation
- Motor symptoms: clumsiness, deep muscle aches and pains, spasm, and loss of strength
- Advanced sensory symptoms: allodynia (painful response to a stimulus that would normally not cause pain, such as the weight of bed sheets on the toes)
- CIPN symptoms more persistent and severe in cancer patients who are also diabetic

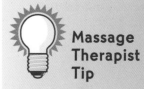

Massage Therapist Tip

Watching for Signs of Dry Gangrene

While diagnosing dry gangrene (the type of gangrene most often experienced by diabetic patients) is well beyond your scope of practice, you will examine your patient's feet before each protocol and should know the warning signs of this serious condition. On the feet, watch for an *extreme* sensitivity to touch, unusually cold patches of tissue, a small area of dark purple tissue, or, more alarmingly, a tiny spot (sometimes the size of a poppy seed) or larger area of black tissue. Any of these signs indicates possible gangrene, and your patient should see her physician immediately.

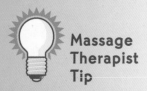

Massage Therapist Tip

Recognizing "Off-Label" Medication

Medications are approved by the U.S. Food and Drug Administration (FDA) for a specific use, such as to eliminate a certain bacterium. However, physicians have found other uses, often not related and not intended, for the same drug to treat very different conditions. This practice is called an "off-label" use of the medication. It is common among physicians, is well within standard medical care, and is often supported by multiple clinical studies showing additional uses for already established medications. Examples of off-label medication use are anticonvulsants and antidepressants to reduce paresthesias associated with DPN and CIPN.

Thinking It Through

Although most Thinking It Through sections in this text guide the therapist to reflect on client care questions, this one prompts the therapist to think through the complicated pathophysiology of peripheral neuropathy. This understanding is paramount if the therapist is to properly perform the protocol and positively instruct the patient in the all-important self-care homework assignments. The therapist must understand that peripheral neuropathies, starting as innocuous and mildly uncomfortable

SIGNS AND SYMPTOMS MASSAGE THERAPY CAN ADDRESS

- The poor blood circulation that is considered the primary cause of both DPN and CIPN can be profoundly improved with careful, localized, systematic, and frequent massage therapy techniques.
- The anxiety, insomnia, and fear that result from an initial diagnosis of diabetes or cancer can be decreased with careful, attentive, and soothing massage therapy.

TREATMENT OPTIONS

Multiple clinical studies focusing on the treatment of DPN indicate that the same protocols can serve as a guide for the treatment of CIPN. Early symptoms of DPN are often treated with physical therapy to address muscle weakness, pain, and the loss of balance, mobility, and strength. Transcutaneous electrical nerve stimulation (TENS) units are recommended for pain control. Physical therapists also teach patients vigilant skin care, and they can attend to open wounds, should the condition progress.

An occupational therapist becomes involved if the patient experiences severe loss of function (following an amputation, for instance) and needs instruction in adaptive skills and equipment.

Acupuncture is an effective tool for pain management in both types of neuropathy. Psychological counseling can help with quality-of-life issues.

Preventive methods include rigorous blood glucose regulation following a DM diagnosis. Monitoring the diet, observing good nutrition, and getting regular exercise are also paramount in preventing DPN. Combinations of B vitamins are often prescribed to reduce early-onset diabetic paresthesias.

No preventive measures have yet been identified for CIPN besides the already mentioned ill-advised decision to cease chemotherapy.

Common Medications: Diabetic Peripheral Neuropathy

Often during the course of pain management, topical creams are prescribed, such as capsaicin cream. Disadvantages include initial pain or discomfort upon application and messiness (it sticks to clothes and socks). These irritations, combined with the necessary four-times-per-day application, make patient compliance a challenge.

The following are medications used in the early stages of neuropathy when symptoms are merely perceived as uncomfortable or annoying:

- Nonsteroidal anti-inflammatory drugs (NSAIDs), such as ibuprofen (Motrin, Advil) and naproxen (Aleve, Anaprox, Naprelan, Naprosyn)

As the neuropathy progresses in severity, simple analgesics are no longer effective. The following off-label medications are then prescribed:

- Tricyclic antidepressants, such as amitriptyline hydrochloride (Apo-Amitriptyline, Endep)
- Selective serotonin reuptake inhibitors (SSRIs), such as paroxetine hydrochloride (Paxil) and sertraline hydrochloride (Zoloft)
- Tricycline antidepressants, such as imipramine hydrochloride (Tofranil)
- Ventricular antiarrhythmics, such as mexiletine hydrochloride (Mexitil)
- Anticonvulsants, such as gabapentin (Neurontin)
- Selective serotonin and norepinephrine reuptake inhibitor (SSNRI) antidepressants, such as duloxetine (Cymbalta)
- Anticonvulsants, such as pregabalin (Lyrica)

Common Medications: Chemotherapy-Induced Peripheral Neuropathy

Because CIPN is considered transient, and because the patient is already receiving so much medical treatment, physicians are generally reluctant to treat it. If the CIPN persists a year or more beyond the regular treatment for cancer, then either Lyrica or Neurontin is usually prescribed.

MASSAGE THERAPIST ASSESSMENT

Assuming the patient has been diagnosed with DPN or CIPN, the oral history taken by the massage therapist will clarify the location and severity of signs and symptoms. The therapist should perform a careful, detailed visual examination of the feet and hands, looking between toes and fingers and inspecting both dorsal and plantar surfaces. Gentle touch should also investigate significant changes in tissue temperature. Pregangrenous tissue can feel alarmingly cold. Gentle pressure is applied to the affected tissue with careful observance of the patient's response. Using the 0–10 pain scale will help the therapist determine the aggressivity with which she can then apply the appropriate protocol.

Charting all observations and responses will prove invaluable as the therapeutic relationship progresses, and in reporting improvement to the patient's physician.

THERAPEUTIC GOALS

It is reasonable to expect that the combination of frequent application of the protocol outlined later in this chapter, combined with daily self-care performed by the patient, can significantly reduce the painful symptoms associated with both DPN and CIPN. Case studies suggest that when the protocol is performed on CIPN patients, symptoms can be reversed, and quality of life enhanced, to the point that medication levels (Lyrica, Neurontin) can be reduced. Case studies involving diabetic patients indicate that pregangrenous tissue can be returned to health, and patients who previously lived with extreme foot pain can experience decreased pain and the full use of pain-free limbs.

MASSAGE SESSION FREQUENCY

- 60-minute sessions once a week for the duration of symptoms, performed by the massage therapist
- 15-minute self-care sessions every day, for each hand and/or foot for the duration of symptoms, performed by the patient
- Infrequent, nondetailed therapy is ineffective

MASSAGE PROTOCOL

This patient comes to you with myriad concerns. Her initial diagnosis of either diabetes or cancer is now complicated by irritating and/or painful neuropathic symptoms. This protocol, however, is aggressive. Although this may seem counterintuitive because the patient already is in a great deal of pain, the protocol starts gently. You must use all of your medical knowledge (be able to explain oxidative debt) and therapeutic massage experience (massage increases circulation), combined with a finely honed diplomacy (explain that you are going to start very, very gently and only progress in work "to her tolerance"), in order for the patient to benefit from this protocol. It often takes several sessions performed with gradual intensity to get the patient to the level that she can experience maximum therapeutic effectiveness.

You must also convince her to perform her homework assignments daily; this is not optional. Cells must be refreshed with richly oxygenated blood frequently, and unless she is willing to visit you every day, she must take on the responsibility of helping to heal herself at home.

Thinking It Through (cont.)

conditions, can lead to life-changing amputations (in the case of diabetic patients) and a severe decrease in the patient's quality of life (in both diabetic and cancer patients). This realization will strengthen the therapist's commitment to perform effectively—and potentially reverse or at least reduce symptoms.

All nerves need an abundance of oxygen to function and survive. One of my most impressive memories from massage therapy school was one instructor's insistence that "A nerve in pain is a nerve screaming for oxygen." He then went on to make the point using sciatic pain as a perfect example.

The exact cause of DPN and CIPN remains multifaceted, yet one cause recurs in most of the literature: oxidative debt or oxidative stress, which occurs when tiny, fragile peripheral nerves have inadequate oxygen.

Remembering one of the greatest benefits of massage therapy—that massage increases circulation—allows the therapist to deduce that (1) if massage therapy increases circulation and (2) if DPN and CIPN are on some level caused by a lack of cellular oxygen (poor circulation), then (3) any techniques that increase circulation to the peripheral nerves should decrease symptoms.

This reasoning enabled me to convince a team of medical oncologists at the Beaumont Hospitals, Rose Cancer Center, in Royal Oak, Michigan, to let me use the protocol found in

Thinking It Through (cont.)

this chapter on hundreds of oncology patients. Furthermore, a grant was written to the Department of Defense (for female veteran cancer patients suffering from CIPN), suggesting this protocol with the approval of the physicians.

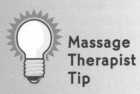

Massage Therapist Tip

Checking the Bottom of the Feet

Diabetic patients are counseled by their physicians to regularly check their feet for signs of skin breakdown or gangrene. Some obese and/or arthritic patients, however, find a foot examination to be challenging. Here's a simple technique to help. Have the patient buy a relatively large two-sided hand mirror, one side magnifying the image and the other side reflecting a normal image. She places the mirror on the floor in front of a chair or at the side of the bed and sits down. She might want to leave the mirror under the chair or the edge of the bed to avoid having to bend down to pick it up each time. She observes the bottom of both feet, one at a time, by positioning the foot over the mirror as the mirror lies on the floor. Ask her to observe both feet in both sides of the mirror.

The protocol itself is quite simple, but the work is extremely detailed, with you working into every crevice of the foot, toes, hand, and fingers. If the 60-minute session includes two feet, you will spend *30 minutes on each foot*. If the session includes both hands and feet, *you will spend 15 minutes on each hand and then each foot*. It may seem incomprehensible that you can work on a foot for 30 minutes, but you are trying to displace, wash out, and return all venous blood from the depths of this foot or hand and allow the body to replace it with freshly oxygenated arterial blood.

Your goal is to massage "to the bone," which means your massage works through all superficial tissue until it pushes against the underlying bone.

Getting Started

Your patient need only disrobe to the extent that the hands and forearms or feet and calves are exposed. Positioning the patient supine on the massage table allows you the best access to perform your work, but the patient can sit in a comfortable chair; you can sit on a rolling stool and gain access to her hands and/or feet without straining your back. (A massage chair is not an option.)

Since the work into the foot includes detailed massage in between the toes and can last for up to 30 minutes, you may want to wash the patient's feet, or ask her to wash them. You can use a basin and towel (do not use soap because the feet may be sensitive to chemicals), or bring one warm, wet towel and one dry towel to the table and cleanse the feet. If this is not possible, you can wear non-latex gloves during the entire procedure, which is another acceptable and effective method for protecting your hands and performing the work. Few patients can feel the difference between skin-on-skin massage and glove-on-skin massage of the feet and hands.

All massage techniques are performed in the cephalic direction, toward the head. Stroke the patient's feet or hands frequently during this protocol to give her a chance to relax from the fear of being hurt and to assess tissue temperature and response.

HOMEWORK

Daily, detailed self-care is essential in order to improve or reverse the tissue damage caused by peripheral neuropathy. The patient can perform these exercises while reading, while watching TV, before bed, upon rising, or while taking a bath. Do whatever is necessary to ensure compliance, even to the point of creating a small check-off calendar for your patient that she shares with you at her next appointment. (The following instructions assume self-care to the feet, but they can be followed for the hands, as well.)

- It's very important for you to make time every day to perform this therapy. You'll be spending at least 15 minutes on each foot.
- Start by lightly massaging both feet. Squeeze and massage as deeply as you can tolerate. Don't cause pain.
- Perform range-of-motion (ROM) exercises at your ankles. "Write out" the entire alphabet in capital letters using your toes and ankle joint.
- Grasp the tip of one toe and massage and squeeze it as deeply as you can without causing pain. Work on the entire toe from top to bottom. Work all toes of both feet. Deeply stroke the skin of both feet *toward your knee* to "clean out" the area.
- Now squeeze and massage all the tissue of your feet in between the toes, on both the front and back surfaces of your foot. Massage as deeply as you can tolerate— squeezing, pressing, and massaging every area you can reach.
- Now aggressively stroke both feet from your toes to your knee, *with strokes moving in the direction of the knee*, to "clean out" the entire foot.
- Massage your calves.
- Repeat the ROM exercises at your ankles.
- Throughout the day, whenever you can, take your shoes off and rub your feet against the floor, bend your toes, and perform ankle ROM exercises. You can also roll a tennis ball under the sole of your bare foot while at work or watching TV.

Step-by-Step Protocol for **Diabetic and Chemotherapy-Induced Peripheral Neuropathy of the Feet**

Technique	Duration
Position the patient comfortably. Cleanse the feet, if desired.	
Gently examine both feet for cold patches, open sores, and reddened or purple blotches while simultaneously applying experimental pressure to determine the patient's pain tolerance.	2 minutes
Stroking, light pressure, using the pressure of your whole hand • Plantar and dorsal surfaces of one foot • Gastrocnemius, tibialis anterior; all tissue below the knee to the toes Repeat on the other foot.	1 minute (Total of 2 minutes)
Compression, light pressure, using the pressure of your whole hand • Plantar and dorsal surface of one foot • Gastrocnemius, tibialis anterior; all tissue below the knee to the toes Repeat on the other foot.	1 minute (Total of 2 minutes)
Stretching, to the patient's tolerance, full ROM • Every toe joint • At the base of the toes • At the ankle Repeat on the other foot and ankle.	1 minute (Total of 2 minutes)
Digital kneading, light pressure, to the patient's tolerance • Each toe from the distal tip to the base of the toe • Work on all toe surfaces, front, back, and both sides. Repeat on the other foot and ankle.	3 minutes (Total of 6 minutes)
Digital kneading, light pressure, to the patient's tolerance • In between each ligament of the foot, working from the base of the toes to the ankle • Knead the ball of the foot. • Knead the arch of the foot. • Knead the heel of the foot. Repeat on the other foot.	3 minutes (Total of 6 minutes)
Repeat the previous digital kneading process of all toes and the entire surface of the foot with your goal being to massage "to the bone." This will take a few sessions before the patient's pain subsides enough to "allow you in." Whether or not she is performing her homework massage will also be directly related to how deep you can get in and how quickly. In each session, progress from light work to massaging as deeply as you can, to her tolerance. This digital kneading takes up the bulk of your protocol. Repeat on the other foot.	10 minutes (Total of 20 minutes)

Contraindications and Cautions

- Neuropathy patients experience good days and bad days. Always perform the protocol to the patient's comfort level; therapy may well be "two steps forward, one step back."
- If there is nonresponsive cold tissue, or you notice any purplish blotches or breakdown of skin, refer the patient to her physician immediately.
- If a cancer patient discusses the possibility of stopping her chemotherapy because of her irritation with CIPN, advise her to speak to her physician.
- Keep orange juice and small candy bars handy when treating diabetic patients.
- Open wounds or sores are contraindications for local massage.
- A high percentage of cancer patients develop foot fungus as a result of a compromised immune system. This is highly contagious and can be picked up by the therapist. It is not wise, even if gloved, to work on a toe that is manifesting fungus until the condition is completely cleared up.

(continued)

Technique	Duration
Effleurage, medium pressure • From the toes to the ankle, around the ankle, to the knee Repeat on the other lower extremity.	3 minutes (Total of 6 minutes)
Effleurage, petrissage, effleurage, deep pressure • From the ankle to the knee Repeat on the other lower extremity.	3 minutes (Total of 6 minutes)
Effleurage, petrissage, effleurage, digital and knuckle kneading, deep pressure • All toes, the plantar and dorsal surfaces of the foot, the ankle and the calf, to the knee Repeat on the other lower extremity.	3 minutes (Total of 6 minutes)
Stroking, using your whole hand • From the toes to the knee, anterior and posterior surfaces Repeat on the other lower extremity.	1 minute (Total of 2 minutes)

Contraindications and Cautions (cont.)

• If the foot has an unusually strong odor, noticeably different from an odor previously noted, this may be a sign of impending gangrene; refer the patient to a physician immediately.

• Although your feet may be tender when you begin this homework, your goal is to work so deeply that you can feel bone underneath your skin. This may take some time. Be patient, and work as deeply as you can each time. Your most important goal is consistent, daily, deep work.

Review

1. Define DPN.
2. Define CIPN.
3. Describe the nerves that are affected by neuropathy.
4. Explain oxidative debt.
5. What are the symptoms of peripheral neuropathy?
6. Describe the symptoms of dry gangrene.
7. Explain how you might convince a patient, who is already in pain, the importance of the work you and she must perform on her feet and hands.
8. What homework assignments you will give your patient? How often must they be performed?

BIBLIOGRAPHY

Dougherty P. What's Causing Your Neuropathy? *COPING.* November/December 2006;16.

Gilbert M, Armstrong T. Understanding Chemotherapy-Induced Peripheral Neuropathy. *COPING,* January/February 2006;26–27.

Polomano RC, Farrar JT. Pain and neuropathy in cancer survivors: surgery, radiation, and chemotherapy can cause pain; research could improve its detection and treatment. *American Journal of Nursing* March 2006;106:39–47.

Rosson GD. Chemotherapy-induced neuropathy. *Clinics in Podiatric Medicine and Surgery* 2006;23:637–649.

Sanders G. Peripheral Neuropathy Support Group Celebrates a Decade of Support. *Daily Sun.* Available at: http://www.thevillagesdailysun.com/news/villages/article_98d99c69-5a85-5ba5-8d72-127972424e00.html. Accessed June 30, 2010.

WebMD, Healthwise, Inc. Understanding Peripheral Neuropathy—the Basics. Available at: http://www.webmd.com/brain/understanding-peripheral-neuropathy-basics. Accessed December 30, 2010.

26

Osteoarthritis

Definition: A noninflammatory condition characterized by a degeneration of joint cartilage.

GENERAL INFORMATION

- Direct cause unknown; correlations to obesity, increased age, previous joint stress or injury, and repetitive joint use; genetic predisposition
- Slow onset, with symptoms usually appearing around age 40 or 50
- Lifetime duration; condition progressive
- Prevalence in people who are obese, older than 40 years of age, female, and those born with malformed joints, or who participated intensively in sports when younger, or who endured an accident
- Higher prevalence in the Native American population
- The most common form of arthritis, usually occurring in the hands, hips, knees, spine; uncommon in the jaw, shoulder, or elbow
- Among older adults, the most common cause of physical disability, especially OA of the knee
- *Not* believed to be an inflammatory condition, despite the medical suffix "itis"
- No cure

Morbidity and Mortality

By age 65, approximately 70% of people X-rayed routinely for nonarthritic conditions will show OA involvement in at least one joint. Only 30% of this population have reported pain or other symptoms, supporting the evidence that OA can be clinically present but remain asymptomatic until after about age 50. OA affects more than 25 million Americans.

Although death from OA is uncommon, annual mortality estimations in the hundreds may be low because of the unreported deaths secondary to gastrointestinal bleed, which is a common side effect of many of the medications prescribed to treat OA.

Gout, rheumatoid arthritis, Paget's disease, and septic arthritis increase the risk of OA. Comorbidities include depression, anxiety, and quality-of-life issues, such as lowered self-esteem, job limitations or loss, and decreased enjoyment of recreational activities.

PATHOPHYSIOLOGY

A joint is composed of at least two articulating bones, the ends of which are covered with cartilage. Cartilage is a shiny, slick, almost rubbery material that contributes to smooth, friction-free joint movement. Surrounding each joint space is a synovial lining, which creates synovial fluid, the nourishing "oil" that lubricates the joint (Figure 26-1). As OA develops, articular cartilage begins to degenerate. The normally smooth, gliding cartilaginous surface is compromised by pits, fragments, and tears as bone spurs develop in the tightly packed space. Eventually, cartilage may wear away to the point that bone grinds against bone.

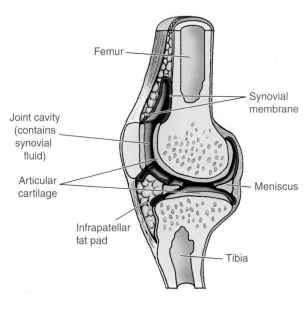

Knee joint

FIGURE 26-1 **The role of cartilage in joint mobility. Cartilage surrounds the distal end of the femur and the proximal end of the tibia in normal knee articulation. Surrounding muscles become hypertonic as they compensate for joint instability secondary to cartilage thinning. From Moore KL, Dalley AF.** *Clinically Oriented Anatomy*, **5th ed. Baltimore: Lippincott Williams & Wilkins, 2006.**

Diagnosis is determined by a combination of the person's medical history and a physical examination, joint X-rays, and laboratory tests. X-ray results, however, can sometimes provide limited evidence of OA because cartilage breakdown is not visible on films. Physicians determine cartilage breakdown, therefore, by measuring joint space narrowing and the presence of bone spurs. Cyst formation and the presence of osteophytes (growths, sometimes called joint mice) further confirm a diagnosis of OA.

People who have OA complain of occasional flares, when joints are unusually painful, tender, and/or warm. These flares are not typical and are fleeting. If they persist and progress, the person should get medical attention.

OVERALL SIGNS AND SYMPTOMS

If symptoms include locally reddened skin, pain and swelling in the joint, and tissue that is hot to the touch, the condition is *not* common OA.

- Joint pain developing slowly, progressing over time
- Joint pain during use, after use, and/or after prolonged inactivity
- Joint tenderness upon light pressure
- Joint stiffness and decreased range of motion (ROM) upon rising and/or after prolonged inactivity
- Bone crepitus (bone-on-bone sensation, crunching, rubbing, or grating sound or sensation)
- Bone spurs or joint mice in and around the affected joint
- Occasional joint swelling, but with no signs of inflammation

SIGNS AND SYMPTOMS MASSAGE THERAPY CAN ADDRESS

- OA sets up perfect conditions for the presence of the pain-spasm-pain cycle, and this cycle can be broken with massage therapy techniques.
- Chronic pain is relieved by skilled massage therapy techniques that decrease trigger points and hypertonicity.
- Palliative techniques relieve anxiety and depression.
- Decreased ROM and stiffness are relieved by the application of deep heat and gentle, passive stretches.

TREATMENT OPTIONS

Although no cure exists for OA, a combination of medical and holistic treatments can reduce pain, increase mobility, slow the progression, and improve the person's quality of life. Treatment for early stage OA focuses on addressing pain level and immobility. Mobility is so important to joint health that some studies indicate underused muscles alone can contribute to much of the pain ascribed to arthritis. Lifestyle adjustments include maintaining good posture; observing a diet high in fruits, vegetables, and whole grains and low in refined sugar; controlling weight; using adaptive devices; and performing regular nonimpact exercise. Taking over-the-counter (OTC) pain medications and applying topical creams are other common, effective treatments.

Treatment for bothersome but not life-altering OA includes resting a painful joint for 12–24 hours, attempting to avoid using the joint for a few minutes every hour; performing regular, gentle exercise; and strengthening and stretching the muscles surrounding the affected joint. At this point, medication may be increased, but it is usually OTC. The use of heat and cold in the early and mild stages can be effective. Heat can be used to relieve stiffness; cold can relieve muscle spasm and more irritating pain. Maintaining ideal weight is highly recommended for all stages of OA.

At any stage, working with a physical therapist or personal trainer can help maintain joint mobility and strength. Adaptive devices, such as padded eating utensils and toothbrushes and pinchers for grasping items off the floor or from high shelves, may prove helpful. Complementary approaches, such as acupuncture, tai chi, yoga, and supplementation with ginger, glucosamine, and chondroitin, have also had limited success in clinical studies.

Joint replacement surgery, bone fusion surgery, the injection of hyaluronic acid derivatives into the joint, and bone debridement are reserved for the most severe cases.

Common Medications

There is a distinction between medications suggested for early-stage OA and those recommended for later stages. OTC medications for early OA include:

- Topical pain-relieving, counterirritant creams, rubs, and sprays, such as Bengay, Aspercreme, Icy Hot, Biofreeze
- Pain relievers, such as acetaminophen (Tylenol)
- NSAIDs, such as aspirin, ibuprofen (Advil, Motrin), or naproxen (Aleve)

As pain and stiffness become more than mildly uncomfortable, begin to compromise the activities of daily living (ADLs), and occasionally flare, the following medication may be prescribed, either alone or in combination with those listed previously:

- Centrally acting analgesics, such as tramadol hydrochloride (Ultram)

For severe OA, prescription painkillers may include narcotics and corticosteroids:

- Mildly narcotic painkillers, such as codeine or hydrocodone and propoxyphene (Darvon)
- Cortisone injections directly into the joint

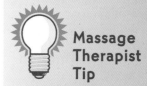

Massage Therapist Tip

Advising Clients in the Use of Hot or Cold

People with OA are often confused about when to apply hot or cold packs to their aching joints. Here's how to help. If the joints are in excruciating, unrelenting pain, it is time to apply ice. If the joints are dully aching, the kind of pain most OA clients experience on most days, it is best to apply heat.

Thinking It Through

Clinical studies indicate that cartilage responds to exercise, as do muscle and bone; that is, cartilage health can be improved with activity. During exercise, the joint is flushed with fresh blood, waste products are forced out of the joint, lymphatic nodes further pump the joint clean of cellular waste, and bone remodeling occurs in response to even moderate weight-bearing. Conversely, immobility leads to decreased nutrient supply to the joint and hypertonicity to all surrounding muscles. This leads to the pain-spasm-pain cycle, further exacerbating the pain experienced by most people with OA. Exercise also improves mood by releasing neurochemicals in the brain, thereby offsetting the depression and anxiety that often accompany OA.

Taking into account the previous information, the therapist can ask himself the following when planning a massage session and assigning client self-care:

- How exactly is my client affected by his OA?
- What activities can he no longer engage in that he will miss the most?
- Which activities may serve as replacements for those previously enjoyed?
- What are his physical exercise limitations?
- Is he resistant to exercising, and if so, how can I help him overcome that resistance?
- Does he understand that immobility, even when he's in pain, further compromises his affected joints?

MASSAGE THERAPIST ASSESSMENT

Given the pervasiveness of joint pain and stiffness in the aging population, combined with the common medical knowledge surrounding the condition, many clients will present to a massage therapist with a self-diagnosis of OA. Before proceeding, it is best for the therapist to determine the presence of any signs or symptoms of true inflammation. Although a physician's order is not necessary to treat common arthritis, a therapist who discovers a reddened, warm, and/or excruciatingly painful joint should decline treatment and refer the person to a physician.

Questioning the client regarding symptoms should clarify that onset has been gradual. The discomfort or pain should not be debilitating, nor should the client present with joint immobility. Uncomfortable stiffness upon arising or after periods of inactivity should be the norm.

Upon palpation, the joint might feel slightly irregular, perhaps larger than the contralateral joint, but again, no heat should emanate from the tissue. Surrounding musculature is usually hypertonic; trigger points may be found proximal and distal to the joint, and the client may report or display compensatory behavior. ROM is probably compromised. The client should be able to pinpoint the exact location of discomfort, pain, or stiffness, although there may be a dull, achy radiating muscular pain up or down the limb. The symptoms should not reflect systemic malaise or pain.

If a therapist takes the time to understand the client's history, lifestyle, and goals, he will be able to determine an appropriate treatment regimen. Detailed SOAP notes will ensure accurate tracking of progression or digression.

THERAPEUTIC GOALS

The massage therapist's goals are directly related to the client's history, lifestyle, and personal goals. Whether the OA is mild or severe, the therapeutic goals include decreasing pain, increasing or maintaining ROM, decreasing joint stiffness, and reducing depression and anxiety.

MASSAGE SESSION FREQUENCY

For mildly uncomfortable OA:

- 60-minute sessions once a month, for the duration of the condition, performed in combination with diligent self-care

For more severe OA:

- 60-minute sessions once a week, for the duration of the condition, performed in combination with diligent self-care

For the most severe, debilitating OA, which may result in joint replacement or bone fusion surgery:

- 60-minute sessions once a week, immediately before and after surgery (At this point, the therapist is probably performing as part of a health care team.)
- 60-minute sessions every week until the person is pain-free or has reached a plateau of performance and pain

Infrequent massage therapy for all stages of OA will provide merely palliative relief.

MASSAGE PROTOCOL

Treating clients who have OA allows you to create a long-term therapeutic relationship. Since arthritis is progressive and symptoms can be relieved through active therapy, you have a unique opportunity to use all of your persuasive and therapeutic skills. Become familiar with your client's disease progression, and tailor your therapy to his *very specific* goals. Encourage weekly visits and daily homework compliance. Be generous in complimenting even the small successes, and be compassionate with setbacks.

The OA protocol (here focused on the knee since that is the most common form of debilitating OA) uses basic massage therapy techniques to bring blood and nutrients to the damaged joint and flush waste products toward the head. Your therapeutic skills, combined with keen attention to your client's needs, should result in tangible improvement in his quality of life.

Getting Started

Keep hot packs and cold packs ready. Your client will present with different complaints at each session, and you want to be prepared. Experiment with various topical muscle creams. Applying these creams is well within your scope of practice. Read the ingredients aloud, ask the client about possible allergic reactions, and apply the substance deeply *to the affected joint and surrounding tissue only*. These products are not intended for full-body application. If you give the client take-home samples, emphasize that he should rub the cream deeply into his joint and muscles, and remind him to wash his hands before touching his eyes or going to the bathroom.

Position him on the table according to his comfort level; side-lying will require more pillows. He may prefer being seated in a comfortable chair. Awareness of the stage of his OA will help you determine positioning, treatment duration, and aggressivity.

In the following protocol, the client is positioned supine with a bolster or pillow under his knees and a pillow under his head for comfort. Total disrobing may not be necessary if you are focusing on the lower extremities.

Although most massage therapy techniques move *cephalically* or in the direction of venous flow, when attempting to increase localized blood flow, the direction of the therapeutic strokes is often *toward the affected joint*, whether or not this direction is cephalic.

HOMEWORK

Sound research supports the importance of giving your OA client moving and stretching exercises for self-care. Working within your scope of practice, you can develop homework assignments that can make a significant difference in his long-term quality of life. You may want to help him create a pain and/or exercise journal to track his progress.

- Use every opportunity during your day to stretch. While talking on the phone, for example, stretch your neck from side to side, pull your shoulders back, and bend at the waist. While watching TV, extend and contract your lower leg, first while pointing your toe, and then flexing at your ankle as hard as you can. Work all of your joints, not just your painful one.
- Buy a big exercise ball. Place it on the floor next to a wall or couch or a very steady object. While watching TV or anytime during the day, sit on it and bounce. Start by bouncing very slightly, to get your balance. Then work up to bouncing as high as you can, making sure you remain stable, while pushing off of the floor using with your thigh muscles. Note how long you can do this, and try to increase the bounce time every week.
- When you're experiencing a dull, achy joint and muscle pain, apply a *moist* hot pack. A hot water bottle or microwaved gel pack is excellent. Beanbags or rice packs are not effective. Place the pack over a thin layer of clothes and leave it on as long as it is comfortable. Do not go to sleep with the hot pack in place.

Thinking It Through *(cont.)*

- Does he understand that OA is progressive and that every small act of ROM and exercise can lead to a lessening of his pain and immobility?
- How can I clearly explain to him that the health of his bone, joint, muscle, and cartilage directly depends on how much he moves every day?

Contraindications and Cautions

- Do not apply a cold pack to a joint if a client has any circulatory disorder, such as diabetes, congestive heart failure, or edema.

- Do not treat the joint if the client is experiencing a flare; mild whole-body relaxation is an option and will provide palliative relief.

- Do not apply a cold pack to a flared joint without a physician's approval.

- Use caution, reduce the pressure, and limit ROM when treating unstable or slightly swollen joints or those containing bone spurs.

- The normal springy end-feel of a joint may be absent in clients with OA. ROM to the joint is important, but when performing passive ROM, use caution when reaching the presumed end of the joint's movement.

Step-by-Step Protocol for Osteoarthritis of the Knee

Technique	Duration
Apply a moist hot pack to the affected knee and surrounding musculature. Leave in place while performing relaxing techniques anywhere other than the affected limb.	5 minutes
Remove the hot pack. Using first gentle then progressively deeper touch, assess the affected joint and surrounding muscles. Assess ROM.	2 minutes
Compression, using your full hand, evenly rhythmic, medium pressure • Entire thigh and leg, from groin to ankle • Use caution when applying pressure around the knee	2 minutes
Effleurage, petrissage, effleurage, medium pressure, evenly rhythmic, working *toward the knee*. • Entire quadriceps complex; include distal attachments in the superior knee region	4 minutes
Effleurage, petrissage, effleurage, medium pressure, evenly rhythmic, working *toward the knee* • Entire lower leg complex, including tibialis anterior; include proximal attachments in the distal knee region	4 minutes
Effleurage, petrissage, effleurage, evenly rhythmic, deeper, to the client's tolerance • Entire thigh and leg, from groin to ankle, working *toward the knee* from both directions	4 minutes
Digital kneading, medium pressure • Proximal, distal, medial, and lateral patellar surfaces • Attempt to gently move the patella • Be aware of the presence of joint mice (osteophytes). Work around them with caution. • Be aware of hypertonicity in muscles near the knee joint.	5 minutes
Effleurage, deep to client's tolerance • Area around the knee, *work cephalically to begin to mobilize waste*	3 minutes
Digital kneading, medium pressure • All muscle attachments, large and small, in and around the entire joint	5 minutes
Effleurage, petrissage, effleurage, deep to client's tolerance • All muscle attachments of the knee joint, *work cephalically now to cleanse the joint*	5 minutes
Hold the knee in both hands, be still, provide comfort, ask the client how he is doing.	1 minute
Effleurage, petrissage, effleurage, medium pressure then light pressure, working cephalically • The entire thigh and leg	5 minutes

(continued)

Technique	Duration
Reassess ROM and local hypertonicity.	2 minutes
Massage the compensating contralateral leg using effleurage, petrissage, and effleurage. Note any areas of hypertonicity for special attention at the next session.	5 minutes
Relaxation massage techniques per the client's requested area, preferably not on the affected limb(s).	8 minutes

Contraindications and Cautions: (cont.)

- Normal OA symptoms should be relieved at least minimally after four massage therapy sessions. If you cannot achieve at least minimal relief, the client's history (e.g., cancer or another other systemic disease) must be considered as a secondary cause of the joint pain, and the client should be referred to another health care professional.

- When you're experiencing a sharper, more irritating and persistent joint pain, apply an ice or cold pack. A bag of frozen vegetables will do the trick. Apply the cold pack over a thin layer of clothes, and leave it on for not more than 10 minutes. Repeat every 30 minutes as needed.
- Walk with vigor, swim, or ride a bike. Engage in any form of *gentle* but daily cardiovascular exercise. Aim for 30 minutes five times a week, but start out at your own pace.
- Extend your morning shower a little longer if you find moist heat helps. Performing joint stretches in the shower is an excellent idea; make sure you hold onto a bar and stand on a secure mat.
- Consider keeping a journal of your "good days and bad days," especially noting your successes in exercise and movement.
- Breathe deeply throughout the day. Inhale as deeply as you can, hold it for a few seconds, and exhale forcibly.

Review

1. Define OA.
2. Is this an inflammatory condition?
3. Name the signs and symptoms of OA.
4. List the joint symptoms that would indicate a person is suffering from another related condition and should see a physician.
5. Explain the physiology of the importance of exercise and joint movement.

BIBLIOGRAPHY

MayoClinic.com. Available at: http://www.mayoclinic.com/health/osteoarthritis/DS00019. Accessed April 2009. Accessed June 29, 2010.

National Institute of Arthritis and Musculoskeletal and Skin Diseases. NIH Senior Health. Available at: http://nihseniorhealth.gov/osteoarthritis/toc.html. Accessed June 29, 2010.

National Institute of Arthritis and Musculoskeletal and Skin Diseases. Osteoarthritis. Available at: http://www.niams.nih.gov/Health_Info/Osteoarthritis. Accessed June 29, 2010.

Osteoarthritis Health Center. Available at: http://www.webmd.com/osteoarthritis/default.htm. Accessed June 29, 2010.

Rattray F, Ludwig L. *Clinical Massage Therapy: Understanding, Assessing and Treating over 70 Conditions*, Toronto: Talus Incorporated, 2000.

Stacey GS, Basu PA. Osteoarthritis, Primary. EMedicine article. Available at: http://emedicine.medscape.com/article/392096-overview. Accessed June 29, 2010.

Werner R. *A Massage Therapist's Guide to Pathology*, 4th ed. Philadelphia: Lippincott Williams & Wilkins, 2009.

27

Parkinson's Disease

Definition: A chronic, progressive neurodegenerative movement disorder resulting from dopamine insufficiency in the brain.

GENERAL INFORMATION

- Etiology unknown
- Contributing causative (or risk) factors: aging, exposure to pesticides and herbicides, living in rural environments or near industrial plants and quarries, consuming well water, genetic predisposition
- Onset usually between ages 50 and 79; onset before age 40 increasing
- Occurrence second only to Alzheimer's disease in neurodegenerative disorders
- Chronic and progressive
- Prevalence in men
- No cure

Morbidity and Mortality

PD affects about 1 in every 1000 people in the U.S.; about 50,000 new cases are diagnosed annually. The prognosis is directly related to the severity of symptoms and the age of onset. An early-in-life diagnosis usually leads to a more dire prognosis.

Complications include multiple hospitalizations secondary to frequent falls and decreased dexterity and coordination. Comorbidities include constipation, urinary incontinence, sexual dysfunction, and multiple, serious medication side effects. Depression affects as many as 40% of PD patients usually because of chemical changes in the brain, combined with the profound toll the disease takes on the patient and his family. Anxiety, fear, physical restlessness, and the inability to easily change positions in bed lead to insomnia. About 15–30% of Parkinson's patients develop dementia in the later stages of the disease. Other late-stage comorbidities include memory loss, confusion, and hallucinations.

PATHOPHYSIOLOGY

A small, vitally important component of the cerebral cortex is the substantia nigra. As the regulator of smooth muscle movement and coordination, it must be bathed in the neurotransmitter dopamine in order to function properly. When the available amount of dopamine is compromised, smooth muscle movement is directly, progressively, and negatively affected. By the time motor signs emerge, 60–80% of the dopamine-deficient neurons have already been irreversibly destroyed.

Diagnosis is established after a complete physical and mental health history has been taken, followed by neurologic examinations. There are no laboratory or blood tests that confirm a diagnosis. An MRI or CT scan may be performed to rule out stroke or brain tumor.

OVERALL SIGNS AND SYMPTOMS

The following symptoms often occur well before the more obvious motor symptoms:

- A loss of the sense of smell
- Rapid eye movement (REM) sleep disturbances
- Daytime sleepiness
- Constipation

Following the previous symptoms, subtle early stage signs appear:

- Decreased dexterity
- The loss of fine movement coordination
- A compromised full arm swing during normal walking
- The absence of a toe-heel strike during normal walking
- The dragging of one foot along the floor while walking
- A very slight tremor in chin, lips, and/or tongue

As symptoms progress, the cardinal signs of PD appear:

- Asymmetric muscle rigidity, and deeply aching muscles, most commonly in the legs, face, neck, and arms
- Asymmetric tremors in the hands, arms, legs, or head when the person is awake and at rest, with resolution upon movement
- Changes in speech and gait

As the disease progresses, these symptoms compromise lifestyle and function:

- Freezing; a sudden, brief inability to move
- Relentlessly stiffened muscles
- A stooped, head-down, shuffling gait
- Trouble swallowing, leading to choking, coughing, or drooling
- Soft, monotonous speech
- A fixed, blank facial expression
- Dementia

SIGNS AND SYMPTOMS MASSAGE THERAPY CAN ADDRESS

Because of the complexity, severity, and progression of PD, it is strongly advised that a massage therapist work in close conjunction with other members of the health care team.

- The hypertonicity created by unrelenting muscle rigidity can be softened by the application of heat, gentle range-of-motion (ROM) exercises, stretches, and massage therapy techniques.
- The secondary risk of pneumonia and respiratory difficulties created by the head-stoop, forward-bending position can be addressed with intercostal muscle massage, gentle diaphragmatic massage, self-care homework assignments, and deep-breathing exercises.
- Depression, anxiety, restlessness, and insomnia can be reduced with soothing techniquesw that move the patient into a relaxed, parasympathetic state.

TREATMENT OPTIONS

Because PD progresses swiftly if left untreated, treatment is strongly advised as soon as symptoms appear. Although there is no known cure or reversal for the destruction

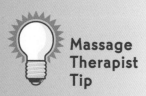

Massage Therapist Tip

Asking About Constipation

Any patient who is taking multiple medications and suffering from debilitating immobility is at risk for constipation. Remember that treating people with this uncomfortable condition is well within your scope of practice. Ask your Parkinson's patient at the beginning of each session if he has had a recent bowel movement. Suggest including a 15-minute colon massage protocol in your treatment to help relieve his discomfort (see Chapter 12).

of nerve cells in the brain, medications and, less commonly, surgery can quiet life-altering symptoms and slow the disease progression.

Thorough treatment depends on the patient's age at onset, overall physical condition, strict medication compliance, and adherence to an exercise and diet regimen. However, since medication side effects themselves can compromise a patient's health, the treatment plan is based on balancing the progressive symptoms of the disease with the profoundly adverse side effects of the medications. Medications are therefore given at minimum dose and often in combinations until symptoms demand a more aggressive regimen. Many physicians will adopt a "wait-and-see" attitude toward minor tremors and muscle rigidity to honor the patient's understandable hesitance about taking medication.

Physical therapy can address muscle rigidity, gait abnormality, and overall stiffness. Since PD profoundly affects muscles and places the patient at a constant risk for contracture, any form of gentle and consistent exercise, such as swimming, water aerobics, biking, walking, yoga, or tai chi, is strongly advised. Occupational therapy can help the patient make lifestyle modifications necessitated by his coughing, choking, or drooling. Speech therapy can address the slurred and/or monotone speech and flat affect that occur in later stages.

A healthy diet consisting of fruits, vegetables, and whole grains is suggested. Increased dietary fiber may help prevent constipation, which results from inadequate fluid intake (because of hand-to-mouth clumsiness) and an overall propensity toward immobility and abdominal tension.

When medications are no longer effective and/or the side effects are intolerable, deep brain stimulation (DBS) surgery can be performed. In this procedure, tiny wires are placed into the brain to electrically stimulate the motor control portions. DBS is not a cure and some symptoms may remain, but usually after the procedure, symptoms subside and the medication level can be reduced.

Individual psychotherapy, family counseling, and support groups are strongly recommended to address the inevitable anger, fear, sadness, and anxiety that accompany such a life-altering condition.

Common Medications

Medications that are prescribed for PD depend on the condition's progression. Taken in combination with many other medications, their efficacy decreases over time. PD medications have severe side effects and must be evaluated at least every 3–6 months by the treating physician.

The goal of PD medications is to try to correct the shortage of dopamine in the patient's brain. Because L-dopa, the primary and most effective Parkinson's drug, also causes the most severe side effects, it is not prescribed until later stages of the disease and/or is given in smaller doses in combination with other medications in the early stages.

The side effects of most PD medications include nausea, vomiting, dizziness, delusions, hallucinations, confusion, excessive daytime sleepiness, sexual dysfunction, irritability, and compromised protein assimilation. Increasing, decreasing, or suddenly stopping any of the following medications can be dangerous.

- Antiparkinson medications, such as pramipexole dihydrochloride (Mirapex), ropinirole hydrochloride (Requip), selegiline hydrochloride (Eldepryl), entacapone (Comtan), trihexyphenidyl hydrochloride (Apo-Trihex), and benztropine mesylate (Cogentin)
- Dopamine agonists, such as rotigotine (Neupro) and rasagiline (Azilect)
- Non-ergoline dopamine agonists, such as apomorphine hydrochloride (Apokyn)

MASSAGE THERAPIST ASSESSMENT

An early stage Parkinson's patient can be seen in a massage therapy setting; however, a later stage patient will most likely be seen in a hospital, rehabilitation institution, or private home. Assessment includes evaluating ROM at affected limbs, palpating for muscle rigidity, determining if inhalation and exhalation are restricted, asking about the presence and level of pain, and determining whether the patient can be comfortably positioned for treatment. A family member may be present to help undress, dress, and reposition or clarify communication.

THERAPEUTIC GOALS

Reducing muscle rigidity can help the patient perform activities of daily living (ADLs). By identifying hypertonic muscles and trigger points, the therapist can help reduce the pain-spasm-pain cycle and modify, although not prevent, postural changes that lead to imbalance and instability. Deeply relaxing techniques can relieve anxiety and help improve sleep patterns. Gentle, persistent ROM exercises can prevent contractures. Deep-breathing exercises and diaphragmatic massage can help prevent pneumonia and respiratory complications. Palliative, gentle relaxing techniques can offset anxiety and reduce cortisol levels.

MASSAGE SESSION FREQUENCY

Since the condition is chronic and progressive, regular massage therapy is essential.

- 60-minute sessions once a week for the duration of the condition

MASSAGE PROTOCOL

Every choice you make to care for this patient must take into account that he feels as if his life is completely out of control. He can no longer perform the simplest acts of daily activity; the medications he is taking destroy clear thinking; he knows no matter what he does, the condition is progressive; and his family members, and his whole support structure, can do little to help. Gentleness, diplomacy, intelligence, and compassion are of utmost importance.

Ideally, you'll see this patient regularly, but he will present with a different set of aches, pains, and concerns at each session. His most pressing concern of the day is your treatment priority. Do nothing to stimulate him. All massage strokes, ROM exercises, and stretches are performed slowly, methodically, and with a keen eye for their effects on his tremors.

Ask about medication side effects so you can be prepared if he gets dizzy easily, is prone to having a sudden drop in blood pressure during position changes, is nauseated, or hallucinates.

Given the previous considerations, the following protocol is not presented in the usual step-by-step process. Instead, several techniques are suggested without recommended duration times. Choose those techniques that address your patient's concerns on any given day.

Getting Started

Positioning will be a challenge, so have plenty of pillows ready. Side-lying may be the best choice. Rearrange the room if his spouse or partner wants to be with him during the massage session. Have towels or tissues available for possible drooling or choking. Keep music and lights very low. Speak slowly but don't be condescending; he can hear you but may not be able to respond quickly and/or be easily understood.

The following protocol includes work on the patient's face. When transitioning to the face, be sure to wash your hands first. Perform all movements slowly and carefully with warm hands.

Thinking It Through

To truly understand the impact of this serious condition, the therapist might take a moment to imagine how uncontrolled motor skills could compromise a person's daily life. She can add to this awareness the knowledge that medications also have serious side effects. The therapist may not ask the following questions aloud, but throughout greeting and assessing and treating the patient, the answers might help her create a more compassionate treatment.

- How severe is his tremor? Does he need help undressing and getting onto the table?
- Can he comfortably reposition himself on the table; how much assistance will he need?
- Since the tremor is worse when he is still and lessens upon movement, what will be the most effective massage strokes that will help calm him?
- What is the muscle's response to continuous movement? Is the pain-spasm-pain cycle ever relieved?
- Can any gentle humor be found in this situation, such as when trying to work on a limb that is constantly moving?
- If the tremors stop and the patient deeply relaxes, and possibly falls asleep, is it possible to accommodate both his schedule and any subsequent massage appointments by allowing him to remain asleep?

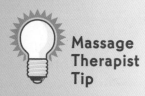

Massage Therapist Tip

Recognizing Contractures

Contractures often develop in the muscles of a patient who suffers from a disease such as PD, or from persistent positioning that immobilizes a part of his body. Muscle that is normally mobile becomes hardened, static, and shortened, and the surrounding joint either has severely limited motion or can no longer move at all. Contractures occur because of unrelenting muscle spasm, fibrosis, sustained loss of muscle balance, muscle paralysis, or loss of movement in an adjacent joint. Contracted tissue has a significantly different feel from extremely hypertonic tissue; prolonged massage on contracted tissue will yield very little tissue softening and almost no increase in movement, whereas the same amount of work on hypertonic tissue will yield significant pliability and movement.

Step-by-Step Protocol for Parkinson's Disease

The performance of all the following techniques depends on the patient's symptomatic presentation at each session. Techniques that soften tissue are listed first and should always be applied before mobilizing tissue or performing ROM exercises. There is no correct order for the techniques. Duration may be from a few seconds, at which time you might determine a technique that brings on tremors and must be stopped, to several minutes. Patient tolerance and symptoms are your guides. Unlike other protocols, further instructions or precautions may be provided for each technique.

Technique	Duration*
Place your open, flat hands softly on any area of the body. Quiet your thoughts and note the level of tremors under your hands. Slowly assess each muscular portion of the body, looking for spasms, tremors, hypertonicity, skin sensitivity, and resistance to touch. The "entire body" instructions listed as follows refer to any part of the body tolerated by the patient.	
Compression, light pressure, move slowly, using your whole hand • The entire body, including the face	
Compression, firmer pressure, move slowly, using your whole hand • The entire body, including the face	
Effleurage, light-to-medium pressure, using your whole hand, slow even strokes • The entire body, including the face	
Effleurage, petrissage, effleurage, light-to-medium pressure, slow even strokes • All major muscles • Include trapezius, latissimus dorsi, pectoralis major and minor, deltoids, biceps, arm extensors and flexors, gluteus complex, hamstrings, quadriceps, gastrocnemius, soleus, iliotibial (IT) bands • Abdominal muscles will be extremely hypertonic; try to perform light-to-medium pressure, clockwise effleurage on the abdominal region	
Colon massage, performed slowly and carefully. See Chapter 12 for the entire protocol.	
Digital kneading, slow, rhythmic strokes, medium pressure • Intercostals from sternum to spine • Diaphragm, working up under the bottom of the rib cage • When intercostals massage is complete, ask the client to take a few very deep breaths.	

(continued)

Technique	Duration*
If you find a joint contracture, ask the patient's permission to *gently* work on this area. Effective measures to help reduce further contracture and/or bring pain relief to the contracted area: • Apply a moist hot pack for 5 minutes. • Effleurage the area and palpate deeply to determine the extent of tissue stiffness. • Digitally knead, using medium pressure, around and into all muscles and bones that comprise the affected joint. • Effleurage, petrissage, effleurage the muscles distal and proximal to the joint. • *Gently* attempt to mobilize the joint and muscles. This may not be possible, but often after the application of heat and detailed massage, the contracted joint can move even a quarter of an inch. Be vigilant in watching the patient's reactions.	
Passive ROM, being careful not to initiate a tremor near end-feel • All joints easily accessible given the patient's symptoms and position on the table	
Gentle resistance and stretching • Laying your hand flat first on the plantar and then the dorsal surfaces of each foot, ask the patient to push against your hand to his tolerance. • After he's performed this a few times, gently stretch all muscles, tendons, and bones of the foot and ankle. • Perform ROM exercises at the ankle joints.	
Digital kneading, gentle stripping, cross-fiber friction, using ample lubricant • Sternocleidomastoid (SCM) muscle, bilaterally • Scalenes • Superior trapezius • Occipital ridge	
Place your hands on either side of the client's face as if to embrace it. Rest for a moment. Then, digital kneading, light-to-medium pressure, circling clockwise and counterclockwise. • All facial muscles • Work along bony ridges including the mandible and zygomatic arches, around the eyes, and at the temporomandibular joint (TMJ) • Finish the digital work with long, slow, medium pressure strokes to the entire face	
At the end of your session, perform deep relaxation techniques that both you and your patient have determined help him relax. These techniques may include: • Energy work • Long, slow effleurage over the entire body • Rocking • Silence while simply holding various points on the body	

*Durations are not given for work with PD patients because their condition and concerns change from day to day. For further explanation, see text.

Contraindications and Cautions

• Do nothing to stimulate the patient's sympathetic nervous system, speak slowly and clearly, lower the lights, and play music softly. Don't use deep-tissue techniques or vibratory tools.

• Identify hypersensitive areas of his skin, and stay away from them.

• Many PD medications seriously affect blood pressure; be sure to know whether he has high or low blood pressure, and if minor positioning changes make him dizzy or unstable.

• Positioning changes, as well as undressing and dressing, will take more time than usual; make sure he does not feel rushed because that will only exacerbate tremors. Accommodate your other clients' schedules so they are not inconvenienced.

• If your patient has previously experienced hallucinations, do nothing new or unusual during the sessions that you have not told him about ahead of time. As in all massage therapy sessions, prevent cell phones from ringing or unexpected interruptions from destroying the smooth flow of a session.

HOMEWORK

Self-care for a PD patient can help slow, but not stop, the condition's progression. It can bolster his self-esteem, add much-needed humor to his life, and can help relieve respiratory complications. Don't overwhelm him with too much homework, but make sure he goes home from each session with at least one *written and clear* instruction. Gently hold him accountable at your next session.

- Speak the letters A, E, I, O, and U very slowly, greatly exaggerating the pronunciation and trying to stretch every facial muscle. Do this several times throughout the day.
- Hold onto a secure couch or the wall. March in place. Plant each foot securely before you pick up the other foot. Lift your knee up as high as you can; there is no need for speed. Performing this to gently paced music may help you keep moving. Start and stop at will several times during the session.
- Walk with purpose; swing your arms front to back while you walk, lightly bending your elbows. Plant your heel and push off with your toe. Try not to shuffle or take small steps while walking.
- Take very deep breaths several times throughout the day. Inhale deeply, hold it for a few seconds, and then exhale with vigor.
- When you're in bed, slowly roll from side to side several times.
- When you're in bed, roll your head and shoulders in one direction and your hips and legs in the opposite direction. Hold this position for as long as you can. Then roll your head/shoulders and hips/legs in the opposite direction and hold.
- Find ways to relax. Listening to soft music, try to concentrate on something beautiful, like a flower or the ocean. Avoid getting upset if you can.
- Watch funny movies that make you laugh.

Review

1. Describe the purpose of dopamine in relation to muscle movement.
2. Explain the early stage symptoms of PD.
3. Describe the symptomatic progression of PD.
4. Name several side effects of the medications given to treat PD.
5. List the effective measures of keeping a Parkinson's patient in a relaxed, parasympathetic state.
6. Explain several homework assignments that can be effective for these patients.
7. Is PD curable?

BIBLIOGRAPHY

Craig LH, Svircev A, Haber M, et al. Controlled pilot study of the effects of neuromuscular therapy in patients with Parkinson's disease. *Movement Disorders* 2006;21:2127–2133. Available at: http://www.ncbi.nlm.nih.gov/sites/pubmed/17044088. Accessed July 5, 2010.

Frei K, Truong DD, Wolters E. Case studies in the advancement of Parkinson's disease. *CNS Spectrums* 2008;13(12 Suppl 18):1–6. Available at: http://www.ncbi.nlm.nih.gov/sites/pubmed/19179948. Accessed July 5, 2010.

Georgetown University Hospital. Movement Disorders and Parkinson's. Available at: http://www.georgetownuniversityhospital.org/body.cfm?id=1236&gclid=CJ6c8Z2465kCFQJHxwodJ2qRTQ. Accessed July 4, 2010.

Hauser RA, Pahwa R, Lyons KE, et al. Parkinson Disease. EMedicine Specialties, Neurology, Movement and Neurodegenerative Diseases. Available at: http://emedicine.medscape.com/article/1151267-overview. Accessed July 5, 2010.

Hernandez-Reif M, Field T, Largie S, et al. Parkinson's disease symptoms are differentially affected by massage therapy versus progressive muscle relaxation: a pilot study. *Journal of Bodywork and Movement Therapies* 2002;6:177–182. Available at: http://www.massagemag.com/Magazine/2003/issue101/research101.php. Accessed July 5, 2010.

Inkster LM, Eng JJ. Postural control during a sit-to-stand task in individuals with mild Parkinson's disease. *Experimental Brain Research* January 2004;154:33–38. Available at: http://www.ncbi.nlm.nih.gov/pubmed/12961057. Accessed July 5, 2010.

Inkster LM, Eng JJ, MacIntyre DL, et al. Leg muscle strength is reduced in Parkinson's disease and relates to the ability to rise from a chair. *Movement Disorders* 2003;18:157–162. Available at: http://www.ncbi.nlm.nih.gov/sites/pubmed/12539208. Accessed July 5, 2010.

Lou JS. Physical and mental fatigue in Parkinson's disease: epidemiology, pathophysiology and treatment. *Drugs & Aging* 2009;26(3):195–208. Available at: http://www.ncbi.nlm.nih.gov/sites/pubmed/19358616. Accessed July 5, 2010.

MayoClinic.com. Parkinson's Disease. Available at: http://www.mayoclinic.com/health/parkinsons-disease/DS00295. Accessed July 5, 2010.

Miesler D. The Effect of Massage Therapy on Parkinson's Disease. *Massage and Bodywork*. February/March 2002. Available at: http://www.massagetherapy.com/articles/index/php/article_id/289. Accessed July 5, 2010.

National Institute of Neurological Disorders and Stroke. NINDS Parkinson's Disease Information Page. Available at: http://www.ninds.nih.gov/disorders/parkinsons_disease. Accessed April 12, 2009.

Paterson C, Allen JA, Browning M, et al. A pilot study of therapeutic massage for people with Parkinson's disease; the added value of user involvement. *Complementary Therapies in Clinical Practice* 2005;11:161–171. Available at: http://www.ncbi.nlm.nih.gov/sites/pubmed/16005833. Accessed July 5, 2010.

Rattray F, Ludwig L. *Clinical Massage Therapy: Understanding, Assessing and Treating over 70 Conditions*, Toronto: Talus Incorporated, 2000.

WebMD Parkinson's Disease Health Center. Parkinson's Disease Overview. Available at: http://www.webmd.com/parkinsons-disease. Accessed July 5, 2010.

Werner R. Parkinsonism. *Massage Today*. March 2005. Available at: http://www.massagetoday.com/mpacms/mt/article.php?id=13183. Accessed July 5, 2010.

28

Piriformis Syndrome

Also known as:

Pseudo Sciatica, Wallet Sciatica, Hip Socket Neuropathy

Definition: A neuromuscular entrapment syndrome resulting from compression of the sciatic nerve by the piriformis muscle, characterized by pain in the gluteals and along the posterior lower extremity.

GENERAL INFORMATION

- Multiple causes, including compression, irritation, or injury to the proximal sciatic nerve by a spasming or contracting piriformis muscle; hyperlordosis; anatomic abnormalities and/or extreme hypertonicity of the piriformis muscle; traumatic fibrosis; prolonged sitting; vigorous activity that involves explosive bending or twisting
- Often misdiagnosed as clinical low-back pain (LBP) associated with radiculopathy (pain radiating from the spine) secondary to lumbar spinal disc anomalies
- Onset gradual if lifestyle-related, sudden if trauma-related
- Duration of weeks or months
- Risk increased for skiers, tennis players, long-distance bikers, truck drivers, and taxicab drivers
- Prevalence in women

Morbidity and Mortality

Approximately 30–45% of people between the ages of 18 and 55 suffer from some form of LBP. Piriformis syndrome is categorized, along with sciatic nerve entrapment, herniated disc, direct trauma, and muscle spasm, as a leading contributor to LBP. About 50% of people experiencing this condition report a history of direct trauma to the buttock (often from a motor vehicle accident), a direct fall onto the buttock, a difficult childbirth, or a hip/lower back torsion injury. Comorbidities include degenerative lumbar disc disease, ischial tuberosity bursitis, and sciatica. Piriformis syndrome and sciatica are often confused, but they are actually two different (although anatomically related) conditions. (Sciatica is covered in Chapter 35.)

The most serious complications arise from improper diagnosis, which can lead to exacerbation of the symptoms, inappropriate treatments, unnecessary spinal disc surgery, and long-term disability and pain. The prognosis depends on early, accurate diagnosis and treatment. Recurrence is uncommon when rigorous therapy is followed.

PATHOPHYSIOLOGY

Clearly envisioning the anatomy and understanding the physiology of the gluteal complex will aid the therapist in treating this complicated syndrome. Table 28-1 and the figures will help simplify the structures and their functions (Figures 28-1, 28-2, and 28-3).

Hypertonicity of the piriformis and surrounding muscles leads to myofascial trigger points, resulting in nerve compression. Although a common cause of the condition is blunt-force trauma, even low-level, chronic compression over time (such as a wallet positioned in the same pocket for years) on the large but otherwise fragile sciatic nerve can cause piriformis syndrome. As seen in other conditions, such as temporomandibular joint (TMJ) syndrome and the pain-spasm-pain cycle, a nerve

TABLE 28-1	Structural and Functional Components of Piriformis Syndrome		
Anatomic Structure	**Origin and/or Insertion**	**Function**	**Notes**
Sciatic nerve	Formed by nerve roots from lumbar and sacral nerve plexuses (L4-S2), courses through anterior sacrum before passing inferior to piriformis muscle	Supplies both motor and sensory function to skin and muscle of posterior thigh, posterior leg, and lateral and plantar surfaces of foot	Largest nerve in body; starts at lower spine, bifurcates in popliteal space to terminate in foot. Usually passes underneath piriformis muscle, but in 15% of people, passes *through* piriformis, creating greater propensity for nerve complications. Its path through tight bony and muscular spaces contributes to compression injury.
Piriformis muscle	Originates at anterolateral aspect of sacrum and upper margin of greater sciatic foramen; passes through greater sciatic notch; inserts on superior surface of greater trochanter of femur	Assists in *ab*ducting and laterally rotating leg; with hip in extended position, externally rotates hip; with hip flexed, allows hip *ab*duction	Flat, very strong, pyramid shaped; lies deep in gluteal complex
Superior and inferior gluteal nerves	Similar path to sciatic nerve; leaves sciatic nerve trunk, passes through canal above piriformis muscle	Primarily motor function; supplies gluteus medius, gluteus minimus, and tensor fasciae latae	Compression mimics piriformis syndrome
Tendinous bands at edges of piriformis muscle	Help attach muscle to bone		Can contribute to nerve compression

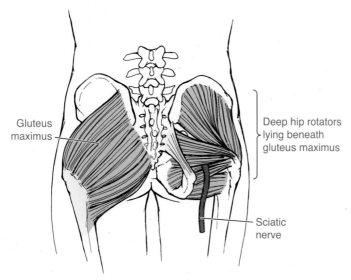

FIGURE 28-1 **Deep hip rotators, gluteus muscles, and the sciatic nerve are all compressed into a compact space. From Hendrickson T. *Massage for Orthopedic Conditions*, Philadelphia: Lippincott Williams & Wilkins, 2003.**

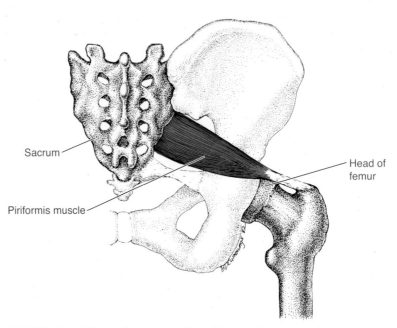

FIGURE 28-2 The piriformis muscle and its attachments on the sacrum
and the head of the femur. Modified from LifeART image. Philadelphia:
Lippincott Williams & Wilkins.

deprived of oxygen through compression or impingement will alert the body of its
need for more oxygen by signaling often surprising pain.

    Diagnosis is based on physical assessment, as well as the patient's neurologic his-
tory and any previous experience with pelvic trauma or childbirth difficulties. A digital
rectal examination (DRE) is often included in the diagnostic process, since the muscle
is directly accessible through the rectum and manual muscle compression will exacerbate the pain, thus confirming the condition. Although there is no single test to confirm

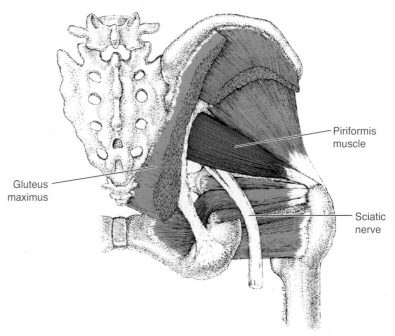

FIGURE 28-3 The piriformis muscle and sciatic nerve lie directly
beneath the gluteus maximus (cut away). Modified from LifeART image.
Philadelphia: Lippincott Williams & Wilkins.

a diagnosis, magnetic resonance neurography is a new diagnostic technique that has demonstrated a high degree of accuracy in pinpointing piriformis muscle asymmetry and sciatic nerve hyperintensity. A physician might order an X-ray, an MRI, and/or nerve conduction tests to rule out other conditions with similar symptoms.

OVERALL SIGNS AND SYMPTOMS

- Pain in the buttocks, coccyx, hip, groin, or posterior thigh
- Numbness or tingling radiating down the posterior leg and/or the lateral foot
- Increased pain with extended periods of sitting, climbing stairs, or squatting
- Spasm and/or hypertonicity in the piriformis muscle
- Weak hip *ab*duction
- A tender gluteal region
- Pain during bowel movements
- Hypomobility of the sacroiliac joint
- A shortened stride length
- A shortened leg on the affected side
- A splayed foot (noticeable lateral rotation) when lying supine

SIGNS AND SYMPTOMS MASSAGE THERAPY CAN ADDRESS

Piriformis syndrome is a soft tissue condition; therefore, it is well within the massage therapist's scope of practice to address many presenting symptoms.

- Nerve compression by surrounding hypertonic muscles can be addressed with layer-by-layer tissue softening.
- Pain, numbness, and tingling of a soft tissue structure secondary to nerve oxygen deprivation can be addressed using multiple massage therapy techniques.
- Muscle tenderness can be addressed with careful muscle-stimulating techniques.
- Anxiety and decreased quality of life can be eased using relaxing techniques that help the client achieve a parasympathetic state.

TREATMENT OPTIONS

The condition's mimicry of common LBP can easily lead the person to several physicians before a correct diagnosis is made and effective treatment begins. A sports medicine or orthopedic physician will most likely treat piriformis syndrome.

Treatment starts conservatively, with physicians or physical therapists (PTs) applying spinal/pelvic traction, introducing progressive stretches and strengthening techniques, carefully increasing range of motion (ROM), applying heat and/or cold, using ultrasound, and modifying the person's activities. A rigorous, daily regimen of home self-care is essential for complete recovery. Corticosteroid injection into the muscle belly is used if all conservative methods are unsuccessful. Surgery is the treatment of last resort.

COMMON MEDICATIONS

- Nonsteroidal anti-inflammatory drugs (NSAIDs), such as ibuprofen (Motrin, Advil)
- Local anesthetics, such as bupivacaine hydrochloride (Bupivacaine) and lidocaine topical (Lidocream, Lidoderm, Xylocaine)

MASSAGE THERAPIST ASSESSMENT

A massage therapist will not assess for the presence of piriformis syndrome but instead will treat the secondary symptoms, which will have been diagnosed by a

Thinking It Through

When a client lies supine, the normal anatomic position of the lower extremities is for the toes of both feet to point toward the ceiling or to *slightly* laterally rotate. When one foot or both feet dramatically splay out to the side (laterally rotate), it is often a strong indicator of the presence of LBP. Thinking through the structural effects of this apparently innocuous splaying will explain this helpful massage therapy assessment tool. The therapist should consider the following points:

- The lateral foot roll will necessarily pull the tibia and thus the knee out laterally.
- The lateral roll of the knee will pull the femur laterally.
- The femur's lateral roll will tug on its articulation at the hip, in the acetabulum.
- Even a gentle, consistent, abnormal pull of the head of the femur laterally out of the acetabulum abnormally stretches the entire gluteal and lumbar spine muscles, bones, discs, ligaments, and tendons.
- As the body attempts to correct and move into proper anatomic alignment, the constant, low-level, soft tissue battle creates hypertonicity in the entire region.

physician. Before planning the massage session, the therapist should ask the following questions while making observational assessments:

- Is the client seeing a sports medicine physician or an orthopedic or chiropractic physician?
- Has she received a corticosteroid or anesthetic injection into the buttocks region in the last 10 days?
- Has she had a rectal examination or treatment in the last 10 days?
- On a scale of 0–10, what is her pain level now?
- What is the exact path of the pain?
- What is the nature of the pain? Burning, numbness, tingling, dull, or achy?
- Is she guarding as she walks?
- Is she walking with an apparent limp, indicating leg shortening?
- Does she brace herself when she sits into or rises out of a chair?

THERAPEUTIC GOALS

Because piriformis syndrome is a soft tissue condition, it is reasonable for the therapist, working closely with a physician and/or PT, to help reduce the compressive force on the affected nerve, to reduce muscle hypertonicity, to facilitate improved posture, and to provide pain relief.

MASSAGE SESSION FREQUENCY

- Ideally: 60-minute sessions twice a week in the early, painful stages
- 60-minute sessions once a week as symptoms begin to subside
- 60-minute maintenance sessions once a month until symptoms are completely relieved

MASSAGE PROTOCOL

Effective treatment depends on clear visualization of the soft tissue structures underneath your hands, and a willingness to begin gently and move, layer by layer, to the depth the client can tolerate.

Although multiple trigger points deep in the piriformis are common with this condition, the step-by-step protocol does not instruct you to use aggressive trigger point techniques. (Trigger points are covered in Chapter 43.) Instead, the protocol leans heavily toward myofascial techniques and warming superficial tissue while working each thick layer of muscle until the piriformis can be palpated and manipulated. (Don't be perplexed by the use of the term "myofascial"; in this context, it indicates that you are working muscle and fascia, and it does not refer to any particular massage therapy method or training.) This can be effectively accomplished by static compression techniques, including the application of compression on a broad area using an open hand and/or forearm. While applying direct, nonmoving (static) pressure, you gently progress from light to deep pressure, waiting for the tissue to release, soften, or move ever so slightly. This movement signals the body's acquiescence and your ability to move even deeper. Use of the elbow (or knuckles or fists) is not suggested, because the untrained elbow, combined with inappropriate body mechanics, will damage the already compromised, fragile sciatic nerve.

Throughout this protocol, remember that the pain of this condition is *due to soft tissue compression*; therefore, your approach must be cautious, intelligent, and performed with constant client feedback. Applying too much pressure in the wrong direction can both alienate your client and exacerbate the condition. Understand the origin and insertions of the surrounding muscles, and work them *in the direction of origin*. This softens the muscle and will help prevent spasm.

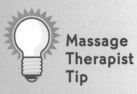

Massage Therapist Tip

Using Discretion When Touching the Gluteal Area

Effective therapy for piriformis syndrome requires detailed and thorough work on the entire gluteal complex. Whether it's the 1st or 10th session with this client, ask permission to touch the gluteal complex before you address this personal area. Be careful not to invade the gluteal fold. Working around binding underwear edges and continuously readjusting underwear will make the protocol clumsy. If you are comfortable and if your state regulations allow, ask the client if she would be comfortable removing her underwear, assuring her that you will keep her snugly draped at all times.

Step-by-Step Protocol for Piriformis Syndrome

Technique	Duration
With the client side-lying, affected side facing up, place a pillow between her knees and ankles. Give her a "teddy bear" pillow to hold, which will help stabilize her rib cage and prevent her from rolling forward.	
Apply cold packs or hot packs as dictated by the tenor of the pain. Leave them in place while you begin distal relaxation techniques.	
Using slaying-the-dragon techniques, massage the shoulders, head, or feet to relax the overall body and help relax the painful site.	5 minutes
Remove the hot or cold packs. Drape snugly to ensure modesty.	
Using no lubrication, tissue mobilization, gentle-to-medium compressions, evenly rhythmic • Entire lumbar spine region from below T-12 to the superior sacrum; do not broach the sacral area or gluteals yet. • Note: Working on a client's lumbar region while she is positioned side-lying presents a body mechanics challenge for the therapist. Try sitting on a rolling stool tableside behind the client or on a large exercise ball, or kneeling, to bring your arms in proper alignment with the client's lumbar region. Do not bend or torque your lower torso awkwardly, or you may cause your own LBP.	6 minutes
Place your open, flattened hands on the hip and simply rest for a moment.	
Using no lubrication, with hands "glued" to the skin, begin moving superficial tissue in first small and then larger circles, moving both clockwise and counterclockwise. • Entire hip region • Entire gluteal complex from PSIS to sacrum, from superior ridge of the posterior pelvis to the ischial tuberosity; do not invade the gluteal fold.	4 minutes
Using lubrication, effleurage, light pressure, evenly rhythmic, superficial tissue only • Entire hip region • Entire gluteal complex from PSIS to sacrum, from superior ridge of the posterior pelvis to the ischial tuberosity; do not invade the gluteal fold.	4 minutes
Effleurage, petrissage, effleurage, deeper pressure, evenly rhythmic • Entire hip region • Entire gluteal complex from PSIS to sacrum, from superior ridge of the posterior pelvis to the ischial tuberosity	5 minutes

(continued)

Contraindications and Cautions

- Modulate your elbow work on trigger points in the gluteal or piriformis complex. The sciatic nerve, and other surrounding nerves, is already compressed, and you can cause serious damage with an ill-placed, aggressive elbow.
- Don't perform cross-fiber friction if the client is taking anti-inflammatory medication.
- Don't perform either active or passive joint ROM. This client has been given a stretching and strengthening regimen by a PT who is working directly with a physician, both of whom know the exact anatomic damage to the area. Without that knowledge, you can cause harm with apparently innocuous joint ROM.
- Don't perform hip ROM on a pregnant woman who has LBP of unknown origin, especially if she is in her third trimester.

Technique	Duration
Cross-fiber friction, medium pressure, working smoothly and calmly, not sporadically, being careful not to overstimulate the tissue • Bony prominence at the PSIS • Bony prominence at the head of the femur • Bony prominence along the lateral edge of the sacrum, including the coccyx • Gluteus maximus and minimus and piriformis muscles origins and insertions and belly	6 minutes
Effleurage, petrissage (using large, almost scooping movements), effleurage, medium pressure, evenly rhythmic • All cross-fibered areas	5 minutes
Jostling, using an open, flat hand, not knuckles or elbows, smoothly energetic but being sure to displace as much tissue as possible • Entire gluteal region	2 minutes
Using the fleshy (ulnar) side of your forearm or your flat, open hand, very slowly compress and slightly push the *insertion* of the piriformis muscle (at the greater trochanter) toward the *origin* (the lateral edge of the sacrum). Keep compressing and slightly pushing the muscle 1 inch at a time. Do not move to the next position until you feel the muscle complex soften under your contact. Your final position will be firmly pushing against the lateral bony prominence of the sacrum.	5 minutes
Petrissage, effleurage, petrissage, medium pressure, briskly • Entire gluteal and piriformis complex	3 minutes
With ample lubricant, effleurage, petrissage, effleurage • Lumbar spine region • Hamstring complex from popliteal fossa to ischial tuberosity • Note: Work the entire leg if the client complains of pain along the entire sacral nerve path, which would include the foot on the affected side.	7 minutes

Getting Started

Have hot packs ready to apply to distal hypertonic tissue and to use if the client complains of dull, aching pain. Cold packs can be applied to quiet a spasm and reduce sharp, stabbing pain. Have plenty of pillows to provide a comfortable side-lying position.

Appropriate draping is paramount since your work involves directly touching the hip and surrounding gluteal complex. You might choose to work through a thin layer of sheet, depending on your comfort and your client's level of trust, but the more effective work will be skin on skin. Your hands must be able to feel even the slightest shift and softening as you apply myofascial techniques.

This client will be in pain and thus holding herself, and she may find it difficult to relax. A soothing approach and environment, combined with suggestions to take a few deep breaths, may help her relax.

To make sure you are working directly on the piriformis muscle, which is deep to the gluteus maximus, use the following technique. With the client side-lying, palpate the posterior/superior iliac spine (PSIS) and the greater trochanter. Lay the heel of your hand on the PSIS and point your fingertips toward the greater trochanter. The piriformis lies deep to the gluteals in that pathway.

HOMEWORK

Although assigning extensive self-care is the norm for most conditions in this text, the fear of doing harm will restrain you from offering more than simple lifestyle suggestions while treating a client with piriformis syndrome. Encourage your client to perform the rigorous regimen she has been assigned by her PT. Here are some suggestions:

- If you must sit for extended periods, consider using a rocking chair with foam padding on the seat.
- If you're driving for any length of time, get out of the car hourly and walk around.
- If your local pain is acute, apply ice. If your local pain is dull and achy, apply heat.
- Before sleep, consider placing a pillow between your knees while on your side and a pillow under your knees while lying on your back. This will take some pressure off your lower back.
- Yoga and tai chi include gentle and effective stretching and strengthening exercises. Be sure to get permission from your physician and PT before beginning a class.

Review

1. List the muscles in the gluteal complex and their anatomic relationship to each other.
2. Describe where the sciatic nerve originates, explain its path, and discuss its function.
3. What other conditions does piriformis syndrome mimic?
4. What level of aggressiveness is appropriate when treating this syndrome?
5. Explain some lifestyle suggestions to help prevent recurrence.

BIBLIOGRAPHY

Dalton E. Low Back, Piriformis and SI Joint Pain. *Massage Today*. May 2007. Available at: http://www.massagetoday.com/mpacms/mt/article.php?id=13628. Accessed July 5, 2010.

Lowe W. Treating Piriformis Syndrome. *Massage Today*. March 2008. Available at: http://www.massagetoday.com/mpacms/mt/article.php?id=13771. Accessed July 5, 2010.

Rattray F, Ludwig L. *Clinical Massage Therapy: Understanding, Assessing and Treating over 70 Conditions*, Toronto: Talus Incorporated, 2000.

Shah S, Wang TW. Piriformis Syndrome. EMedicine article. Available at: http://emedicine.medscape.com/article/87545-overview. Accessed July 5, 2010.

29

Also known as:

Jogger's Heel, Tennis Heel, Policeman's Heel

Plantar Fasciitis

Definition: An overuse injury of the plantar fascia, characterized by mid-heel pain that can radiate toward the toes.

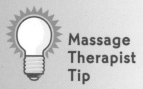

Massage Therapist Tip

Being Aware of Compensation in a Client's Body

When one part of the body is in pain, the person will move in such a way to avoid causing more pain in that region. Those often awkward movements are known as *compensation*. For instance, if you have a sore right wrist from performing too many massages, you may use your right forearm or left wrist more—either of which may be unaccustomed to the extra load. You are compensating for your right wrist pain by using another body part to perform the activity. Often, when clients are in pain, the hypertonicity in the compensating body part also needs treatment. When a client has plantar fasciitis, for example, the act of limping to avoid foot pain places unusual strain on the contralateral foot and the ipsilateral ankle, knee, hip, and lower back. Compensation is an important consideration when you're planning a treatment protocol.

GENERAL INFORMATION

- Multiple causes involving repetitive micro-tearing (sometimes accompanied by inflammation) to the plantar fascia, including improper foot biomechanics, nonsupportive footwear, excessive strain to the plantar fascia, exercise overload, obesity, pregnancy, extremely hypertonic gastrocnemius, arthritis
- Most common cause of heel pain
- Gradual onset
- Acute stage: new, nearly intolerable pain
- Chronic stage following acute: symptoms more bearable
- Duration usually no more than 1 year
- More prevalent in those who participate in high-impact sports, or after increasing the intensity of an exercise program
- More prevalent in diabetics and in people between ages 40 and 60
- Greater risk in people with pes cavus (high arch), pes planus (low arch, excessive foot pronation), increased inversion or eversion
- Occurrence usually unilateral

Morbidity and Mortality

Heel pain affects approximately 2 million Americans annually. About 10% of runner-related injuries and 15% of all foot symptoms requiring professional care involve damage to the plantar fascia. Complications of plantar fasciitis include bruising, swelling, numbness, tingling, and, in rare cases, rupture. When the condition is ignored, complications can arise in the foot, knee, hip, or back as the body compensates for the pain and subsequent abnormal footfall. The prognosis is good, and 80% of cases completely resolve within a year.

PATHOPHYSIOLOGY

The plantar fascia is a very tough aponeurosis (fibrous sheet or flat, expanded tendon that facilitates muscular attachments) located on the foot's deep plantar surface. It functions with every step as it absorbs shock, and serves as a bowstring to hold up the foot's longitudinal arch. It inserts into the base of the calcaneus (large heel bone), weaves into the deep transverse metatarsal ligament, and attaches to the proximal phalanx of each toe (Figure 29-1).

Overuse, combined with biomechanical foot abnormalities, causes straining, tiny tears, and sometimes inflammation of the fascia. This leads to further inflammation, occasional swelling, and persistent, often excruciating, pain. Plantar fasciitis is not technically an inflammatory condition as the "itis" indicates. The pain, previously believed to be inflammatory, often occurs as a result of degeneration of the aponeurosis and may or may not be accompanied by inflammation.

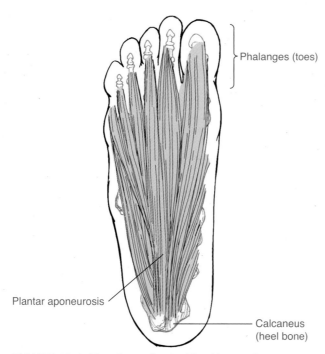

Phalanges (toes)

Plantar aponeurosis

Calcaneus (heel bone)

FIGURE 29-1 **The plantar fascia. This fibrous sheet originates at the medial tubercle of the calcaneus, then spreads out over the bottom of the foot to insert onto the proximal phalanges and flexor tendon sheaths. From Hendrickson T.** *Massage for Orthopedic Conditions*, **Philadelphia: Lippincott Williams & Wilkins, 2003.**

Diagnosis is usually confirmed with a verbal history of physical activity, gait assessment, visual observation of the feet and shoes, and palpation and stretching of the plantar surface of the foot. X-rays are not necessary but may be ordered to rule out fracture.

Although heel spur is used to be synonymous with plantar fasciitis, it has been clinically proven that while the two conditions sometimes coexist, they are two distinct conditions. Heel spur pain can mimic the discomfort of plantar fasciitis, yet a heel spur is often painless. Plantar fasciitis is never asymptomatic.

OVERALL SIGNS AND SYMPTOMS

- Heel pain, described as stabbing, burning, or deep aching
- Plantar surface pain radiating from the heel to the base of the toes
- Worse heel pain in the morning, easing for a while, worsening as the day progresses
- Increased heel pain after long periods of sitting
- Pain upon plantar surface palpation
- Plantar surface pain after, not usually during, exercise
- Mild swelling in and around the heel

SIGNS AND SYMPTOMS MASSAGE THERAPY CAN ADDRESS

- Compensatory hypertonicity can be treated with multiple routine massage therapy techniques.
- The local increased blood supply and subsequent tissue cleansing that are essential for healing can be initiated with careful, layer-by-layer tissue softening.

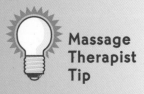

Massage Therapist Tip

The Effects of Prolonged Nonsteroidal Anti-Inflammatory Drug Intake

Since plantar fasciitis is usually treated outside of a medical setting and may last up to a year, your client may be taking an NSAID or aspirin. Although these medications can reduce the inflammation and pain, prolonged use of any medication should be medically supervised. Ask your client to be aware of the side effects of daily or frequent intake of even the most common OTC medication. If he complains of stomach burning, nausea, or ringing in his ears, refer him to his physician.

- The exquisite pain of the acute stage and persistent pain of the chronic stage can be addressed with cold and heat applications, respectively.
- The fact that this condition usually often persists for months gives the massage therapist an ideal opportunity for multiple, effective, client self-care assignments.

TREATMENT OPTIONS

Most patients who receive appropriate and prompt care will respond to conservative treatment. The first step is rest. The offending impact on the plantar surface of the foot must be relieved if healing is to begin. High-impact exercise regimens should be replaced by swimming, cycling, yoga, or another low-impact activity. It's interesting to note, however, that immobilization is *not* advised (except for the occasional night splint prescribed by a physician for specific biomechanical corrections) because it can lead to debilitating stiffness and increased pain. Ice massage and/or ice packs can reduce pain and inflammation. Custom-made or over-the-counter (OTC) orthotics and/or heel pads that support the arch and protect the heel are commonly used.

If conservative treatment, combined with taking nonsteroidal anti-inflammatory drugs (NSAIDs), does not completely resolve the condition, ultrasound physical therapy is used to decrease inflammation and promote healing. Anti-inflammatory injection directly into the heel is a painful, temporary treatment that carries the risk of breaking down the heel's fat pad, and exacerbating heel pain. Studies indicate that extracorporeal shock wave therapy (ESWT), which directs high-velocity sound waves at the painful heel, may stimulate healing. Surgery to detach the plantar fascia from the calcaneous is a rare treatment of last resort.

Preventing a recurrence includes moderating the exercise program, maintaining ideal body weight, wearing supportive shoes, stretching before and after exercise, and performing foot and ankle exercises to maintain strength and flexibility.

Common Medications

NSAIDs are used to reduce symptoms and prevent complications. No healing medication has been found.

- NSAIDs, such as ibuprofen (Motrin, Advil)

MASSAGE THERAPIST ASSESSMENT

It is best for a massage therapist to perform an assessment of a client presenting with heel pain as a reconfirmation of a physician's diagnosis. However, plantar fasciitis is so common; few people will seek a physician's care but instead will self-diagnose after a quick online search. With a sound clinical understanding of the signs and symptoms, the therapist can accurately assess for the presence of plantar fasciitis and then move ahead with an effective treatment plan. If the condition gets worse and does not respond to conservative treatment, a referral to a physician is necessary.

The first step is to determine whether the condition is acute or chronic. The acute stage is characterized by a relatively recent onset of exquisite pain, whereas the chronic stage is determined by the classic symptoms of morning pain that eases and then progresses. Clients in both stages usually report initial onset related to a specific activity, or to having spent an unusual or sustained amount of time on their feet.

The therapist observes the client's gait, checking for signs of limping. She asks the client to stabilize himself and then instructs him to carefully hop up and down on the affected foot. The pain should reproduce immediately. She tells him to stop as soon as he feels pain. The therapist asks to see the condition of the client's shoe(s) and checks for uneven wear, indicating inefficient gait mechanics. She also notes whether his shoe provides adequate or inefficient support. She notes any compensatory movements that add duress to the ankle, knee, hip, and/or lower back.

With the client clothed but shoes and socks removed, he is positioned comfortably either prone or supine on the massage table. The therapist gently palpates for the presence of fibrotic thickenings and adhesions along the plantar (bottom) surface of the foot. Holding the foot in one hand so it can remain relaxed, she grasps the toes with the other hand and slowly bends the toes up toward the knee. This should reproduce the pain of plantar fasciitis. She immediately stops the passive stretch when the client indicates pain. She then observes and palpates for any slight swelling around the heel, gently palpating the heel and the entire aponeurosis, into the base of the toes. She watches the client's reaction, which will indicate the exact location of pain and tenderness. The therapist asks him to point his toes and flex his foot, bending the toes back toward his knee, and notes when pain is reproduced. Trigger points in the soleus muscle, along with other plantar flexors, commonly refer pain into the heel and plantar surface of the foot; therefore, calf palpation is performed during the assessment. The therapist asks about compensatory pain, his exercise or work regimen, and the kind of shoes he normally wears.

THERAPEUTIC GOALS

Since plantar fasciitis is a chronic condition lasting up to 1 year, in an effective long-term therapeutic regimen, the therapist can expect to reduce pain, reduce the hypertonicity of compensating structures, help heal the plantar fascia, instruct the client in the all-important daily self-care techniques, and help the client return to normal, pain-free activity.

MASSAGE SESSION FREQUENCY

In the acute stage:

- 30-minute sessions directly on the foot twice a week
- Followed immediately by 30 minutes of work to compensating structures or for relaxation

In the chronic stage:

- 60-minute sessions once a week until the pain is completely managed
- 60-minute sessions every other week as the pain lessens and the client takes on the responsibility of daily self-care
- 60-minute monthly maintenance sessions

MASSAGE PROTOCOL

Protocols for both acute and chronic stages of plantar fasciitis are included. Because the acute pain can be almost unbearable, the protocol will address the foot for only 30 minutes, with Swedish relaxation techniques used for the remaining time. Treating the chronic stage will require a full 60-minute session, with 30 minutes spent on the affected foot and the remaining time on compensating structures.

Many of the techniques used in the protocol mimic the self-care assignments. Read the Homework section of the chapter before beginning your protocol. You can then educate your client in both the technique and the reasoning behind your work.

When properly treating chronic plantar fasciitis, you will work down to the depth of the bone. This may seem counterintuitive, given the fact that the client is already

Thinking It Through

The *gait cycle* is a term that describes the biomechanics of leg and foot movements while walking, and it's worth reviewing in the context of determining an effective treatment plan for plantar fasciitis. A thorough understanding of the anatomy and physiology of the muscles used during walking and running will lead to a better understanding of the pain of plantar fasciitis. The terminology might seem awkward at first, but if the therapist stands and takes the steps directed as follows, the terms will become self-explanatory. The gait cycle includes a stance phase and a swing phase.

Stance Phase:

- *Loading response* is when the foot makes contact with the ground; usually, the heel strikes first.
- *Midstance* begins when the center of gravity is directly over the foot.
- During *terminal stance*, the heel leaves the ground and the foot is in a toe-off position.
- *Pre-swing* is the contralateral foot's stance as soon as the toe-off occurs.

Swing Phase:

- *Initial swing* indicates that the contralateral toe has left the ground (after toe-off) and the foot is ready to swing forward.
- *Midswing* is the period of maximum knee flexion.
- *Terminal swing* is the point at which the step has moved out as far as it biomechanically can swing, and the body is preparing for the next step.

Contraindications and Cautions

- If the client complains of numbness and tingling through the lower extremity, nocturnal pain, heat, or swelling anywhere in the leg, he should see a physician.

- Cross-fiber friction should be avoided if the client suffers from painful inflammation or if he is taking anti-inflammatories or anticoagulants.

- Deep work to the heel is contraindicated if the client has received an injection to the heel within the last week. (This does not mean you cannot treat the rest of the plantar fascia and/or compensating structures.)

- Frequent monitoring of the pain level by using the 0—10 pain scale will help you modify your work.

Step-by-Step Protocol for	Acute Plantar Fasciitis	
Technique		**Duration**
Do nothing more than hold the foot. Because of his acute pain, the client will resist any therapeutic attempts if trust is not initially established. While holding the foot, let him talk about his symptoms and discomfort.		1 minute
Continue holding the foot, and slowly and gently apply a cold pack. Tell the client what you are going to do; apply it gently and position it securely so the cold contacts the plantar surface. Tell him you're going to leave it in place for 5 minutes or until the discomfort from the cold is unbearable. Once the pack is secure, use compression, slow effleurage, petrissage, effleurage, medium pressure. • Entire gastrocnemius and soleus muscles • From the Achilles tendon to just below the popliteal fossa		5 minutes
Remove the cold pack. Gentle finger compression, squeezing, and ROM. Make no contact with the plantar fascia yet; do not tug on the plantar fascia. • Every toe		1 minute
Stroking, using your whole, flat hand, working in all directions, slowly with gentle pressure (not too light, to avoid a sympathetic response) • Entire plantar surface of the foot • Entire dorsal surface of the foot • All toes • Malleoli		2 minutes
Using lubricant, effleurage, using your whole, flat hand, working in all directions, slowly, with more depth than the previous step but not moving to a firm pressure yet. Carefully gauge the client's response; do not cause pain. • Entire plantar surface of the foot • Entire dorsal surface of the foot • All toes • Malleoli		3 minutes
Replace the ice pack. Return to the gastrocnemius. Effleurage, petrissage, effleurage, gentle tugging from proximal to distal while gripping the belly of the muscle, firm pressure, working slowly, but creating no discomfort. • Entire gastrocnemius and soleus muscles • From the Achilles tendon to just below the popliteal fossa		5 minutes
Remove the cold pack. Effleurage, petrissage, effleurage, compressions, slow, medium pressure • Hamstring complex		
Long, slow, smooth, effleurage, firm pressure, working cephalically • From the Achilles tendon to the ischial tuberosity		2 minutes

(continued)

Technique	Duration
Long, slow, smooth, stroking using light but full hand pressure (avoiding a sympathetic response), stroking cephalically • From the Achilles tendon to the ischial tuberosity	2 minutes
Stroking, using fingertips only, slowly, very lightly, working in a cephalic direction • In the popliteal fossa only	1 minute
Instruct the client to perform ROM exercises at his ankle, point and flex his toes, point and flex at the ankle, bend his toes toward his knee just to the point of pain, and then release. Teach him how to deeply massage his calf muscles.	3 minutes
Effleurage, with as much pressure as he can tolerate, a little more briskly • Entire plantar fascia	1 minute
Simply hold the foot.	1 minute

experiencing pain. Remember, though, that your work is slow and careful, warming layer by layer well before you reach the bone. At the point when you finally palpate the deep fascia and the underlying bone, the client should be sufficiently relaxed and trusting to allow you to do the necessary deep work.

Your goal is to bring blood to the micro-tears in the plantar fascia and surrounding tendons. Recall from basic anatomy that fascia and tendons are not as sanguinous as muscle, so your work must be thorough and creative in your attempt to increase local blood supply. Flushing the area after treatment is important for ridding the tissue of accumulated metabolites. When treating chronic cases, half of your session will be dedicated to addressing proximal hypertonicity.

Getting Started

Have cold packs ready to treat the acute stage and moist warm packs ready for the chronic stage. Your inclination may be to ask the client not to disrobe completely since you "are only working on the foot." However, remember your hands will find compensatory hypertonicity, which will lead you to work on the lower back, hips, and knees, in addition to the obvious footwork. Place pillows and bolsters under the knees (if supine) or ankles (if prone). Since the client will probably remain awake during this protocol, you might offer him a pillow to use under his head (if supine) or to hold (if prone) so he can "see" you as you work and instruct him.

HOMEWORK

Homework assigned for plantar fasciitis addresses both prevention and treatment. The goals are to reduce impact injury to the damaged fascia, to decrease inflammation, and to rebuild and stretch weakened foot and calf muscles.

• Before getting out of bed in the morning, deeply massage your affected foot. Perform range-of-motion (ROM) exercises at the ankle. Deeply massage your calf. Stretch your leg out, point your toes straight out and then back toward your knee (gently flexing the foot).

Step-by-Step Protocol for   Chronic Plantar Fasciitis

Technique	Duration
Apply a moist warm pack to the plantar surface of the client's foot. Leave in place as you perform the next step.	
Effleurage, petrissage, effleurage, medium pressure, slow, evenly rhythmic. Follow with gentle jostling. • Gastrocnemius from the Achilles tendon to just below the popliteal fossa	5 minutes
Remove the warm pack. Chat about whatever the client is interested in as you simply hold the foot. Do nothing but hold the foot.	1 minute
Passive but full ROM • At the ankle • At every toe	1 minute
Active and full ROM. (Ask the client to trace the alphabet, using capital letters, while performing active ankle ROM.) • At the ankle	1 minute
Compression, squeezing, cross-fiber friction, ROM, deep effleurage • Every toe	2 minutes
Compression, squeezing, effleurage, petrissage, effleurage, cross-fiber friction, slowly rhythmic, light pressure • Entire plantar fascia	3 minutes
Compression, squeezing, effleurage, petrissage, effleurage, cross-fiber friction, little more quickly, medium pressure • Entire plantar fascia	3 minutes
Passive ROM, gently, slowly • Each toe • At the ankle	1 minute
Compression, squeezing, effleurage, petrissage, effleurage, cross-fiber friction in all directions, moving very briskly and with as much depth as the client will tolerate	5 minutes
Effleurage, to the client's tolerance, slowly and firmly, moving cephalically, in the direction of the knee • Plantar and dorsal surface of the foot	2 minutes
Effleurage, petrissage, effleurage, medium pressure and speed, working cephalically • Entire gastrocnemius and soleus complex	2 minutes
Foot jostling, muscle, tendon and ligament stripping, deep compressions, hacking and brisk but careful passive ROM • All structures below the malleoli	4 minutes

(continued)

Technique	Duration
Gentle, slow, deep effleurage, working cephalically • Plantar fascia	1 minute
This completes the first 30 minutes of this protocol, the direct work on the plantar fascia. The remaining 30 minutes is spent on compensating hypertonicity with the usual effleurage, petrissage, compression, jostling, muscle stripping, and passive and active ROM that you would use to address any hypertonic region of the body.	30 minutes

- While sitting with bare feet, place a small, thin towel on the floor beneath your foot. With your toes only, gather up as much of the towel as you can and pick it up off the floor.
- Put an ice cube or ice pack on a thick towel, and place them both on the floor beneath your foot. Starting with light pressure and working progressively deeper, rub the sole of your foot over the ice. Periodically stop and hold your foot in one position on the ice, and gently press your foot into the cold. Hold it until the pain is very uncomfortable, and then begin moving your foot over the ice's surface. (You can perform this exercise while holding an ice cube or ice pack, but this can become uncomfortably cold to the skin of your hand.)
- Stand and stabilize yourself on the edge of a stair or a curb. Wriggle so just the balls of your feet rest on the edge of the step/curb. Raise yourself up on your toes; lower yourself so your heel moves slightly below the edge of the step/curb. Repeat until your calves tire.
- Sit with one leg crossed on your knee so you can reach the bottom of your affected foot. Gently bend your toes up toward your knee. With the thumb, knuckles, or fingers of your other hand, slowly push on the entire sole of your foot, moving from point to point, and working from your heel to the base of your toes. At very painful points, back off for a moment, *but then return into the painful area and gently press until the pain seems to lessen.* Bend your toes back the other way toward your heel, and deeply massage the sole of your foot. Repeat this several times a day, especially before you get out of bed, if that's when your symptoms are at their worst, if you have to stand for long periods throughout the day, and before and after exercise.
- Sit or stand. Place a tennis ball underneath your bare or socked foot. Roll the tennis ball along the bottom of your foot. Slowly increase the pressure you apply to the ball. Curl your toes to try to keep the ball underfoot. When the ball escapes, use your foot and toes to retrieve it, and continue the rolling.
- Grip the calf of your affected leg and deeply massage it. Massage all the way up to just below the back of your knee and all the way down until you can feel your heel bone.
- Monitor the intensity of your existing or new exercise program.
- Wear properly fitting and supportive shoes not only while exercising, but also if you stand for long periods.
- Avoid walking barefoot on hard surfaces.

Review

1. Explain how plantar fasciitis occurs.
2. What is compensation?
3. Describe the gait cycle.
4. Explain the difference between acute and chronic plantar fasciitis.
5. Outline suggested homework assignments for the typical client who has chronic plantar fasciitis.

BIBLIOGRAPHY

Charrett M. Care Options for Plantar Fasciitis. Available at: http://www.dynamicchiropractic .ca/mpacms/dc_ca/articles.php?id=53734. Accessed July 5, 2010.

Gage JR. An overview of normal walking. *Instructional Course Lectures* 1990;39:291–303.

Digiovanni BF, Nawoczenski DA, Malay DP, et al. Plantar fascia-specific stretching exercises improves outcomes in patients with chronic plantar fasciitis: a prospective clinical trial with two-year follow-up. *The Journal of Bone and Joint Surgery* 2006:88;1775–1781.

Mayo Clinic. Plantar Fasciitis. Available at: http://www.mayoclinic.com/health/ plantar-fasciitis/DS00508. Accessed July 5, 2010.

Medline Plus. Plantar Fasciitis. Available at: http://www.nlm.nih.gov/medlineplus/ency/ article/007021.htm. Accessed July 5, 2010.

Plantar Fasciitis Organization. Plantar Fasciitis, Heel Spurs, Heel Pain. Available at: http://www.plantar-fasciitis.org. Accessed July 5, 2010.

Rattray F, Ludwig L. *Clinical Massage Therapy: Understanding, Assessing and Treating over 70 Conditions*, Toronto: Talus Incorporated, 2000.

Singh D, Silverberg M, Milne L. Plantar Fasciitis in Emergency Medicine. Available at: http://emedicine.medscape.com/article/827468-overview. Accessed July 5, 2010.

Sportsinjuryclinic.net. Plantar Fasciitis (Heel Spurs). Available at: http://www .sportsinjuryclinic.net/cybertherapist/front/foot/plantarfasciitis.htm. Accessed July 5, 2010.

WebMD. Plantar Fasciitis. Available at: http://www.webmd.com/a-to-z-guides/ plantar-fasciitis-topic-overview. Accessed July 5, 2010.

30

Post-Polio Syndrome

Also known as:

PPS

Definition: A progressively debilitating neuromuscular condition occurring decades after recovery from acute poliomyelitis.

GENERAL INFORMATION

- Possible causes: long-term nerve damage and nerve overcompensation; long-term stress of aging, weight gain; enterovirus infection of polio survivor's motor neurons
- Onset gradual, approximately 30 years after acute polio
- Lifelong duration
- Increased risk related to severity and age of initial polio infection, and people who underwent intense physical rehabilitation following polio infection
- Spread through oral–fecal contamination
- No cure

Morbidity and Mortality

Until the 1950s, polio killed or disabled thousands of people, predominantly children. Of approximately 440,000 polio survivors in the U.S., 25–50% may be affected by PPS. Some researchers believe that if polio survivors are tracked long enough, all of them will develop signs of the condition. The prognosis is good; the condition is rarely life threatening. Symptoms are slowly progressive and can remain stable for 3–10 years. The Salk vaccine and Sabin oral vaccine eliminated polio in the U.S., and there have been no new polio cases in decades.

PATHOPHYSIOLOGY

Muscle movement is possible only when motor neurons (nerve cells) originating in the spinal cord provide stimulation, which produces movement. One of the most accepted theories of the pathophysiology of PPS is as follows: When the polio-virus attacks, it causes a paralytic disease that destroys nerve cells. Surrounding neurons try to compensate by generating new motor connections to the still working, but potentially orphaned, nearby muscles. After years of overwork, the nerve cells weaken, resulting in muscle weakness. Another theory posits that the normal aging process is accompanied by a decrease in functioning motor nerves. One final theory relates an autoimmune response triggered by the body's initial illness to the onset of PPS.

A firm diagnosis is often difficult because the symptoms mimic those of arthritis, tendonitis, fibromyalgia, cartilage damage, Lou Gehrig's disease, multiple sclerosis, and the aches and pains that accompany aging. Diagnosis is confirmed if decades have passed since the initial onset of poliomyelitis, if symptoms persist for 1 year, and if positive signs of nerve damage are indicated on an electromyograph (EMG). The results of an MRI and/or CT scan, blood tests, and a spinal tap will rule out conditions that mimic the syndrome.

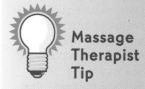

Massage Therapist Tip

Reassuring Clients that Post-Polio Syndrome Is Not a Recurrence

A client suffering from PPS will often compound her diagnosis with a high level of anxiety over the fear that she again has polio. Her memories of isolation (because of the highly contagious nature of the disease) and the struggle with assistive devices, such as crutches and braces, may bring back painful memories and put her at risk for depression. You can assure your PPS client that she is not experiencing a recurrence of her original polio diagnosis. The syndrome rarely progresses to the severity of the original disease, she cannot "spread" her condition, and she certainly does not have to live in isolation, as was the case in her youth.

Thinking It Through

A variety of assistive devices may be prescribed to help stabilize clients with PPS. When treating a body restricted by braces, a cane, crutches, a walker, or a wheelchair, the therapist has the opportunity to address compensating pain and hypertonicity resulting from the use of such devices. The therapist might ask himself the following questions:

- *Cane use:* How hypertonic is the arm/shoulder that is clutching the cane? Are there blisters/calluses on the gripping hand? How has her gait changed due to cane use? Why is she using the cane? What other areas of her body are compensating?
- *Back brace use:* Can I safely remove the brace during treatment? If I remove it, does she need help putting it back on? Is the brace rubbing any skin, causing blisters or calluses? Is her breathing restricted? How have her neck muscles adapted? Have the back muscles become hypotonic or hypertonic?
- *Leg brace use:* How hypotonic or hypertonic are the braced leg's muscles? How is the contralateral leg compensating? How have the gluteal complex and lumbar spine compensated for the gait change? What is the condition of the foot muscles? Are there blisters or calluses around the brace? Can it be removed during massage treatment?

OVERALL SIGNS AND SYMPTOMS

Use of the word "new" in the context of muscle weakness indicates symptoms in muscles unaffected by the earlier diagnosis of polio. PPS symptoms can be so subtle and gradual that it is common for a firm diagnosis to be made only after a symptomatic retrospective of 15–50 years.

- New muscle weakness, fatigue, pain
- Deep aching myofascial pain
- Weakness in originally affected muscles
- Muscle wasting
- Joint pain
- Gait disturbance
- Exhaustion
- Difficulty swallowing, breathing, chewing
- Cold intolerance

SIGNS AND SYMPTOMS MASSAGE THERAPY CAN ADDRESS

- Given the musculoskeletal and myofascial nature of the condition, the massage therapist can treat most PPS symptoms.
- Compensatory muscular hypertonicity and pain can be relieved by the most ordinary massage therapy techniques.

TREATMENT OPTIONS

A person with PPS will experience lifelong intermittent symptomatic remission and progression. Treatment aims to control symptoms and maintain strength and endurance. Physicians may use regular MRIs, CT scans, neuroimaging tests, and electrophysiologic studies to track muscle decline and stabilization. An ongoing team of medical specialists may include a neuromuscular disorder physician, a neurologist, a physiatrist (rehabilitation specialist), and an orthopedist. The treatment plan will optimally include referral to a physical therapist (PT) and/or occupational therapist (OT). PT will teach the delicate balance between sufficient exercise and overexertion, as well as instruct the use of appropriate assistive devices, when necessary. OT will address potential swallowing, choking, and chewing difficulties and help adjust the home environment to adapt for any disability.

Rest, ice, heat, massage, pain medication, a healthy diet, and weight reduction further help the person maintain a near-normal lifestyle. No treatment has been found to prevent the progressive nerve cell deterioration of PPS.

Common Medications

Currently, there is no effective pharmaceutical treatment for PPS. Several drugs, including high-dose steroids and interferons, have not proven to be clinically significant in improving function or reducing symptoms. Over-the-counter (OTC) pain medications, such as nonsteroidal anti-inflammatory drugs (NSAIDs), are often suggested, but they provide pain relief only and do not address causes.

- NSAIDs, such as ibuprofen (Motrin, Advil)

MASSAGE THERAPIST ASSESSMENT

Since PPS manifests over a period of decades and the symptoms mimic common medical conditions, a therapist may treat a client with PPS without either her or the client realizing it. The two keys for appropriate assessment are being aware of the client's childhood history of acute polio, and noticing her present clinical symptoms.

While being careful not to diagnose, the therapist may be the precipitating factor in nudging the client toward a firm medical evaluation, if she combines these two pieces of information and believes the condition to be PPS.

Assessing for treatment, with or without a firm diagnosis of PPS, includes taking a detailed history about muscle and joint pain, gait disturbance, fatigue, and cold intolerance. Appropriate and effective treatment can proceed, with or without a physician's confirming diagnosis, since all of the earlier mentioned symptoms are safely treated by multiple, noninvasive massage therapy techniques.

THERAPEUTIC GOALS

Since PPS symptoms mimic those of many musculoskeletal conditions treated effectively by massage therapy, it is reasonable to expect these benefits: decreased hypertonicity, increased joint range of motion (ROM), decreased pain, increased balance, and reduced anxiety.

MASSAGE SESSION FREQUENCY

Once diagnosed, PPS persists for the remainder of the client's lifetime. Massage therapy should therefore become an integral part of the client's long-term medical care and self-care.

- Ideally: 60-minute sessions twice a month
- Helpful: 60-minute monthly maintenance sessions
- Minimally: Infrequent sessions when the client is experiencing pain or discomfort

MASSAGE PROTOCOL

You can feel completely comfortable addressing the symptoms associated with this long-term condition. Remember that you may be treating PPS without knowing it because your client might present with symptoms resembling fibromyalgia, arthritis, or other musculoskeletal complaints. Your primary frustration, however, could be that your client's symptoms might significantly vary from session to session, and she may never seem to completely recover or progress. Your key to pinpointing that you are caring for a client with PPS is her history of acute poliomyelitis.

Given that your client will be older, you can approach her with the same care and precautions you'd use with any client in her age group. Be aware of the skin's condition, the limited ROM, the reduced endurance, the fear of losing control and falling, the expected mild depression, and the frustration that accompanies a chronic condition.

Do not work energetically or with any techniques resembling sports massage. Use slow, long, careful, and precise strokes that do not stimulate or fatigue a muscle set or the person herself. You'll find plenty of hypertonicity and compensating structures, and each session will present you both with a different challenge. Keep excellent SOAP notes, documenting the client's progression and digression.

Remember this is mainly a neurologic condition, and the muscles will benefit from *gentle* stimulation. Since only motor nerves are affected, your client will be able to provide accurate sensory feedback.

Be perceptive in your questioning of the client before each session. Many aspects of her life may be compromised because of her PPS. Include questions about balance, the efficiency of her assistive devices, her mood and overall energy, and her compliance with homework assignments.

Getting Started

Have hot packs ready if the client regularly experiences dull, aching pain. If she uses assistive devices, rearrange your room and waiting area accordingly. You may need

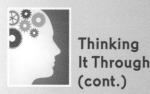

Thinking It Through (cont.)

- *Crutch use:* Are the crutches fitted properly? Is she leaning too far forward during her crutch-assisted gait? How hypertonic are her forearms, arms, and shoulders? Does she have low-back pain? How are her neck and abdominal muscles affected? Can I safely position her to get on and off the table?

Contraindications and Cautions:

- Avoid vigorous, quick, or too deep massage techniques.
- Use cold packs only for short periods and only if the client complains of unrelenting and intolerable short-term local pain.
- The client's balance may be compromised; use caution when positioning on and off the table and maintain physical contact when repositioning.
- Other than the usual contraindications for musculoskeletal work—avoiding open sores and rashes, not treating during fever of unknown origin, and so forth—the contraindications for treating a client diagnosed with PPS are rare.

Step-by-Step Protocol for Post-Polio Syndrome (Bilateral Lower Extremities)

Technique	Duration
Position the client comfortably and securely supine. Provide sufficient pillowing under her shoulders to maintain comfortable breathing and under her knees to relieve low-back tension.	
Begin by providing long, slow, steady, light-to-medium pressure, effleurage while applying ample lubrication. • Bilateral feet • Bilateral legs • Bilateral knees • Bilateral thighs • Abdomen (ask permission) • Bilateral superior pectoralis major and minor • Bilateral arms • Bilateral shoulders • Neck and occipital ridge	15 minutes
Gently grasp one foot at the ankle. • Perform full passive ROM. • Place your palm against the plantar surface of the foot. Instruct the client to push against your hand as you offer gentle resistance to her tolerance. Hold a few seconds. • Hook your hand around the front of the foot. Instruct the client to push against your hand as you offer gentle resistance to her tolerance. • Repeat on the contralateral foot.	3 minutes
Ask her to point her toes as hard as she can and hold to fatigue. Ask her to point her toes toward her knee as hard as she can and hold to fatigue. (You are trying to engage the gastrocnemius.) Perform on the contralateral leg.	2 minutes
Grasp the client's leg gently but firmly so that you can move the knee joint. • Perform gentle, repeated extension and flexion at the knee joint. • With her leg bent, place the client's foot flat but positioned a few inches up off the table. Gently grip her ankle and ask her to "kick out" against your resistance. (You are trying to engage and strengthen the muscles surrounding the knee.) Hold to fatigue. • Repeat on the contralateral knee	2 minutes
Grasp the client's leg gently but firmly so you can mobilize the hip joint. • *Very* gently perform ROM at the client's hip. Watch for signs of discomfort. • With the client's hip rotated laterally as far as she can comfortably hold, place your hand on the medial surface of the thigh and ask her to "squeeze inward" as you offer gentle resistance. Hold to fatigue. • Repeat on the contralateral hip.	4 minutes

(continued)

Technique	Duration
Ask the client to place both feet flat on the table. • Place your hand on her lower abdomen. • Ask her to "tighten her abs" so you can feel the movement with your hand. Hold to fatigue. Repeat several times.	
• While in the same previous position, ask the client to gently push her hips up off the table a few inches. Hold to fatigue. Repeat several times.	3 minutes
Effleurage, petrissage, effleurage, slow, evenly rhythmic, medium pressure • Bilateral feet • Bilateral legs • Bilateral knees • Bilateral thighs • Abdomen • Bilateral superior pectoralis major and minor • Bilateral arms • Bilateral shoulders • Neck and occipital ridge	10 minutes
Ask her to inhale as deeply as she can. *Very gently* place your open hands against her rib cage and offer slight resistance as she exhales. Ask her to inhale again, this time against your *gentle* pressure. Repeat this 3 times. Stop if she becomes light-headed.	3 minutes
Digital kneading, effleurage, petrissage, effleurage, medium pressure • All compensating upper extremity structures • Bilateral hands, forearms, arms, and shoulders	15 minutes
Effleurage, long, slow, sweeping strokes, evenly rhythmic, light-to-medium pressure • Any area that will provide profound relaxation according to the client's request	3 minutes

to remove throw rugs, move a chair in your treatment area to provide more maneuvering room, and lower your table for easier on-and-off access. If her breathing is compromised, be sure to provide sufficient pillowing for a comfortable supine or side-lying position. Prone positioning might not be possible.

Since most PPS symptoms manifest in the lower extremities, the following protocol treats bilateral legs for an older client who uses an assistive walker. The techniques can be adapted to any region of musculoskeletal discomfort. Allow for additional session time at the beginning and end of the appointment to accommodate challenges in dressing, undressing, furniture movement, and stabilizing the client on the walker.

HOMEWORK

As with any musculoskeletal and neuromuscular condition, homework is essential in order to keep the client working up to her personal potential. A regular routine of physical activity is essential. Your suggestions may repeat those of the client's PT or OT, but they are worth reinforcing.

- Take full, deep breaths several times throughout your day. Inhale as deeply as you can, hold for a few seconds, and then exhale forcibly.
- Perform gentle ROM exercises every day, especially at particularly stiff joints.
- Check with your PT and confirm that you can sit and bounce on a large exercise ball. This will increase both your balance and your leg strength. Make sure you hold onto something secure during your bouncing.
- If you can do nothing else, go for a walk. Try to use more energy than a stroll would require, but do not work to the point of exhaustion. Swing your bent arms back and forth with a little vigor.

Review

1. Describe the incidence, spread, and cure of acute poliomyelitis.
2. Describe symptoms of PPS.
3. This syndrome mimics what other medical conditions?
4. Explain the adaptations to a massage therapy treatment area required to accommodate various assistive devices.
5. Are there medications or a cure for PPS?

BIBLIOGRAPHY

Easter Seals Disability Services. Understanding Post-Polio Syndrome. Available at: www.easterseals.com/site/PageServer?pagename=ntl_understand_post_polio. Accessed July 5, 2010.

Golonka D. Post-Polio Syndrome–Topic Overview. Available at: http://www.webmd.com/brain/tc/post-polio-syndrome-topic-overview. Accessed July 5, 2010.

March of Dimes. Post-Polio Syndrome. Available at: www.marchofdimes.com/professionals/14332_1284.asp. Accessed July 5, 2010.

MayoClinic. Post-Polio Syndrome. Available at: www.mayoclinic.com/health/post-polio-syndrome/ds00494/dsection=symptoms. Accessed July 5, 2010.

Muniz F. Postpolio Syndrome. Available at: http://emedicine.medscape.com/article/306920-overview. Accessed July 5, 2010.

National Institute of Neurological Disorders and Stroke. Post-Polio Syndrome Fact Sheet. Available at: http://www.ninds.nih.gov/disorders/post_polio/detail_post_polio.htm. Accessed July 5, 2010.

Post-Polio Health International. Available at: www.post-polio.org. Accessed July 5, 2010.

Werner R. Post-Polio Syndrome. *Massage Today*. January 2008;08. Available at: http://www.massagetoday.com/mpacms/mt/article.php?id=13741. Accessed July 5, 2010.

31

Post-traumatic Stress Disorder

Also known as:

PTSD (historically: Shell Shock, Battle Fatigue, Soldier's Heart)

Definition: An anxiety disorder triggered by a traumatic event.

GENERAL INFORMATION

- Caused by altered brain chemistry in response to witnessing or experiencing an event that instills fear, helplessness, and horror
- Contributing factors: inherited predisposition to psychiatric illness, anxiety, or depression; intensity of trauma experienced since or during early childhood; individual temperament
- Increased risk with severity, intensity, and/or duration of the event, and with lack of emotional support after the event
- Onset typically within 3 months or even years after the event
- Occurs in people of all ages and in women four times more than men
- Prevalence among survivors of combat, imprisonment, torture, torment, and stalking
- Higher prevalence among African Americans than Caucasians
- Unclear why some experience PTSD and some do not

Morbidity and Mortality

Approximately 60% of men and 50% of women will experience a traumatic event in their lifetime, and about 8% of them will experience PTSD. About 7.7 million American adults suffer from PTSD annually. Experts believe that 30% of Vietnam veterans, 10% of Gulf War veterans, 6–11% of those returning from Afghanistan, and about 12–20% of Iraq War veterans will experience PTSD.

Psychological comorbidities include depression, relationship difficulties, drug and alcohol abuse, eating disorders, and suicide. Physical comorbidities include cardiovascular disease, chronic pain, autoimmune disorders, and musculoskeletal conditions.

The prognosis is poor for those who do not receive treatment, and it is significantly improved for those who receive both therapy and medications. Although troubling memories continue, they lose their power to significantly alter behavior and function.

PATHOPHYSIOLOGY

It is normal to experience temporary discomfort, or even dysfunction, after a traumatic event. A physiologic chain of events sends powerful hormones from the brain to every organ in the body in response to any perceived or real trauma. A car accident, a natural disaster, the death of a loved one—any of these can produce anxiety, lack of focus, sleeping or eating changes, bouts of crying, and even nightmares and recurrent, unwelcome thoughts. After the event passes, the level of "fight-or-flight" response hormones decreases and returns to normal.

The expected response to trauma and loss is to experience strong emotions, coupled with some physiologic reactions, talking about the experience with family and friends, perhaps seeking short-term counseling, and eventually regaining composure and control over a functioning life. (See references to the body's response to stress in Chapter 38.) If, however, symptoms persist in severity and become life- and routine-altering, the person could be experiencing PTSD. Research using MRI and PET (positron emission tomography) has shown on scans that PTSD actually changes the brain's biochemistry and the way memories are stored. Scientists do not know whether the condition is reversible.

Diagnosis is confirmed by a mental health professional who reviews signs and symptoms and performs a psychological evaluation after symptoms have persisted for at least 1 month. PTSD is listed in the *Diagnostic and Statistical Manual of Mental Disorders (DSM)*, published by the American Psychiatric Association, and criteria for a diagnosis are confirmed by the signs and symptoms listed as follows. This step in categorizing the condition as a recognized mental disorder gave PTSD the credibility it did not have previously.

OVERALL SIGNS AND SYMPTOMS

Signs and symptoms are categorized according to the age at which the disorder manifests. They do not appear linearly, that is, from immediately post-event and then dissipating in the future. Instead, signs and symptoms are transient and changing in both frequency and intensity, taking the person by surprise, and often accompanying periods of stress unrelated to the original trauma. Symptoms can become severe enough to place the person at risk for endangering himself or others. Children may experience symptoms that include passivity, feelings of helplessness, and regressive behaviors, while adults, especially men, may manifest much more aggressive and destructive behavior. The signs and symptoms are grouped into three categories:

Intrusive memories:

- Flashbacks, lasting minutes, hours, or days
- Nightmares

Avoidance and emotional numbing:

- Avoiding thoughts about the event
- Avoiding any intense feelings (positive or negative)
- Feeling hopeless
- Difficulty concentrating
- Difficulty maintaining relationships

Increased anxiety and emotional arousal:

- Overwhelming anger, irritability, guilt, or shame
- Self-destructive behavior, including drug and/or alcohol abuse
- Insomnia
- Being easily startled or frightened
- Auditory or visual hallucinations
- Irrational fear for one's own or another's safety

SIGNS AND SYMPTOMS MASSAGE THERAPY CAN ADDRESS

- Many massage techniques induce the parasympathetic state, and these modalities are appropriate for the client suffering with PTSD.
- PTSD is a mental disorder. Symptoms are unpredictable and can be agonizing and/or violent. The normal listening skills and compassionate approach most massage therapists use must be finely honed to prevent transgressing into psychotherapy.
- Massage therapy for a client with PTSD must approach the *muscular hypertonicity* that classically accompanies stress and anxiety *and nothing more.*

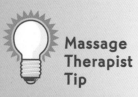

Massage Therapist Tip

Preventing Your Client from Falling Asleep

If a client suffers from PTSD, especially if he has recently returned from active combat, he may experience unexpected and violent flashbacks. These usually occur while falling asleep or during sleep. It is wise, in your work on such a fragile client, *not to allow him to fall asleep.* Although you want to perform techniques that let him relax, if he falls asleep, he may experience a flashback that you are not trained to handle. You can prevent sleep by periodically asking him how he is doing, asking him if the strokes are relieving tension in his muscles, playing music that is slightly more upbeat than the usual soothing massage music, and asking a few questions about one of his favorite topics.

- Advanced training in emotional-release techniques and close supervision by a mental health professional are essential if the therapist is to perform more than the most rudimentary massage techniques.

TREATMENT OPTIONS

Several forms of therapy are recommended to treat PTSD; their effectiveness depends on the person's age and the severity of the symptoms. Cognitive therapy is a talk therapy that helps identify and change painful thought patterns. Exposure therapy, another talk therapy, teaches the safe confrontation of the person's worst nightmares and how to effectively cope. Eye movement desensitization and reprocessing (EMDR) is a series of guided eye movements that helps the brain process traumatic memories. Cognitive behavioral therapy teaches positive behavior after unhealthy beliefs are identified.

Group therapy can be helpful by providing support from like-minded trauma sufferers. Family therapy can help significant others work through their concerns. Any safe and nonaddicting therapy that can help the person achieve a relaxed, parasympathetic state can be highly effective in relieving anxiety and stress and thus lessening the attendant symptoms. (PTSD sufferers must be vigilant not to use alcohol or recreational drugs to mask their pain.)

No therapeutic techniques have been found that can prevent PTSD for those directly affected by trauma. However, immediate debriefing, followed by counseling and peer support, have been proven effective in preventing the disorder from occurring in firefighters, police officers, rescue workers, medical personnel, and volunteers who respond to trauma.

Common Medications

- Selective serotonin reuptake inhibitors (SSRIs), such as fluoxetine hydrochloride (Prozac), paroxetine hydrochloride (Paxil), and sertraline hydrochloride (Zoloft)
- Antipsychotics, such as risperidone (Risperdal), olanzapine (Zyprexa), and quetiapine fumarate (Seroquel)
- Anticonvulsants, such as lamotrigine (Lamictal) and tiagabine hydrochloride (Gabitril)
- Antiseizure medications, such as divalproex sodium (Depakote)

MASSAGE THERAPIST ASSESSMENT

The therapist assesses the client for muscular hypertonicity *only*. A psychological intake is not done because that is beyond the scope of practice. Ideally, the therapist should be made aware that the client has been diagnosed with PTSD or that he has recently experienced a traumatic event. It will help her treat the client more effectively—and safely—if the client offers a short, historical perspective to explain his stress level and muscular tension. The therapist should *not inquire about any psychological symptoms or the initial event.*

THERAPEUTIC GOALS

Reducing muscular hypertonicity that accompanies stress and anxiety, stopping the pain-spasm-pain cycle, and inducing a mild—not deep—parasympathetic state are appropriate treatment goals.

MASSAGE SESSION FREQUENCY

- Ideally: 60-minute sessions once a week
- Minimally: 60-minute sessions every other week
- Infrequent, intermittent 60-minute sessions can provide relief

Thinking It Through

The massage therapist might be the professional who first helps identify that her client is, indeed, suffering from PTSD. Well-reasoned suggestions for the client to seek counseling or medical help may save him and his family from further agony. Referring him to the professional associations listed at the end of this chapter could guide him in the right direction. It may be very difficult for the therapist to remain within her scope of practice, and she can ask herself the following questions as she maintains professional boundaries while simultaneously being of service:

- Am I focusing on the musculature alone? How can I keep myself clearly focused on the muscular hypertonicity and addressing that which I do best?
- What should my responses be if he starts to talk about his traumatic event?
- What will I say if he asks me if I think he has PTSD?
- What will I say if he wants to talk about the conflict in which he was engaged?
- What will I do if he suffers a flashback?
- What is my intention as I treat this client?
- Do I have a list of mental health professionals I can offer him—if he asks for help?
- How can I offer compassionate support while maintaining professional boundaries?

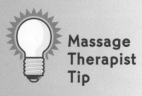

MASSAGE PROTOCOL

The Massage Protocol section of this chapter varies from the usual setup because of the preponderance of necessary precautions. Two possible optional techniques are provided.

The moment you lay your hands on a client's body with a helping intention, the healing process begins. That process is best facilitated if the client reaches a deep parasympathetic state. Before proceeding with the following techniques, both of which induce deep relaxation, make sure that your client does *not* tend to have nightmares or flashbacks. These techniques can be used at the end or the beginning of a session. They can also be ideal for a home or hospital setting, where you do not have the luxury of providing a full 60-minute treatment, and are effective on either a clothed or a disrobed body.

Slow-Stroke Back (or Front) Massage

This protocol assumes that the client is positioned prone, but in many cases (as in a hospital or nursing home environment), the patient may be able to lie supine only.

- Stand at the side of the hospital bed or massage table, facing the client's head. Lay your *non-lubricated* hands (either directly on the client's skin or over the client's clothes) at the base of the client's neck (see Figure 22-1). Using only the weight of your hands (no lighter, because this will be stimulating to the body, and not deeper, because your intent is not to massage muscle) and maintaining full hand (not fingertip) contact, slowly slide your hands down the client's back to the sacrum. It should take you about 1 minute to travel the length of his spine.
- When your hands reach the sacrum, slowly "brush off" your hands to either side of the body.
- Return to the base of the neck immediately and repeat. *This work is unidirectional—running down the spine only.*
- Duration is 15–20 minutes.

Hold and Stroke

This technique can be performed with the client lying in any comfortable position.

- Facing the massage table, standing at about the location of the client's waist, gently place one of your hands on your client's shoulder and the other on his hand. Simply rest *for a full minute*. Focus and determine your intent. Breathe slowly and evenly. Do nothing. Do not speak.
- Once you are focused, begin stroking *down* the arm with the *nonlubricated* hand that was holding your client's shoulder. Use the weight of your full, open hand; do not use your fingertips. Move slowly. This work is performed to the depth at which you would normally apply lubricant and goes no deeper than superficial fascia.
- Repeat three times on one arm.
- Move silently to the contralateral upper extremity and repeat.
- Use slow-stroke back (or front) techniques to the trunk of the body.
- Moving to the lower extremities, place one hand near the head of the femur and the other as far down the leg as you can comfortably reach. Again, center yourself and focus in silence.
- Repeat the slow stroking down the leg.
- Silently move to the other lower extremity and repeat.
- Finish for about 5 minutes of slow-stroke back (or front) massage.
- Duration is 15–30 minutes.

Routine muscle-relaxing techniques are outlined in the step-by-step protocol that follows. Before beginning, ask the client to identify specific areas of hypertonicity; this protocol focuses on the neck and shoulders.

Step-by-Step Protocol for Post-traumatic Stress Disorder

Technique	Duration
With the client positioned comfortably prone, compression, light pressure, using your whole hand • Entire posterior surface of the body	3 minutes
Effleurage, petrissage, effleurage, medium pressure, evenly rhythmic • From the occipital ridge to the sacrum	5 minutes
Digital kneading, medium pressure • In the laminar groove, on either side of the spinous process, from the occipital ridge to the sacrum	3 minutes
Effleurage, slightly deeper pressure • Entire back	2 minutes
Rolling petrissage, kneading, compression, digital kneading, effleurage. Work deep to the client's tolerance. • Bilateral superior trapezius	10 minutes
Turn the client supine, and sit on a stool near his head. Effleurage, deep to his tolerance, working both sides simultaneously. • From the superior deltoids, into the base of the neck, and then up to the occipital ridge	3 minutes
Digital kneading, deep to his tolerance • Occipital ridge	3 minutes
Effleurage, petrissage, effleurage, deep to his tolerance • Superior trapezius	5 minutes
Digital kneading, deep to his tolerance • Laminar grooves, next to the spinous process of the cervical vertebrae	5 minutes
Effleurage, slow, medium pressure • Entire shoulder and neck region	5 minutes
Cleanse your hands. Ask permission to touch the client's face. Digital kneading, medium pressure; slow, evenly rhythmic. • Bilateral temporomandibular joint (TMJ) • Entire mandible	5 minutes
Ask permission to touch the client's scalp. Deep digital kneading, slow, being careful not to tug hair • All scalp muscles	5 minutes
Ask the client to get dressed. Demonstrate door stretching or other appropriate stretches to help relieve hypertonicity.	6 minutes

Contraindications and Cautions

- Do not ask questions about the precipitating traumatic event.
- Use caution when asking about PTSD symptoms. Focus on the secondary musculoskeletal symptoms.
- If the client is mentally unstable, touch may not be an appropriate therapy.
- If at all possible, and only with the client's permission, work with the counseling therapist to coordinate your care and discuss the results you are seeing.

HOMEWORK

You can offer gentle reminders regarding relaxation and self-care to a client whose emotional and psychological state causes constant stress. Stretching tight muscles will help alleviate hypertonicity. Here are some appropriate homework assignments:

- Before sleep, starting at your toes, tighten and release every major muscle group in your body. Tighten and then relax the muscles in your feet, calves, thighs, abdomen, shoulders, neck, and face. Take a few deep breaths once you complete the exercise.
- Throughout the day when you feel anxious, stop what you're doing and take some very long, slow, deep breaths.
- Find small activities that help you relax, such as lighting a candle and playing soft music, working a jigsaw puzzle, doing a crossword puzzle, or watching a relaxing, upbeat movie.
- Be sure to perform the stretching exercises that were demonstrated at the end of your massage session.

Review

1. Define PTSD.
2. Explain several signs and symptoms.
3. Who is at an increased risk for this condition?
4. Describe various appropriate therapies for treating PTSD.
5. Explain, in detail, ways you might unintentionally cross your professional boundaries when treating a client suffering from PTSD.

BIBLIOGRAPHY

American Psychiatric Association. *Diagnostic and Statistical Manual of Mental Disorders*, 4th ed. (*DSM-IV*). Washington, DC: American Psychiatric Association, 2000.

Fitch P, Dryden T. Recovering Body and Soul from Post-Traumatic Stress Disorder. Available at: http://pamelafitch-rmt.com/docs/soul.pdf. Accessed April 5, 2011.

Foote C. What is Post Traumatic Stress Disorder—Part I: The Causes. March 17, 2000. Available at: http://www.suite101.com/article.cfm/womens_ptsd/35615. Accessed July 16, 2010.

Foote C. What is Post Traumatic Stress Disorder—Part 2: The Symptoms. March 31, 2000. Available at: http://www.suite101.com/article.cfm/womens_ptsd/36173. Accessed July 16, 2010.

MayoClinic.com. Post-traumatic stress disorder (PTSD). Available at: http://www.mayoclinic.com/health/post-traumatic-stress-disorder/DS00246. Accessed July 16, 2010.

National Center for PTSD, Department of Veterans Affairs. What is PTSD? Available at: http://www.ptsd.va.gov/public/pages/what-is-ptsd.asp. Accessed July 16, 2010.

Upledger J. The Role of CranioSacral Therapy in Addressing Post-Traumatic Stress Disorder. *Massage Today*. November 2001;01. Available at: http://www.massagetoday.com/mpacms/mt/article.php?id=10353. Accessed July 17, 2010.

Wanveer T. Post-Traumatic Stress Disorder and Cell Patterns. *Massage Today*. January 2008; 08. Available at: http://www.massagetoday.com/mpacms/mt/article.php?id=13737. Accessed July 17, 2010.

WebMD. Post-Traumatic Stress Disorder (PTSD). Available at: http://www.webmd.com/mental-health/post-traumatic-stress-disorder. Accessed July 17, 2010.

32

Raynaud's Phenomenon

Also known as:

Primary Raynaud's (or Raynaud's Disease); Secondary Raynaud's (or Raynaud's Syndrome)

Definition: Chronic, episodic peripheral vasoconstriction (blood vessel narrowing), usually precipitated by an extreme response to cold temperatures.

GENERAL INFORMATION

- Primary Raynaud's: cause unknown
- Secondary Raynaud's: caused by disease, injury, or repetitive impact damage to arteries and nerves in hands and feet, exposure to vinyl chloride (a plastic component), frostbite, or medications that narrow arteries or affect blood pressure
- Primary Raynaud's onset: age 15–25; secondary Raynaud's onset: after age 40
- Increased risk from nicotine inhalation; migraine medications containing ergotamine; cancer medications, such as cisplatin and vinblastine; beta-blockers; contraceptive pills; and over-the-counter (OTC) cold, allergy, and diet pills
- Primary Raynaud's more common, less severe than secondary Raynaud's; affects people of all ages
- Fingers usually affected, toes less frequently, usually bilateral; nose, ears, lips rarely
- Possible genetic link
- Primary Raynaud's prevalence: women age 30 or younger who live in a cold climate, or have a family history of the disorder
- Lifetime duration
- No cure

Morbidity and Mortality

About 5% of the U.S. population and 3–20% of the worldwide population have some form of Raynaud's phenomenon. Primary Raynaud's can be so mild that it presents neither medical nor lifestyle challenges. Secondary Raynaud's, however, coexists with underlying conditions, making it more difficult to manage and thus causing substantial medical and life-altering challenges. Comorbidities of secondary Raynaud's include rheumatoid arthritis, atherosclerosis, scleroderma, lupus, carpal tunnel syndrome, and Sjögren's syndrome.

Tissue damage or limb disability does not usually result from lifelong Raynaud's, but occasionally repeated, severe episodes can lead to skin sores and gangrene (death or decay of body tissues). Although there is no cure, both forms of the condition can be successfully managed and controlled.

PATHOPHYSIOLOGY

When the body is exposed to cold, the normal physiologic response is a redirection of blood flow from the periphery (hands and feet) to the core. A similar response occurs during episodes of anxiety or stress, and as a side effect of taking certain medications. During a Raynaud's attack, which is usually triggered by exposure to cold, and sometimes by emotional upset, the body overreacts by severely constricting blood vessels that feed (and thus warm) the hands and feet, leaving the affected areas with a longer-than-usual sensation of extreme cold. The initial cause of this physiologic reaction remains unclear.

Diagnosis is confirmed by medical history and physical examination, combined with a cold simulation test, during which the hands or feet are briefly placed in ice water in an attempt to trigger Raynaud's symptoms. A nail fold capillaroscopy, to examine microscopic nail cells, can help confirm a diagnosis and differentiate between the primary and secondary forms. No simple tests exist that can absolutely confirm Raynaud's. Blood tests, arterial Doppler studies, and arteriograms help rule out other circulatory disorders.

OVERALL SIGNS AND SYMPTOMS

Signs and symptoms, although they share the same physiologic basis, differ significantly in primary and secondary Raynaud's. Primary Raynaud's symptoms can be so mild and fleeting that a firm diagnosis is never made and treatment is never sought. The frequency and intensity of secondary Raynaud's, however, often prevent normal daily activities, and the condition is sufficiently distressing to require medical attention. Attacks can begin in one finger or toe and thereafter move to other digits. The same toes or fingers are not affected every time. Attacks vary in length from 1 minute to several hours and can occur daily or weekly. Typically, the following signs and symptoms occur sequentially in the fingers and/or toes:

- Skin turning white, then blue
- Numbness, coldness, pain
- Skin turning red
- Throbbing, tingling, burning
- Severe pain and/or discomfort, and/or difficulty with hand or foot function

SIGNS AND SYMPTOMS MASSAGE THERAPY CAN ADDRESS

- Because Raynaud's phenomenon involves compromised peripheral circulation, massage therapy, which increases circulation, can successfully address this condition.
- When symptoms result from comorbidities, the therapist must address the coexisting condition *first* and then attend to the circulatory challenges.
- When anxiety and/or stress are known triggers, massage techniques that induce a parasympathetic state are effective in increasing circulation and instilling a sense of calm.

TREATMENT OPTIONS

The treatment of Raynaud's depends on its classification. Primary care physicians and internists will treat both forms of Raynaud's while aiming to reduce the number and severity of attacks, prevent tissue damage, and address underlying medical conditions.

Prevention and self-care include keeping the body warm, maintaining a room temperature higher than 68–70°F, avoiding exposure to cold, using hand warmers, exercising regularly, and massaging the hands and feet. Clients are also counseled to reduce anxiety, stop smoking, and avoid caffeine, nicotine, and certain medications that trigger attacks. Pragmatic lifestyle adaptations include wearing gloves while removing frozen items from the freezer, drinking hot liquids, warming the hands under *warm* (not hot) running water, and swinging the arms in a large circle to temporarily increase peripheral blood flow.

Ginkgo biloba has been shown to reduce the number of attacks, and several ongoing studies support the use of this herb in the treatment of Raynaud's. Fish oil

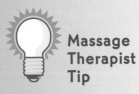

Massage Therapist Tip

Curbing the Power of Your Handshake

You may be seeing a client who is experiencing a current Raynaud's attack, and her hands might be painfully throbbing. If your usual approach includes a warm, firm handshake, you may want to forgo this greeting until you are sure your Raynaud's client is pain-free. Even if she has only mild Raynaud's, her hands may be constantly sensitive, in which case she may be guarded. A warm, verbal greeting is the best approach.

supplements, evening primrose oil, and ginger have also been used with varying levels of success. In rare cases, nerve-blocking surgery is necessary.

Common Medications

Medication is not generally prescribed to treat primary Raynaud's. The use of vasodilating medications is common only for secondary Raynaud's. Prescription skin creams can address local circulation and treat compromised and damaged tissue.

- Antianginals, such as nifedipine (Adalat) and diltiazem hydrochloride (Dilacor)
- Antihypertensives, such as prazosin hydrochloride (Minipress)

MASSAGE THERAPIST ASSESSMENT

The client will most likely present to a massage therapist after a physician has diagnosed either primary or secondary Raynaud's. Primary Raynaud's symptoms will be mild, may be visible and palpable by the therapist, and rarely pose a therapeutic challenge. However, comorbidities associated with secondary Raynaud's will require the massage therapist to speak directly with the physician. Questions about the underlying disease, the possibility of the presence of tissue damage, lurking deep vein thrombosis (DVT), or potential gangrene must be addressed before the therapist proceeds.

Since primary Raynaud's is far more common, the succeeding protocol addresses treating these signs and symptoms. A protocol is not given for secondary Raynaud's because the array of comorbidities is too numerous.

In either case, the therapist's assessment includes questions about the frequency and duration of the attacks—whether the hands, feet, or, more rarely, the nose and lips are affected—and the pain level. Asking about what causes an attack (cold temperatures, emotional upset) further helps determine the therapy's focus.

Gentle palpation of the affected tissue will help identify the extent of tissue damage, if any. Palpation will also determine sensory and motor function and pain tolerance. The therapist can safely proceed with treatment at any time before, during, or after an episode.

THERAPEUTIC GOALS

Therapeutic goals for treating Raynaud's include increasing local circulation and inducing a deep parasympathetic state. As mentioned, with secondary Raynaud's, the goals must be appropriate to the treatment of the underlying medical condition.

MASSAGE SESSION FREQUENCY

Primary Raynaud's: With a chronic yet episodic circulatory condition, it is best if the client routinely receives massage therapy as part of her self-care regimen, rather than wait for the episodes to cause distress and discomfort, which can further exacerbate the condition.

- Ideally: 60-minute sessions every other week
- Minimally: 60-minute sessions once a month

Secondary Raynaud's: Addressing this condition is possible only after treating the underlying medical condition. The therapist determines session frequency and duration based on the client's medical history, and treats secondary Raynaud's concurrently.

Thinking It Through

As always, empathy leads to more effective massage therapy. Although it may be tempting to think that a medical condition that merely produces cold hands and/or feet is somehow less severe than other, more dramatic conditions, awareness might be increased if the therapist performs the following exercise.

- Fill a large container with cold water and ice cubes.
- Wear a buttoned shirt. Place some pins or other small items on a nearby surface.
- Place both of your hands in the container until the sensation of cold is intolerable.
- Remove and dry your hands.
- Now, try to unbutton and button your shirt.
- Try to pick up the small items.
- Be aware of how long it takes your hands to return to normal sensation and function, and of the uncomfortable sensations along the way.
- Think about how your life would be affected if these symptoms appeared whenever you were even mildly cold or emotionally upset.

Step-by-Step Protocol for Primary Raynaud's (Bilateral Hands)

Technique	Duration
Perform relaxing techniques, anywhere the client requests, to bring the body into a parasympathetic state.	10 minutes
With the client positioned supine, effleurage, petrissage, effleurage, medium-to-deep pressure • Bilateral superior trapezius	5 minutes
From this point forward, perform the techniques on one arm only before moving to the contralateral side. Effleurage, petrissage, effleurage, medium-to-deep pressure • Entire anterior, medial, and posterior deltoid	3 minutes
Effleurage, petrissage, effleurage, kneading, long, deep strokes performed from elbow to shoulder • Biceps and triceps • Flexors and extensors	5 minutes
Digital kneading, ROM followed by long, deep strokes from wrist to elbow • Carpals	2 minutes
Hold the client's hand in both of yours. Ask her to relax so all muscles are loose and easy to get to. Working *cephalically*, use your thumbs and fingers to deeply and broadly spread and massage all tissue. • Carpals • Palmar and dorsal surface of the hand • Each finger	4 minutes
Still holding the hand, digitally massage, deep to the client's tolerance, each section of every finger, beginning distally, working proximally, and massaging *cephalically*.	5 minutes
Effleurage, deep to the client's tolerance • From the fingertips to the wrist • From the wrist to the elbow • From the elbow to the deltoids	2 minutes (Total for one arm: 21 minutes)
Repeat the previous steps to the contralateral arm, forearm, and hand.	21 minutes
Perform relaxing techniques, at the client's request, to ensure the client leaves the table in a parasympathetic state.	8 minutes

MASSAGE PROTOCOL

The following protocol addresses primary Raynaud's. Even with mild symptoms, affected extremities must be approached with care and attention. After a thorough visual and manual examination, you will most likely spend significant time deeply massaging the *proximal* region of the affected limb, after which you will approach the affected area. Work will be detailed, specific, localized, and intelligent as you attempt to soften and spread affected tissue, increase local circulation, and return waste products to the proximal limb. Your work will be not only therapeutic but also possibly preventive. An important element of your work will be teaching self-massage to your client.

Getting Started

Determine which limbs you will focus on, and be prepared to pillow and position the client accordingly. Your main focus will most likely be on the bilateral arms and hands, but the feet can also be affected. Rarely will you have to address both upper and lower extremities. Because you do want to bring the body into a parasympathetic state, the client will need to disrobe if you intend to perform relaxing Swedish techniques before you begin your localized work.

HOMEWORK

The ease of reaching one's own hands and feet proves to be advantageous when instructing your Raynaud's client about self-care massage. Although she has been warned by her physician to be vigilant about handling cold items and exposing herself to cold temperatures, it is well within your scope of practice to offer supportive advice in this area also. Here are some recommended homework assignments:

- Massage your hands and/or feet frequently and deeply, but not to the point of pain. Work from your fingertips to your wrists, or from your toes to your ankles—stroking, pulling, and tugging in the direction of your elbow or knee.
- Shake your hands or feet vigorously after you massage them.
- Swing your arms in vigorous big circles several times each day.
- Run your hands or feet under *warm* water if you feel an attack coming on.
- Keep gloves near the refrigerator, and don't take anything out of the freezer with your bare hands.
- Stay warm at all times.
- Try to avoid becoming anxious or overly stressed.

Review

1. Define Raynaud's phenomenon.
2. Distinguish between primary and secondary Raynaud's.
3. Which form is more common and less severe?
4. Explain the physiology of Raynaud's phenomenon.
5. Describe your challenge as a massage therapist when treating secondary Raynaud's clients.

BIBLIOGRAPHY

Davis V. Conservative Management of Raynaud's Disease. *Dynamic Chiropractic* 1995;13. Available at: www.chiroweb.com/mpacms/dc/article.php?id=40166. Accessed July 17, 2010.

Estrad S. Raynaud's Phenomenon—Topic Overview. Arthritis WebMD. Available at: http://arthritis.webmd.com/tc/raynauds-phenomenon-topic-overview. Accessed July 7, 2010.

Ginkgo Biloba (yin xing yi) [Article] MassageToday.com. Available at: http://www.massagetoday.com/topics/herbcentral/ginkgo_biloba.php. Accessed July 7, 2010.

Rattray F, Ludwig L. *Clinical Massage Therapy: Understanding, Assessing and Treating over 70 Conditions*, Toronto: Talus Incorporated, 2000.

Raynaud's Disease. MayoClinic.com. Available at: http://www.mayoclinic.com/health/raynauds-disease/DS00433/DSECTION=causes. Accessed July 17, 2010.

Raynaud's Phenomenon. NIAMS article. April 2009. Available at: http://www.niams.nih.gov/Health_Info/Raynauds_Phenomenon/default.asp. Accessed July 17, 2010.

Werner R. *A Massage Therapist's Guide to Pathology*, 4th ed. Philadelphia: Lippincott Williams & Wilkins, 2009.

What is Raynaud's? [Article] NHLBI Disease and Conditions Index. Available at: http://www.nhlbi.nih.gov/health/dci/Diseases/raynaud/ray_what.html. Accessed July 17, 2010.

33

Rheumatoid Arthritis

Definition: A chronic, inflammatory, and autoimmune disease affecting both the connective tissue and the synovial membrane of multiple joints.

GENERAL INFORMATION

- Etiology unknown; compromised immune system possible contributing factor
- Gradual onset
- All ages affected; most common between ages 25 and 50
- Women affected three times more often than men
- Remission usual in pregnant women with RA; high occurrence in women immediately postpartum
- Affects about 1% of the U.S. population
- Genetic predisposition

PATHOPHYSIOLOGY

RA results from many factors; there is no single genetic cause, as previously thought. The immune system's involvement in the development of RA is indicated by the presence of an antibody called rheumatoid factor (RF) in most cases. The body normally creates a specific antibody for every recognized invader. In an autoimmune disorder, the body mistakenly perceives part of its normal functioning to be invasive and sets up a defensive response against itself. RA is an example, and its inflammatory reaction can be powerful.

The disease triggers attacks on the joints' synovial fluid (necessary for normal joint movement), creating an inflammatory environment characterized by heat, swelling, pain, and stiffness. Multiple inflammatory chemicals are present during the disease's flare stage, thereby causing a domino effect of pain and swelling: (1) The presence of inflammatory chemicals leads to joint capsule fluid accumulation; (2) the synovial membrane thickens and swells, causing more fluid accumulation; (3) further internal joint pressure and pain trigger more inflamed tissue; (4) the cascading damage cyclically continues until bone and cartilage are also damaged.

Bilateral hand and wrist joints are commonly affected initially (Figure 33-1). The disease can progress to the knee, ankle, and foot joints. In severe cases, spinal involvement (C-1 and C-2) results in seriously compromised neck range of motion (ROM).

Progression is usually gradual, but it can occasionally be fast, followed by periods of flare and remission. RA can affect various joints mildly and not get worse for years and then drop into remission with only occasional flare-ups. In some cases, it progresses unremittingly from a mild state to frequent flares and severe debilitation.

Diagnosis is determined by various tests. Blood serum tests indicating the presence of RF, in approximately 75% of the diagnosed cases, reveals that the body is waging an autoimmune battle. However, some who suffer from RA do not have RF and some who have RF do not manifest the disease. A medical history is taken, along with X-rays of painful joints. Because RA can mimic other skeletal and musculoskeletal disorders, a firm diagnosis is often not made until four of the following symptoms

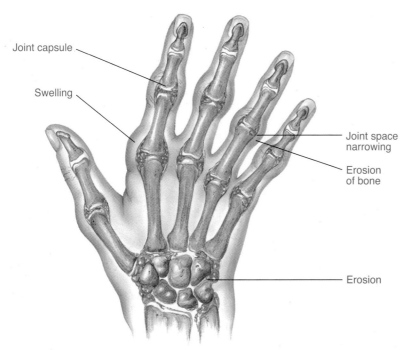

FIGURE 33-1 **Joints typically affected by rheumatoid arthritis. Asset provided by Anatomical Chart Co.**

persist: (1) rheumatoid nodules (firm, nontender, and subcutaneous joint nodules), (2) arthritis in three or more joints, (3) morning stiffness that persists for at least an hour, (4) arthritis of the fingers and wrist, (5) bilateral involvement, (6) a positive blood test for RF, and (7) X-rays indicating bony involvement.

If complete remission occurs, it is usually within the first 2 years of the disease. The prognosis varies; some clients live a mildly compromised life, while others may become wheelchair-bound. In rare cases, RA clients die from pulmonary and/or renal compromise.

OVERALL SIGNS AND SYMPTOMS

Symptoms manifest, with dramatically varying degrees of severity, depending on whether the disease is in the early stages, or if the client is experiencing a flare or a remission. During remission, the signs of RA continue but the painful inflammatory response is absent. Moderate RA is characterized by several flares followed by remissions. In severe RA, however, the inflammation is chronic and remissions are infrequent.

Early stage:

- Malaise
- Vague muscle aches and pains
- Gradual worsening, becoming joint specific
- Low-grade fever
- Appetite loss
- Anemia

Remission (subacute) stage:

- Stiffness after long periods of immobility
- Stiff, often deformed, swollen bilateral joints
- Shiny, tightly stretched skin over affected joints
- Puffy joints

- Achy affected extremity
- Malaise
- Anemia

Flare (acute) stage:

- Red, hot, painful, and swollen joints
- Restricted, painful ROM
- Improved movement with mild stretching
- Anemia

SIGNS AND SYMPTOMS MASSAGE THERAPY CAN ADDRESS

- Research indicates that massage decreases stress hormones and depression, increases natural painkilling endorphins, improves sleep and immune function, and eases muscle pain.
- Since persistent stress triggers pain and persistent pain triggers stress, both of which initiate the cascading effects of inflammation, any relaxation technique that reduces pain and stress can help address the deteriorating effects of this inflammatory disease.

TREATMENT OPTIONS

Early, aggressive treatment, which is often based on multiple medications, is supervised by a rheumatologist. This approach has recently replaced the more passive "wait and see" family physician approach of the past. The treatment goals are reducing pain and inflammation, minimizing joint damage, and improving well-being and overall function. A medication regimen focused on the specific RA stage, combined with diet alteration, exercise, stress reduction, massage, and sometimes surgery, can help meet these treatment goals.

Beneficial self-management techniques include hot showers to relieve morning stiffness, consistent yet moderate exercise, and massage during the remission stage. Acupuncture can release natural anti-inflammatory endorphins and can ease pain.

Various highly effective surgical options can significantly make the difference between a client living with intolerable pain and/or being wheelchair-bound or living a near-normal existence. Synovectomy removes the diseased joint lining, thereby reducing inflammatory tissue. Arthroscopic surgery determines the extent of bone and joint damage and simultaneously repairs tears. Joint replacement surgery reconstructs or replaces highly compromised joints. Arthrodesis fuses two bones together leading to limited movement but decreasing joint pain and increasing stability.

Common Medications

A medication cocktail is often the most effective pharmaceutical approach in treating this multi-symptomatic, systemic condition. Several categories of medications may be prescribed based on disease progression and the extent of systemic involvement. Nonsteroidal anti-inflammatory drugs (NSAIDs) help reduce inflammation and pain. Analgesics reduce pain but don't affect inflammation. Steroids slow joint damage caused by inflammation. Biologic response modifiers quiet the overreaction of the immune system in an autoimmune disease. Examples of commonly used medications are as follows:

- Salicylate nonopioid pain relievers, such as aspirin (Ecotrin, Empirin, Astrin)
- Nonopioid pain reliever and fever reducers, such as acetaminophen (Tylenol, Feverall, Anacin, Panadol)

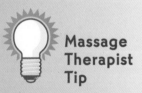

Massage Therapist Tip

Being Aware of Medication Side Effects

Your RA client will most likely be taking multiple medications, most of which have significant side effects. Question your client about the duration, frequency, timing, and severity of her medication side effects. You may need to adapt your massage session to accommodate for dizziness, bathroom trips, and nausea. It is not beyond your scope of practice to sit down with your client and make a small chart of her medication side effects, so you can adjust your sessions accordingly.

- Anti-inflammatory immunosuppressants, such as methylprednisolone (Medrol)
- Heavy metal antagonist antirheumatics, such as penicillamine (Cuprimine)
- Immunosuppressants, such as azathioprine (Imuran) and abatacept (Orencia)
- Antimalarial amebicides, such as chloroquine (Aralen)
- Antimalarial anti-inflammatories, such as hydroxychloroquine (Plaquenil)
- Anti-inflammatories, such as sulfasalazine (Azulfidine) and infliximab (Remicade)
- Antirheumatics, such as etanercept (Enbrel) and adalimumab (Humira)
- Human monoclonal antibodies, such as golimumab (Simponi)

MASSAGE THERAPIST ASSESSMENT

Assessing an RA client includes the following:

- Observing compensatory movement and affected joints
- Intelligent, compassionate querying about ROM and about joint and muscle pain
- Gentle, cautious palpating of joint and muscle
- Thoroughly listing all medications and side effects
- Determining, with the client's help, whether she is experiencing a flare or remission

The therapist must approach an RA client with caution because serious damage can result from overzealous therapy.

An RA client will be under a physician's care and may be seeing a physical therapist. It is best for the massage therapist to create a working relationship with both.

THERAPEUTIC GOALS

When the RA client is in early stages of the disease or is in remission, it is reasonable to expect that massage therapy can improve joint mobility, maintain connective tissue health, increase or maintain ROM, and reduce the pain and stress that often exacerbate the condition.

MASSAGE SESSION FREQUENCY

- 60-minute sessions once a week for the duration of the disease (except when the client is experiencing a flare)
- Infrequent therapy provides only temporary, palliative relief

MASSAGE PROTOCOL

Because of the autoimmune, systemic, and inflammatory nature of RA, the body's lymphatic and immune systems will be compromised. Any gentle, cephalic, effleurage-like techniques will help stimulate and cleanse these systems. Gentle proximal (to the affected joint) ROM will also stimulate lymph nodes.

Gentle exploratory palpation will help you determine the presence of swollen joints and rheumatoid nodules. Remember to proceed gently and to establish trust early to enable you to work with the appropriate depth as the session proceeds. Never work to the point of pain or even mild discomfort.

Techniques, such as skin rolling, compression, and dry effleurage that move and shift the ever-weaving but most likely profound stuck myofascia will also help eliminate waste products and increase ROM. Never use jostling or excitatory techniques that could risk moving your client into a sympathetic state.

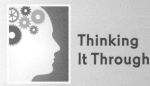

Thinking It Through

Extensive research, ranging from studying the electro-encephalographs (EEGs) of meditating monks to analyzing the heart rates of frustrated rats, repeatedly proves the profound healing that takes place in the body during the parasympathetic state. The cascading neuronal effects of a sympathetic ("fight-or-flight") response can last for hours or days and can exacerbate any systemic disease. However, the parasympathetic state, a state of deep physiologic rest, significantly reduces the effects of pain and stress. With this in mind, the therapist can ask himself how he maintains a calm mental state during a massage therapy session, and how he can affect others by helping them relax.

- What is my mental or emotional state as I approach my clients?
- If I am presently ill at ease, what can I do to erase my personal irritations so I can focus calmly on this client?
- What does my body feel like when I'm irritated or upset?
- What does my body feel like when I'm profoundly relaxed?
- Which techniques have I learned that can help my client reach a parasympathetic state?
- Where in the protocol should I include relaxation exercises?
- What are the signs that my client is not relaxing?
- Have I thought deeply about the mind-body connection and its effects on every aspect of my client's life?

Contraindications and Cautions

- Since RA symptoms are exacerbated during a flare, all bodywork during this painful stage is absolutely contraindicated.

- Heat is never appropriate on tissue that is inflamed or swollen.

- Cold should be used judiciously and only after receiving permission from the attending physician or physical therapist.

- The end-feel of affected joints may not have the "bounce" of a normal joint; use caution during ROM exercises and stop immediately upon meeting resistance.

- RA medications may thin the client's blood or dull her pain perception. Do not work so deeply that you cause bruising.

Step-by-Step Protocol for **Rheumatoid Arthritis of Bilateral Wrists and Fingers**

Technique	Duration
Before beginning, palpate both wrists and hands for the presence of tenderness, nodules, and inflammation. If the joints are warm to the touch and/or appear red, do not proceed until the client is no longer in a flare.	
With the client positioned comfortably, place a hot pack on the left wrist and hand. Perform "slaying-the-dragon" techniques (general comforting techniques) anywhere on the body except the upper extremities.	5 minutes
Remove the hot pack, reheat it, and place it on the right wrist and hand. Watch the clock while performing the next step, and remove the hot pack after 5 minutes.	
Compression, light-to-medium pressure • The entire left upper extremity, begin proximally, work to the wrist and fingers. Be sure to include detailed compression on each digit.	2 minutes
Wringing, light-to-medium pressure • Biceps, triceps, flexors, extensors (*Do not wring affected joints.*)	2 minutes
ROM to end-feel • Shoulder • Elbow (spend extra time at this joint) • Wrist • Every joint of each digit	2 minutes
Compression, medium-to-deep pressure, a little more briskly • The entire left upper extremity, begin proximally, work to the wrist and fingers	2 minutes
Effleurage, petrissage, effleurage, medium pressure • Left biceps and triceps • Left flexors and extensors	4 minutes
Any combination of detailed effleurage, plucking, friction, petrissage, compression, digital kneading, and medium pressure • Around each left carpal bone • Around and between each knuckle joint • Into the palmar and dorsal hand surface	10 minutes
ROM to end-feel (noting if range has improved) • Wrist • Every joint of each digit	2 minutes
Effleurage, deep to tolerance • Start proximally at shoulder, work to end of digits	1 minute (Total time 25 minutes)
Repeat protocol to right arm, wrist, and hand.	25 minutes
Finish with relaxation techniques performed per the client's request.	5 minutes

GETTING STARTED

Have hot packs and cold packs ready. Provide plenty of pillows and be inventive with positioning to accommodate your client's limited ROM. Be sure to offer her a bathroom break sometime during the session. If she uses a cane, walker, or wheelchair, rearrange your working space and reception area for easy and safe access. You may need to help her on and off the table and with undressing and dressing.

HOMEWORK

Your client will most likely be seeing a physical therapist (PT) or a personal trainer along with her attending physician. She certainly has been instructed to exercise, breathe deeply, and maintain her ROM. You can frequently and diplomatically remind her that even though she is in pain, if she does not continually use her muscles and joints, she will lose movement and will experience even more pain. Joints that are swollen and painful, however, should not be worked. The following homework assignments are well within your scope of practice and can provide the added support your client needs to maintain a desirable lifestyle. Detailed strengthening exercises are best left to a trained PT.

- Before exercising, apply heat via a hot pack or a hot shower.
- Move gently at the start of your exercise regimen to warm the joints and muscles.
- Move every joint of your body, not just your affected ones, into full ROM every day.
- Avoid keeping your joints in the same position for long periods.
- Avoid long periods of grasping and pinching.
- Breathe deeply at least three times a day.
- Practice progressive relaxation exercises. Lying down or sitting comfortably progressively tighten and relax every major muscle set of your body. Work from your toes to your nose. Imagine all the stress leaving each muscle as you relax it.
- Drink plenty of water. Your muscles and joints will benefit, and adequate hydration will help your liver efficiently process your medications.

Review

1. Define rheumatoid arthritis.
2. Describe the symptoms during remission and during a flare.
3. In which joints does RA usually initially occur?
4. Which connective tissues may also be affected by RA?
5. Describe the various classifications of medications an RA client may be taking.
6. Explain the massage therapy contraindications for an RA client.
7. What is the prognosis for a client who has an RA?

BIBLIOGRAPHY

Anderson RB. Researching the Effects of Massage Therapy in Treating Rheumatoid Arthritis. *Massage Today*. November 2007;7(12). Available at: http://www.massagetoday.com/mpacms/mt/article.php?id=13716. Accessed January 4, 2011.

Arthritis Foundation. Overview: Common Therapies to Consider. Available at: http://www.arthritis.org/common-therapies-to-consider.php. Accessed January 4, 2011.

Arthritis Foundation. Rheumatoid Arthritis. Available at: http://www.arthritis.org/disease-center.php?disease_id=31. Accessed January 4, 2011.

Food and Drug Administration. FDA Approves Monthly Injectable Drug for Treating Three Types of Immune-Related Arthritis. April 24, 2009. Available at: http://www.fda.gov/NewsEvents/Newsroom/PressAnnouncements/ucm149569.htm. Accessed January 4, 2011.

MayoClinic. Rheumatoid Arthritis Pain: "Tips for Protecting" Your Joints: Use These Joint Protection Techniques to Help You Stay in Control of Your Rheumatoid Arthritis. Available at: http://www.mayoclinic.com/health/arthritis/AR00015. Accessed January 4, 2011.

National Institute of Arthritis and Musculoskeletal and Skin Diseases (NIAMS). Rheumatoid Arthritis. May 2004. Available at: http://www.niams.nih.gov/Health_Info/Rheumatic_Disease/default.asp. Accessed January 4, 2011.

Rattray F, Ludwig L. *Clinical Massage Therapy: Understanding, Assessing, and Treating over 70 Conditions*. Toronto: Talus Incorporated, 2000.

Relaxation Response Can Influence Expression of Stress-related Genes. *Massage Magazine*. July 2, 2008. Available at: http://www.massagemag.com/News/massage-news.php?id=2830&catid=16&title=relaxation-response-can-influence-expression-of-stress-related-genes. Accessed January 4, 2011.

Werner R. *A Massage Therapist's Guide to Pathology*, 4th ed. Philadelphia: Lippincott Williams & Wilkins, 2009.

34

Scars

Definition: Irregular fibrous tissue that replaces normal tissue following injury or incision.

GENERAL INFORMATION

- Caused by lacerative trauma, burns, surgery, and breaches in the dermis
- Can occur anywhere on the body
- Onset within hours of injury; ongoing formation
- More prevalent in younger people

PATHOPHYSIOLOGY

The following scenario outlines the body's physiologic response to any localized injury, including the chemical reaction of scar formation. The explanation also reinforces the thinking behind the massage protocol. When a finger is accidentally cut by a knife, bleeding immediately ensues from lacerated capillaries. Multiple alert signals to the brain indicate something akin to, "Oh no, the body is bleeding, we've got to act fast to close up this wound!" Chemicals rush to the area to cauterize capillary ends, thereby stopping the bleeding. Tissue regrowth starts immediately to close the skin rupture. Because the skin barrier was breached, there is a possibility of infection, and macrophages flood the site to combat infectious organisms. The process is efficient and swift, but not tidy. A microscopic view would reveal a messy network of collagen and fibroblasts knitting tissue back together quickly to heal the breach and avoid infection. Next comes the pathophysiology of scar formation.

When an insult or injury happens to the body from a surgical incision, a burn, a trauma, or a severe dermatological condition, a natural healing process begins, involving an inflammatory response and a complex chemical domino effect. The result is wound healing, scar formation, and the avoidance of infection. Here are the basic steps in this cascading process:

1. Inflammation and vascularization
2. Epithelium rebuilding
3. Tissue granulation
4. Fibroplasias and matrix formation
5. Wound contraction
6. New vascularization
7. Matrix and collagen remodeling

The entire process can last from a matter of weeks to as long as 2 years.

Matrix and collagen remodeling is of particular interest to the massage therapist because this is a process that can be directly affected by massage techniques. *Therapists should note that localized inflammation and the presence of macrophages are important, ongoing elements in the formation of healthy, pliable scar tissue. This will become evident during the protocol discussion later in this chapter.*

Although all scars diminish in size and color over time, the final scar tissue is different from, and weaker than, the original skin. The previously symmetrical collagen and fascia are replaced by an irregular web of tissue that is only about 80% as strong as the preinjured site. Sensation may be lost, and sweat pores or hair follicles are gone. A person's metabolism, activity level, vitamin and mineral intake, insulin delivery, immune system efficiency, ethnic background, and age can directly affect wound healing and scarring.

Other forms of compromised tissue not addressed in this chapter, but directly related to scarring, include the following:

- *Adhesion:* Plates, strands, or localized scar tissue that typically form in the chest, abdomen, or pelvis after surgery or radiation
- *Fibrotic adhesion:* Plates, strands, or localized scar tissue that form secondary to ongoing chronic inflammatory conditions affecting joints
- *Hypertrophic scar:* Scar tissue overgrowth that remains within the boundaries of the original insult but involves tissue deep into the dermis; often associated with second- and third-degree burns
- *Keloid scar:* Scar tissue overgrowth outside the boundaries of the original injury; often characterized by a gnarled, noticeably ropy appearance, and most often found in dark-skinned people
- *Contracture:* Shortened connective tissue, usually around a joint, formed after prolonged immobility

OVERALL SIGNS AND SYMPTOMS

Wounds and scars are classified into characteristic stages of acute, subacute, and chronic. Depending on the severity of the injury, the wound or scarring process can last from a matter of weeks to as long as 2 years.

Acute scarring (earliest):

- Redness
- Raised appearance
- Hypersensitivity
- Continuous weeping of serous fluid

Subacute scarring (wound healing begun):

- Pink or pale appearance
- Flat or slightly puckered appearance
- Possible lost sensation

Chronic scarring (wound healing complete):

- Slightly raised, puckered, or sunken appearance
- A white line in lighter skin and a dark line in darker skin
- Taut, probably insensitive tissue surrounding the scar
- Usually not problematic or painful
- Coolness compared to surrounding tissue
- Possible stiffness or pulling if the scar lies close to or on a joint

SIGNS AND SYMPTOMS MASSAGE THERAPY CAN ADDRESS

- Massage therapy can loosen restrictive fibrous tissue, increase localized circulation, and facilitate healing.
- Since the matrix and collagen remodeling phase can last for months, during which time tensile strength—the rebounding, responsive, soft but resilient

nature of normal skin—is being restored, the final appearance and integrity of scarred skin can be improved by massage therapy techniques.

TREATMENT OPTIONS

Although scarring cannot be completely eliminated, the goals of treatment are to minimize scar appearance, speed up tissue healing, and improve tissue mobility. Some products applied topically can reduce unsightliness, but more research is needed to validate the effectiveness claimed by their advertising.

Invasive and minor surgeries can alter a scar's appearance and increase tissue mobility. Dermabrasion removes built-up skin, and chemical peels and laser resurfacing even out color and texture. Grafting healthy skin from another part of the body and attaching it to extensively burned or injured areas can help control or prevent long-term regional stiffness and immobility. Cortisone injection may effectively reduce the appearance of keloid or hypertrophic scarring.

Common Medications

Prescription or over-the-counter (OTC) medications applied directly to a healing wound or postoperative site can facilitate repair, increase the rate of epithelial tissue growth, and decrease infection. The following is a list of prescription and OTC medications formulated to help treat keloid scars, minimize surgical scars, minimize old scars, and reduce burn scars. Before any of these medications are used, a physician should be consulted about the manufacturer's promised results. (Note: Most of these kinds of medicines are known primarily by their brand name, so they are listed that way.)

- MEDscar
- Dermatix Ultra
- Talsyn-CI

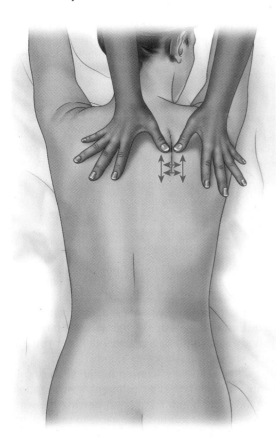

FIGURE 34-1 **Cross-fiber friction for scar work. The technique is performed with the thumb or fingertips, with deep strokes perpendicular to the scar and no farther than 1 inch away from the scar's border.**

Thinking It Through

An essential element of the massage therapist's scar work protocol is to purposely create an area of localized inflammation. During the intensely focused, digital, cross-fiber friction technique (Figure 34-1) performed to trigger the inflammatory response, the therapist can think through the physiologic benefits of creating such a temporary irritant:

- The scar is not merely the visible line but the erratic "rope" of tissue deep to the scar. I must carefully palpate so my work directly affects the subcutaneous tissue.
- The cross-fiber friction techniques must be extremely localized, deep, consistent, and of sufficient duration to create hyperemia (reddening of the skin).
- When the skin is reddened, I know I have "tricked" the body into an inflammatory response, and the immune system will send macrophages to fight the mock battle.
- When the macrophages appear on the scene, they begin eating away *deep into the ropy scar, which is exactly where I want the erosion to occur.*
- After I work the appropriate amount of time, it would be physiologically irresponsible to "walk away" from this battlefield without "cleaning out" the results of the "hardworking" macrophages. Centripetal effleurage will flush waste from the area and aid the infusion of arterial blood.

Thinking It Through (cont.)

- In conclusion: I must set up a mini-battlefield of macrophages to help me perform scar work by using the body's normal inflammation process to further reduce the scar and increase local tissue mobility.

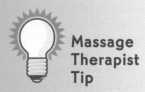

Massage Therapist Tip

The Timing of Scar Work Following Surgery or Injury

As effective as scar work is, you must use caution before beginning this aggressive treatment. Although most surgeons will tell a patient that the surgical seal should be healed in 4–8 weeks, this does not give you free rein to begin aggressive work. The scar work mantra is: "The newer the scar, the lighter the work." You could begin scar work after 2 months, but the approach would be very light, even cautious. Remember, the scar is not merely the closed-up line visible on the skin's surface; it is the damaged subcutaneous tissue that has endured assault. Scar work is highly effective and can remodel damaged tissue, even if begun weeks or months after the wound occurrence. Erring on the side of caution is the wisest course in deciding when to begin.

- ZENMED
- Kelo-Cote
- PreferON
- Scar Esthetique
- Bio-Oil
- Scar Zone
- Mederma

MASSAGE THERAPIST ASSESSMENT

A visual inspection will reveal tissue that appears paler than surrounding tissue, and/or a distinct darkened line, and/or a wavy or puckered patch of shiny or discolored skin. In any case, the scarred tissue will be easily identifiable. Digital palpation will indicate that the affected skin is slightly cooler to the touch. Tissue immediately deep to the scar may feel ropy or tough. Careful, sensitive probing into the scar may reveal varying regions of lumpiness intertwined with a tough smoothness. If the palpation causes any discomfort for the client, the massage therapist should not proceed with scar work until pain-free probing can be performed.

THERAPEUTIC GOALS

Reasonable goals for scar work performed on the mature scar during the subacute or chronic stage are remodeled scar tissue, followed by increased tissue and/or joint mobility in the immediate and surrounding areas.

MASSAGE SESSION FREQUENCY

Expert, focused scar work must initially be performed by a massage therapist. However, if a client is willing and able to learn the protocol—and to perform it several times a day—impressive results can be achieved after one instructional professional session. If the client is unwilling or unable to perform intensive, daily self-care, improvement will rest in the hands of the therapist.

- Ideally: 15- to 30-minute localized sessions at least once a week. For larger or complicated scars involving a joint, the localized work might last 30–45 minutes. (The remainder of the session can include other requested therapeutic or relaxation techniques.) These sessions must be followed by daily self-care performed by the client.
- Infrequent scar work results in no improvement in appearance and no increase in tissue mobility, other than that which occurs over time.

MASSAGE PROTOCOL

Before starting this protocol, it is important that your attitude toward the client's scar be one of positive acceptance. Many people who bear physical scars think of them as unsightly or embarrassing. Scars often also carry an unpleasant emotional history. As you release surrounding adhesions and diminish the scar's physical appearance, be aware that you are helping return the body to its highest function—not that you are in any way eradicating something that is wrong with the client's body.

Your work will be focused, detailed, and aggressive. In order to achieve the localized inflammatory process that is essential for true scar diminishment, pay attention to the effects of your work on both the local tissue and the person bearing the scar. You may cause discomfort during this protocol, but it is not acceptable to cause pain.

Step-by-Step Protocol for	Postoperative Scar Following Knee Replacement Surgery

Technique	Duration
After determining the level of disrobing and comfortably positioning the client to allow for your easy access during the protocol, apply a hot pack to the scar site. Leave it in place while you perform relaxation techniques to another part of the client's body.	5 minutes
Compression, wringing, jostling, medium pressure, slowly and *non*rhythmic. Begin proximally, working within a few inches of the scar but *not engaging the scar tissue yet*. • Quadriceps, adductors, tibialis anterior, anterior soleus	2 minutes
Compression, wringing, jostling, pressure deep to the client's tolerance, more quickly *non*rhythmic. Begin proximally, working within a few inches of the scar but *not engaging the scar tissue yet*. • Quadriceps, adductors, near but not on the knee, tibialis anterior, anterior soleus	2 minutes
Range of motion (ROM), to the client's tolerance, moving to end-feel and holding the stretch • Knee joint	1 minute
Place both of your hands on either side of the knee and pull the tissue *toward the scar*. Reposition your hands in several points around the perimeter of the knee, and continue to attempt to stretch tissue *toward the scar*.	1 minute
Plucking, gentle hacking, more wringing • Tissue surrounding the scar	1 minute
Lubricate the entire knee and scar region. Effleurage, petrissage, digital kneading, medium-to-deep pressure, briskly rhythmic • All muscles, including the quadriceps, adductors, tibialis anterior, that attach at or around the patella	3 minutes
Cross-fiber friction, medium pressure, directly over and within 1 inch of the borders of the scar. Attempt to create hyperemia (redness).	3 minutes
Cross-fiber friction, deep pressure, to the client's tolerance, directly over and within 1 inch of the borders of the scar. Attempt to create further hyperemia.	3 minutes
Small circles, made by digital kneading, tracing from about 1 inch away from the scar border and circling back in *toward* the scar	3 minutes
Cross-fiber friction, deep pressure, to the client's tolerance, directly over and within 1 inch of the borders of the scar	3 minutes
ROM, moving to the client's tolerance, to end-feel. Hold the stretch. • Knee joint	1 minute

Contraindications and Cautions

- Wounds from incompletely healed incisions, with remaining stitches, or that appear red, puffy, swollen, or seeping should not be touched.
- Friction on a newer (yet healed) wound is performed more lightly than a completely healed scar site that is months or years old.
- Friction on a keloid scar is not beneficial and can unnecessarily irritate surrounding tissue.
- Do not use friction, which purposefully sets up a site of localized inflammation, on a client taking anti-inflammatory medication or blood thinners.

(continued)

Technique	Duration
Effleurage, brisk, deep • From above the knee working just short of the inguinal area	1 minute
Effleurage, slower, light pressure, almost feathering • From above the knee working just short of the inguinal area	1 minute (30 minutes, including hot pack application)
Use the remaining time to perform either therapy or relaxation techniques per the client's request. *Do not replace the hot pack on the scar.*	30 minutes

Ample warming and stretching techniques, before and after the protocol, will ensure that the tissue (and the client) can tolerate the deep techniques.

Throughout the protocol, keep one anatomic principle and one physiologic process in mind. You are attempting to stretch, move, and remodel the fascia while simultaneously causing a "false" localized inflammatory response. If you let each of these concepts underlie your techniques, your protocol will yield very positive results.

Getting Started

Have a hot pack ready for localized application before you begin. Although your initial thought might be that the client doesn't need to completely disrobe, the scar work protocol itself may last for only 15–30 minutes, leaving ample time to perform an overall relaxation massage, or work on tight shoulders or lower back. Discuss with the client the "after scar work" needs before determining the extent of disrobing.

HOMEWORK

For scar remodeling to occur, the tissue must be consistently stimulated and stretched. Weekly or biweekly massage therapy sessions will not provide adequate improvement. Encourage your client to perform self-care mini-massage sessions, ideally using vitamin E oil, at least once a day and up to six times daily for optimum improvement and tissue health. (You may find a highly motivated client willing to do anything to reduce the scarring, but overzealous work can do harm, thus the earlier discussed limitation.)

- To soften the scarred area, apply a hot water bottle, run warm water over it, or begin work directly after your shower. This step is advantageous but not essential.
- Do not work to the point of pain or discomfort. This is not a "no pain, no gain" endeavor.
- After drizzling an ample amount of vitamin E oil directly onto and immediately surrounding the scarred area, gently massage *the surrounding tissue* first, making 100 deep, firm circles. Imagine you are trying to bring blood to the scarred area, and make your circles to achieve this (Figure 34-2).
- Now, make 100 deep firm circles *directly on the scarred area.* You might feel some ropy tissue deep underneath the scar, *and this is the area you ultimately want to massage into.*
- Firmly, with an open palm, massage and rub the entire area, stroking in the direction of your heart.
- Move and stretch the limb.

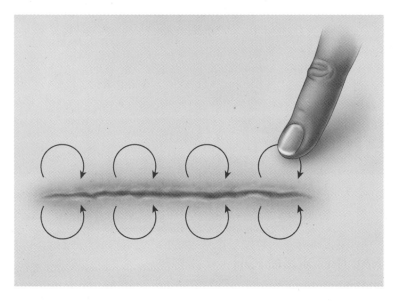

FIGURE 34-2 **Massaging a scar: Make deep, small, localized circles with the fingertips, as if pushing blood *toward* the scarred area.**

- Feel free to perform this exercise up to six times every day. It helps if the area you are working on becomes reddened, but do not work to the point of pain.

Review

1. What is a scar?
2. What is an adhesion?
3. What is a keloid scar, and in which populations do they most typically occur?
4. List the contraindications and cautions for scar work.
5. Explain the physiologic process behind setting up a localized area of inflammation during the treatment protocol.

BIBLIOGRAPHY

Adhesions, General and After Surgery. WebMD. Available at: http://www.webmd.com/a-to-z-guides/adhesion-general-post-surgery. Accessed July 30, 2010.

Brook M. The Importance of Scar Tissue Release Therapy. *Massage Today*. June 2009;09. Available at: http://www.massagetoday.com/mpacms/mt/article.php?id=14020. Accessed July 30, 2010.

Deodhar AK. Surgical Physiology of Wound Healing: A Review. *Journal of Postgraduate Medicine*. 1997;43. Available at: http://www.jpgmonline.com/article.asp?issn=0022-3859;year=1997;volume=43;issue=2;spage=52;epage=6;aulast=Deodhar. Accessed July 30, 2010.

Forbis R. Overview of Scars and Adhesions. Available at: http://www.edgarcayce.org/are/holistic_health/data/prscar3.html. Accessed July 30, 2010.

Phillips N. Surgical Adhesions: The Ties That Bind. Nurse.com. Available at: http://ce.nurse.com/CE573/Surgical-Adhesions-The-Ties-That-Bind. Accessed July 30, 2010.

Rattray F, Ludwig L. *Clinical Massage Therapy: Understanding, Assessing and Treating over 70 Conditions*, Toronto: Talus Incorporated, 2000.

Singleton C. What You Need to Know About Scars. Scar Treatment Association Review Site. Available at: http://www.scartreatmentassociation.com/review.html?gclid=CKfo_bGGv5wCFRlcagodg3skoQ. Accessed July 30, 2010.

Werner R. *A Massage Therapist's Guide to Pathology*, 4th ed. Philadelphia: Lippincott Williams & Wilkins, 2009.

35

Sciatica

Radiculopathy (spinal disc extrusion compressing a lower back nerve root)

Definition: Pain in the lumbar spine region radiating from the buttock down the back of the leg to the foot.

GENERAL INFORMATION

Sciatica is not a condition unto itself; it is a collection of secondary symptoms indicating one of several possible primary etiologies.

- Causes: secondary to conditions that compress or irritate the sciatic nerve as it exits the spinal cord
- Most common cause: herniated disc in the lumbar spine
- Other causes: degenerative disc disease, piriformis syndrome, degenerative arthritis, gluteal muscle spasms, spinal stenosis, vascular abnormalities in and around the spinal cord, trauma, spinal tumor, infection, inflammation, and injury to the sacroiliac ligaments, or the gluteus medius or maximus muscles
- Risk factors: advanced age, occupations that demand constant back twisting, carrying heavy loads, or driving long distances
- Possible sudden onset
- Duration of days or weeks
- Prevalent in adults age 30–50

Morbidity and Mortality

Statistics indicating occurrence are difficult, if not impossible, to determine because of the varied etiology of the condition. It is estimated, however, that millions of Americans suffer from sciatica at some point during their lifetime secondary to a herniated disc.

Most people completely recover without treatment. Permanent damage, which rarely occurs, can be related to trauma, infection, or tumor. Possible complications are loss of feeling or movement in the affected leg and, most seriously, loss of bowel or bladder function.

PATHOPHYSIOLOGY

A short anatomic review will help elucidate why the longest nerve in the body is so often injured. The sciatic nerve originates in the lower back at lumbar vertebra L-3, where it runs through the bony canal in the spine. A pair of nerve roots exit the spine, then come together to form the true sciatic nerve, which then runs the length of the posterior leg. At the popliteal fossa, the large nerve branches into two smaller nerves called the peroneal and tibial nerves (Figure 35-1).

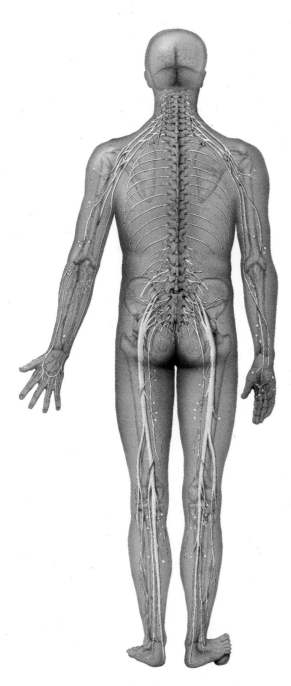

FIGURE 35-1 **Spinal nerves, including the largest, the sciatic nerve. It originates in the lumbar spine and travels posteriorly down the leg and bifurcates (branches) in the popliteal fossa. Asset provided by Anatomical Chart Co.**

The sciatic nerve is actually a bundle of five separate spinal nerves—at L-3, L-4, L-5, S-1, and S-2—and each one innervates a distinct path of sensory and/or motor function down the leg, thus explaining the wide variety of symptomatic presentations. Symptoms are directly related to *which segment* of the nerve is compressed or irritated. Because the nerve is so large, and since it runs through major, strong muscle masses and often lies up against bony prominences in the posterior pelvis (Figure 35-2), it is easy to see why sciatica is so pervasive.

Diagnosis is aided by a medical history, combined with a physical examination and muscle strength and reflex testing. The physical exam is followed by X-rays and an MRI and/or CT scan to determine the precise location of the sciatic nerve involvement. A confirmed diagnosis is often difficult because injury to the lower back and gluteal nerves, ligaments, and muscles can cause referred pain that mimics sciatica.

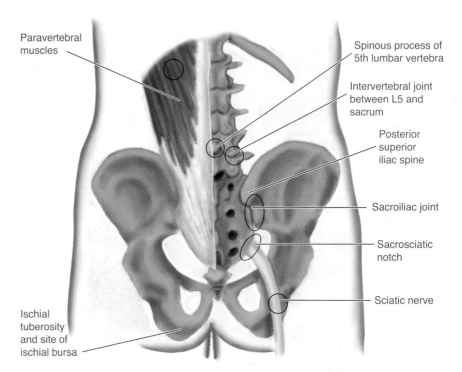

FIGURE 35-2 The location of the spinal nerve, nestled between large gluteal muscles and often running over or near bony prominences, makes it especially vulnerable for compression, injury, and inflammation. From Bickley LS, Szilagyi P. *Bates' Guide to Physical Examination and History Taking*, 8th ed. Philadelphia: Lippincott Williams & Wilkins, 2003.

OVERALL SIGNS AND SYMPTOMS

Symptoms and onset are very specific to the function of the strand of the sciatic nerve affected. For example, impingement at L-5 causes weakness in the big toe and perhaps foot drop. Or, if the sciatica is secondary to a herniated disc at L-4/5 or L-5/S-1, the symptoms will be exacerbated by squatting, sneezing, side bending, coughing, or laughing. Pain is usually unilateral and *referred*, which means that the cause of the pain originates in one location but is felt in another, usually distal, location. Symptoms include:

- Mild, achy discomfort to sharp, burning, excruciating, and shooting pain
- Numbness or muscle weakness in the foot or leg
- Burning sensation or tingling in the posterior/lateral thigh and/or leg
- Pain originating in the gluteal complex, running down the back of the leg
- Nagging, cramping sensation in the thigh
- Rarely, a loss of bladder or bowel control

SIGNS AND SYMPTOMS MASSAGE THERAPY CAN ADDRESS

- If sciatica is secondary to nerve root compression, massage therapy can provide comfort but cannot relieve the cause of the pain.
- If, however, sciatica is secondary to a tendon, ligament, or muscle injury, massage techniques can provide relief and decrease symptoms.
- If the etiology is degenerative disc disease, muscle spasm, piriformis syndrome, or trigger points, massage therapy can provide relief (see Chapters 13, 24, 28, and 43, respectively).

TREATMENT OPTIONS

Sciatica responds well to moderate, conservative treatment that attempts to both relieve pain and prevent further recurrence. Self-care, physical therapy (PT), and over-the-counter (OTC) medications are the most effective and pervasive treatments for this usually transient but irritating condition. Self-care techniques include hot or cold pack application, exercise, stretching, and building core strength, along with taking medications. If self-care techniques fail, PT is used for rehabilitation where necessary, to correct poor posture and/or lifelong improper body mechanics, combined with stretching, strengthening, and flexing the core and back muscles. Surgery, the treatment of last resort, is performed if symptoms progress, pain is intractable, and/or bowel or bladder dysfunction occurs. Surgeries include microdiscectomy, discectomy, and lumbar laminectomy to remove the compressing disc or relieve pressure on the nerve.

Prevention includes maintaining ideal weight, exercising regularly for overall back health and core strength, maintaining proper posture and body mechanics, changing position often when driving or sitting, adjusting hip and leg position while not overextending to reach the gas and brake pedals while driving, and lifting and bending properly.

Common Medications

There are no medications targeted to treat sciatica; instead, several categories of medications are given alone or in combination in order to address the etiology and severity of discomfort and pain.

- Nonsteroidal anti-inflammatory drugs (NSAIDs), such as ibuprofen (Motrin, Advil)
- OTC pain and anti-inflammatory medications, to address minor symptoms
- Oral steroids, to decrease inflammation and mid-range pain
- Locally injected steroids, to reduce more severe pain
- Muscle relaxants, to address muscle spasm
- Narcotics, for intractable pain
- Antidepressants in combination with any of the preceding medications, to address chronic pain that affects lifestyle

MASSAGE THERAPIST ASSESSMENT

Although many clients will present to a massage therapist with classic signs of sciatica, it is not appropriate for her to either assess or begin work based on a verbal report from a client alone. The therapist must have a firm diagnosis of the *cause* of the sciatica before proceeding with treatment. Although a simple muscle spasm or twisting event can, in fact, cause sciatic pain, the same symptoms can also accompany a bulging disc, in which case a massage therapist could unintentionally do a great deal of harm with minimal therapy. Sciatic symptoms appear secondary to conditions as benign as muscle spasm or as serious as osteoporosis, fracture, cancerous tumor, or nerve root infection.

There are times, however, when a client is in pain and is astute enough about his own body to report something like this: "Oh, this happens every few months, it's just my sciatica acting up again." In this situation, a massage therapist's assessment of sciatica is done by asking the client to physically point out the exact origin, route, and ending point of the pain and confirm that injury or trauma *is not a possible cause for onset*. The client's response must indicate a *posterior* and sometimes slightly *lateral* path of pain and tingling/numbness. If the client indicates *anterior* thigh or leg pain, or numbness or symptoms on the dorsal (front) of the foot, the therapist is not dealing with sciatica.

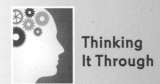

Thinking It Through

Except for the earliest stages of sciatica when pain may be intolerable and bed rest or immobility is prescribed, movement is an essential treatment for this condition. Although encouraging movement when a client is in pain may seem counterintuitive, thinking through the physiology of healing and muscle spasm will clarify the importance of encouraging your client *not to remain on the couch* when suffering from sciatic pain. The therapist can consider these points:

- Remember the pain-spasm-pain cycle (see Chapter 3). Fresh, oxygenated blood to hypertonic muscles is essential to reduce both spasm and pain.
- Movement helps exchange nutrients and fluids within the spinal discs. This ebb and flow of nutrients and waste products keeps the discs lubricated, pliable, and healthy. Immobility decreases this important exchange and stiffens the discs.
- Movement increases lymphatic cleansing, thus reducing the accumulated waste products that often accompany pain, immobility, and inflammation.
- Movement can increase the production of endorphins—the body's natural painkillers.

THERAPEUTIC GOALS

It is reasonable to expect spasming muscles to relax, localized blood circulation to improve, and endorphin flow and overall mobility to increase as a result of effective and careful massage therapy techniques.

MASSAGE SESSION FREQUENCY

If pain is severe (therapy not contraindicated):

- Ideally: 60-minute sessions twice a week
- Minimally: 60-minute sessions once a week

If pain has subsided:

- Ideally: 60-minute sessions once a week

Used preventively:

- Ideally: 60- to 90-minute sessions once a month

MASSAGE PROTOCOL

The massage protocols for degenerative disc disease in Chapter 13, muscle spasm in Chapter 24, piriformis syndrome in Chapter 28, and trigger points in Chapter 43 will help you determine an appropriate protocol for treating sciatica. In addition, once you are sure of the etiology of your client's pain, any combination of the following techniques used on the gluteal complex, thoracolumbar myofascia, sacroiliac joints, proximal hamstrings, and entire lumbar spine region should relieve pain and increase mobility.

- Stimulation will increase local circulation.
- Application of hot and/or cold packs will increase or reduce circulation.
- Muscle relaxation techniques will reduce spasm.
- Relaxing techniques will release endorphins.
- Myofascial release will soften the tissue in order to allow you to work deeply.
- Trigger point work (used with caution and only if you've been appropriately trained) will release acute hypertonicity.
- Basic holding and stretching will relax muscles, release joints, and improve lymphatic flow.
- Basic Swedish techniques will soothe and relax.

Getting Started

Although therapy to the gluteal region to address sciatic problems is most often very beneficial, it takes diplomacy, tact, and patience to "get in." Most clients are understandably initially hesitant to allow prolonged work directly on such a private area. They will "hold" themselves or resist your work, which will frustrate a successful outcome. Before the client is undressed and gets on the table, it's wise to counsel him about exactly which techniques you will be using. Let him know that he'll remain draped to his comfort level. Perhaps explain a little anatomy so he understands the route of the sciatic nerve and how it must be released and, thus, your therapeutic rationale for working on his gluteals. Most clients suffering from sciatica are desperate to achieve relief and will allow you to proceed after your careful and compassionate explanation.

Step-by-Step Protocol for   Sciatica

Technique	Duration
Begin myofascial stretching techniques with the client positioned comfortably prone. Work over the entire surface of the back from the base of the neck to the sacrum. Include use of your two flat hands pushing in opposite directions, deep compression, or skin rolling. Start superficially, work deep to the client's tolerance.	5 minutes
Once the client is relaxed and the back muscles have been softened, ask permission to work on the gluteus muscles. You can work over the sheet if modesty and your place of employment demands, but working directly on the skin is most effective.	
Facing your client's head, place your body-side forearm lateral to the gluteus maximus and medius. Push in the direction of the sacrum and slightly up the back. Remain stationary as your forearm firmly stays above the ischial tuberosity but deep around the bony ridges of the posterior pelvis. Rest here for a minute. You are trying to displace as much gluteal tissue as possible and help release any restrictions around the sciatic nerve while not pushing the nerve into any underlying bone. Ask your client to relax, because his natural inclination when someone works deep on the gluteals will be to hold his breath. Release after about 1 minute and continue planting and pushing your forearm along the lateral border of the gluteus maximus and medius until you have moved the entire gluteal complex. Remember, you are not gliding with this technique, but planting your forearm, pushing it deep into the tissue and then holding the tissue.	5 minutes
Repeat on the other side.	5 minutes
With a soft fist, jostle the entire gluteal complex from the posterior/superior iliac spine (PSIS) to the ischial tuberosity. If the client has experienced pain in his hamstrings, include jostling of the hamstrings. This is firm, deep, and fairly rapid work. Engage all gluteal tissue.	5 minutes
Repeat on the other side.	5 minutes
Knead, firm to deep, all gluteal tissue. Include the hamstring insertions on the ischial tuberosity.	5 minutes
Repeat on the other side.	5 minutes
Effleurage, petrissage, effleurage, medium to deep, slow and purposeful to the entire gluteal and hamstring complex.	5 minutes
Repeat on the other side.	5 minutes
Effleurage, petrissage, effleurage, all muscles of the back. Move briskly.	5 minutes
Final jostling of the gluteal complex.	5 minutes
Slow, purposeful, medium deep stroking of the entire posterior surface of the body from the occipital ridge to the hamstrings.	5 minutes

Contraindications and Cautions

- Unless the client has a history of chronic sciatica and reports that he is sure of the etiology, do not proceed in treating this condition without a firm diagnosis indicating the primary cause of the symptoms.

- Cross-fiber friction techniques are not appropriate if the etiology is inflammatory.

- Deep work is not appropriate if the etiology is a tumor or suspected cancer.

- Hip adduction, abduction, flexion, and extension stretches are best supervised by a PT, with regard to treating this condition.

- Do not perform direct work proximal to, distal to, or near an injection site (such as for a steroid injection) for at least 24 hours after the injection.

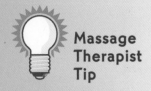

Massage Therapist Tip

How to Ice an Injury

Inflammation often accompanies musculoskeletal injuries. To reduce inflammation, ice is most effectively applied locally within the first 48 hours of an acute injury or anytime during a flare-up of an acute or chronic inflammatory condition. Here are three safe and effective ice application techniques: (1) Perform ice massage with an ice pop. Freeze water in a paper cup into which you've placed a popsicle stick; peel the paper off the frozen pop before use. Constantly move the ice pop in a wide area around the affected area. (2) Place a few ice cubes and a little water in a plastic, sealable bag and lay the bag over the affected area; be sure to place the bag over the sheet, not directly on the skin. (3) Use a bag of frozen vegetables or fruit and follow the same instructions as in (2). Never ice for longer than 15 minutes. Allow the tissue to return to normal sensation and warmth, waiting at least an hour, before reapplying ice. Reapplication of ice is appropriate and safe if you follow these guidelines.

HOMEWORK

While remaining well within your scope of practice, you can encourage your client with sciatica to keep moving and to carry out the following homework assignments. It would serve both you and your client well to work in conjunction with his PT.

- Unless you are in acute pain or have been instructed by your physician to remain immobile, keep moving, because even limited movement is important.
- Do low-impact exercise routines that incorporate strengthening and stretching without aggravating your symptoms, such as water aerobics and/or the stationary bicycle.
- Use cold packs or ice to reduce inflammation or intolerable pain.
- Use hot packs when your pain is dull and achy.
- When taking a long drive, move your hips, rotate your pelvis, and stretch safely; stop hourly to get out and move around.
- Rather than sitting for long periods, stretch, get up, and walk around.
- Before getting out of bed, gently stretch your entire body, moving all joints, focusing on gentle stretching of your hip joints.

Review

1. Define sciatica.
2. List several common causes of sciatica.
3. Describe some contraindications for massage therapy with a client who has sciatica.
4. Name effective self-care techniques for a client with chronic low-back pain.
5. How frequently would you see a client suffering from an acute (not disc-related) attack of sciatica?
6. Why are aggressive hip stretches not appropriate when a client who has sciatica is on your table?

BIBLIOGRAPHY

Benjamin B. Sciatica. *Massage Today*, May 2008. Available at: http://www.massagetoday.com/mpacms/mt/article.php?id=13802. Accessed July 30, 2010.

Cutler N. A Preferred Approach to Sciatica. Institute for Integrative Healthcare Studies. Available at: http://www.integrative-healthcare.org/mt/archives/2007/05/a_preferred_app.html. Accessed July 30, 2010.

Hildreth CJ, Lynm C, Glass RM. Sciatica. *Journal of the American Medical Association* 2009;302:216. Available at: http://jama.ama-assn.org/cgi/content/full/302/2/216?maxtoshow=&hits=10&RESULTFORMAT=&fulltext=sciatica&searchid=1&FIRSTINDEX=0&resourcetype=HWCIT. Accessed July 30, 2010.

Hochschuler SH. What You Need to Know About Sciatica. Spine-Health. Available at: http://www.spine-health.com/conditions/sciatica/what-you-need-know-about-sciatica. Accessed July 30, 2010.

MayoClinic.com. Sciatica. Available at: http://www.mayoclinic.com/health/sciatica/DS00516. Accessed July 30, 2010.

Miller RS. Sciatica Exercises for Sciatica Pain Relief. Spine-Health. Available at: http://www.spine-health.com/wellness/exercise/sciatica-exercises-sciatica-pain-relief. Accessed July 30, 2010.

36

Scoliosis

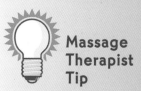
Definition: An abnormal lateral curvature of the spinal column.

GENERAL INFORMATION

- Cause in infants and adolescents: unknown
- Common causes in adults: sudden pressure on spinal discs; abnormal, persistent wear and tear on the spinal column; exacerbation from childhood scoliosis
- Less common causes in adults: degenerative disc disease, lumbar spinal stenosis, piriformis syndrome
- Rare causes: infection, tumor
- *Not caused* by poor posture, poor diet, or the use of backpacks
- Gradual onset, categorized as infantile, juvenile, adolescent, adult
- Possible lifetime duration
- Can worsen during growth spurts
- More prevalent in young girls than young boys
- Genetic predisposition
- No cure

Morbidity and Mortality

Scoliosis of unknown cause (idiopathic) accounts for 80–85% of all scoliosis diagnoses in the U.S.. The condition affects about 3% of the general population and about 10 in every 200 children between ages 10 and 15. Degenerative scoliosis usually occurs after the age of 40 and is often associated with osteoporosis. Although rare, severe complications secondary to scoliosis do occur; the more severe the initial curvature, the more likely the condition is to progress and worsen. Most instances of scoliosis, however, do not progress, and the condition is not usually life altering.

A normal spine has a curvature of 0–10 degrees. In curvatures greater than 70 degrees, the rib cage may press against the lungs and heart, substantially compromising the functioning of both. Complications from misshapen bones can include nerve irritation. Severe scoliosis can decrease a child's life expectancy from reduced pulmonary function.

PATHOPHYSIOLOGY

Scoliotic curvature can occur in either the thoracic or the lumbar spine, or both (Figure 36-1). It is generally categorized as functional, neuromuscular, or degenerative.

- *Functional scoliosis:* Characterized by a medically normal spine in which a curve is caused by a functional abnormality somewhere else in the body, such as one leg being shorter than the other or a habitual, uneven standing position.
- *Neuromuscular scoliosis:* Results from faulty bone formation often secondary to a medical condition, such as muscular dystrophy, cerebral palsy, or a birth defect.
- *Degenerative scoliosis:* Occurs in older adults and secondarily to changes in the arthritic or osteoporotic spine.

Massage Therapist Tip

Labeling Spinal Curvatures

This brief review will help you correctly identify normal and abnormal spinal curvatures. All spinal columns have a slight thoracic *kyphosis*, a normal forward bending (the spine curves posteriorly). A hunchback or pronounced forward thoracic curvature is termed *hyperkyphosis*. All backs also have a slight lumbar *lordosis*, a normal backward bending. A swayback or pronounced posterior lumbar curvature is appropriately termed *hyperlordosis*. *Scoliosis* is an abnormal, S-shaped curvature of the spine.

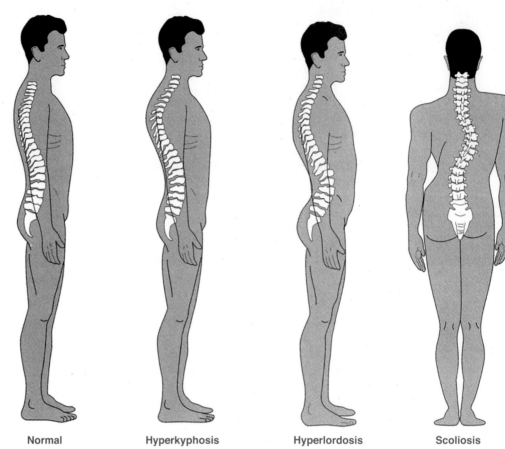

| Normal | Hyperkyphosis | Hyperlordosis | Scoliosis |

FIGURE 36-1 (A) Normal spinal curves include gentle kyphosis and lordosis. (B) Hyperkyphosis. (C) Hyperlordosis. (D) Scoliosis. Adapted from Willis MC. *Medical Terminology: The Language of Health Care*, 1st ed. Baltimore, MD: Lippincott Williams & Wilkins, 1996.

In response to scoliosis, the back muscles surrounding the spine attempt to hold the spinal column upright and straight. This constant (losing) battle creates muscular hypertonicity (the tense, bunched muscles will appear convex on one side of the spine) and hypotonicity (the lax, weakened muscles will appear concave on the contralateral side of the spine).

Diagnosis is confirmed by observing the person in standing and forward-bending positions. Palpation will also reveal abnormal spinal curves and musculature adaptations. X-rays and sometimes a CT scan and/or an MRI will help determine the exact position of the curvature and the effects on surrounding tissues and nerves. Questions about individual medical history will address pain progression, injuries, surgeries, bowel and bladder function, and leg pain. Scoliosis in children is now usually identified by routine school screening programs. Mild scoliosis in adults often goes undiagnosed until found by a massage therapist, physical therapist (PT), personal trainer, or astute partner.

OVERALL SIGNS AND SYMPTOMS

The pain associated with scoliosis ranges from mild to moderate to severe; it can be temporary or lifelong or it can be completely absent. Pain is most common in adults with severe or degenerative scoliosis and in children with a severe curve. This abnormal spinal curvature is often asymptomatic or mildly symptomatic in both children and adolescents. Adult signs and symptoms can be subtle and difficult to determine, because years of miniscule muscular and spinal adjustments often cause aches and pains that are considered "normal." Usually, the more advanced the age and progressive the condition, the more prevalent the pain. An actual abnormal spinal curvature is, of course, the single most pervasive sign. Other signs and symptoms include the following:

- One shoulder or hip appearing higher than the other
- One shoulder blade protruding more
- One leg appearing longer
- One arm hanging lower
- The upper body tilting to one side
- The head appearing off-center
- A hump appearing on one side of the thoracic spine when bending forward
- A hump appearing on one side of the thoracic spine when lying prone
- Hypertonicity and hypotonicity in spinal and surrounding muscles
- Back pain
- Weakness, numbness, and/or pain in the lower extremities
- In rare cases, breathing problems, fatigue, or heart failure

SIGNS AND SYMPTOMS MASSAGE THERAPY CAN ADDRESS

- No matter what form the scoliosis takes or at what age it becomes a problem, massage therapy's focus on relieving muscular pain and discomfort can substantially help a physician's or PT's treatments.
- In cases of functional scoliosis, the massage therapist can work to help correct habitual muscular adaptations and compensations that have led to scoliosis.
- In cases of neuromuscular and degenerative scoliosis, massage therapy can address the muscular hypertonicity and hypotonicity, joint pain, and stress that accompany any precipitating medical condition.

TREATMENT OPTIONS

The level of treatment is directly related to the degree of spinal curvature, the overall symptomatic picture, and the person's age. Treatment at any age usually cannot reverse the curve, but it can help slightly straighten a spine, slow the progression, and relieve pain and discomfort. Beginning conservatively, ongoing observation at any age is considered the baseline treatment for scoliosis. Treatment then moves to bracing and/or PT as necessary, and finally to surgery, as a last resort.

About 90% of infantile scoliosis cases resolve without treatment. Bracing, PT, exercise, and sometimes medications are recommended for curvatures of 40 degrees or less. Curves greater than 40 degrees may require surgery. In adults with osteoporosis and scoliosis, the osteoporosis is treated conservatively with exercise and medication for pain relief. Conservative treatment for adult scoliosis will not reverse the curve but can slow progression while reducing pain and discomfort.

Surgery is appropriate only for those experiencing severe pain or breathing difficulties, or for people in whom the progressive deformity is significantly compromising the lifestyle. Surgery for scoliosis involves spinal fusion with the insertion of rods and other hardware, which remain in place for a lifetime.

Common Medications

Since pain may or may not accompany scoliosis, and because any pain could be due to muscular and joint abnormalities, organ dysfunction, nerve involvement, or a tumor, there is no single medication suggested for the condition.

- Nonsteroidal anti-inflammatory drugs (NSAIDs), such as ibuprofen (Motrin, Advil)

MASSAGE THERAPIST ASSESSMENT

Although it is outside the massage therapist's scope of practice to diagnose scoliosis, she can assess the severity of the curvature, its effects on the rest of the body, and the extent of the muscular concavity (hypotonicity) and/or convexity (hypertonicity) in order to determine an effective treatment protocol. It would be ideal for the therapist to work with a PT or a physician who is caring for the client, and even more helpful to have written reports of the X-rays and MRIs to help determine the extent of the curvature, as well as an indication of affected organs and nerves. In the absence of these diagnostic confirmations, and in cases where a client will say, "I've had scoliosis since I was a kid, it's not really serious but my back always hurts, please do something," the therapist can assess to help determine the most effective treatment plan.

- When the client walks in, the therapist notes her posture, whether one shoulder is lower, or one shoulder rolls forward. In the presence of pronounced muscular hypertrophy (enlarged muscle cells), the muscles of the back may abnormally protrude under the shirt.
- When the client is on the table, positioned prone, the therapist stands at her head and looks down the spine. One side of the spine will probably look rounded and raised (the hypertonic/convex side of the spine) compared to the other side.
- Again with the client prone, the therapist palpates down the spine by using her thumbs running along the transverse processes. A palpable spinal curve will be revealed. The hypertrophic muscles will feel much more hypertonic, and the contralateral/hypotonic/concave side will feel substantially different.
- In the supine position, the client's shoulders may not evenly rest on the table due to the abnormal spinal muscle hypertrophy.

THERAPEUTIC GOALS

The staggering number of specific muscles that are affected by scoliosis highlights the need for creating realistic goals. The client's age and onset of scoliosis further affect treatment goals. Over time, with continuous therapy, the therapist can help stretch shortened muscles, relieve hypertonicity and spasm, remove myofascial restrictions, increase breathing capacity and restricted range of motion (ROM), relieve constipation and headaches, increase circulation to hypertonic muscles, and remove waste from underused muscles.

MASSAGE SESSION FREQUENCY

Scoliosis is a lifelong condition. The client might present in childhood or adulthood, with or without pain, while actively being treated by a physician or never having seen one. The complexity of the muscular and bony involvement makes estimating the frequency of massage sessions impractical. Once begun, however, weekly massage therapy sessions will prove much more effective than sporadic work. Therapy should continue for as long as the symptoms persist, which is usually the client's lifetime.

MASSAGE PROTOCOL

As massage therapists, we are trained to look at the client holistically. This is never more important than when treating scoliosis. Because the body's basic supporting structure is compromised, therefore, everything attached to that structure is also compromised. A one-size-fits-all protocol does not exist. Instead, each client must be viewed for her particular set of aches and pains and adaptations. Using your anatomy book to review the layers of back muscles and how each of them connect to the head, abdomen, and lower extremities will give you a much clearer picture of which treatment to choose.

Your work will be spot work, localized for each session. You could cause massive reactive spasms if you attempt to release and loosen all hypertonic back muscles at one time. Map out the client's symptoms and pains and determine a step-by-step approach to her therapy that includes her understanding of what is going on in her body and how you will both address her discomfort. Include some relaxation techniques in each session so the client is not overwhelmed with too much detailed, localized therapy.

Excellent SOAP charting will help you track progression, digression, areas treated, and the client's reaction to each session. You have a rare opportunity to treat this client for life, so your best efforts at diplomacy and patience, combined with intelligent skills, will go a long way toward making a significant difference in her quality of life.

Rather than the usual step-by-step process for treating one condition, the protocol outlined subsequently provides suggestions for more localized work, which will be your approach in treating scoliosis. Localized, sequential, carefully thought-out massage therapy performed and then assessed by the client is the best plan of action for this complicated yet seemingly simple condition. That said, there may be sessions where the client simply wants moderately firm work to her entire back, "just to relax." This will help, but be careful not to work deeply on an entire scoliotic back; spasms will result as the back's muscles unnaturally relax and then fight to right themselves again.

Although there has been a substantial amount written about how massage therapy can structurally correct scoliosis, it is not my belief that this is possible. Put in its simplest anatomic light: Bone wins out over muscle. If the (hard) bone is pulling on (soft) muscle unrelentingly, it's plain to see which structure will "win." It is up to you, the massage therapist, to understand that you cannot alter bony formations (well outside your scope of practice) but can substantially and sometimes profoundly affect the muscle's reaction to that bony abnormality. Unless the scoliosis is purely functional (secondary to bad posture), the condition cannot be corrected by massage therapy alone. It is in that spirit and with this understanding, combined with many years of clinical practice, that the following protocol suggestions are offered—in an attempt to relieve pain, discomfort, and stress and allow the body to heal to its greatest extent.

Getting Started

Positioning for client comfort is extremely important, so be sure to have plenty of pillows ready. Have hot packs and cold packs prepared. Remember to call your client the day after the first few sessions to make sure your work has not caused reactive spasms.

HOMEWORK

In an adult who is enduring mild, lifelong scoliosis, the following suggestions can help relieve pain, headaches, and/or stress. In a child with bracing or an adult with comorbidities, homework assignments are best left to the treating PT, chiropractor, or physician.

- Avoid postures that worsen your condition. Carry a backpack (making sure to keep your back upright) rather than a heavy purse on one shoulder.
- If your job demands that you sit all day, make sure your chair provides adequate support.
- If you stand all day, ask a physician about a supportive back brace.
- Breathe deeply throughout the day.
- Stretch your back daily. Go to a PT and get a set of back exercises that will help stretch your tight muscles and strengthen your weak muscles.

Contraindications and Cautions

- Although the client will experience multiple areas of fascial and muscular restrictions, it is best not to overwork any one body part, attempt to work the entire back, or worse, work multiple regions randomly. You and the client should determine one localized region to be worked at each session.

- Resisted breathing techniques that attempt to hold and release the rib cage should not be performed in the presence of osteoporosis, fused vertebrae, or rib hypermobility or hypomobility.

- Applying heat or cold to a spine in which metal rods have been implanted is contraindicated because the metal could retain the applied temperature.

- Scoliosis of unknown origin that causes nerve or radiating pain might be related to an infection or tumor, and the client should be referred to a physician before massage therapy treatment.

Step-by-Step Protocol for **Adult Idiopathic Scoliosis of About 20 Degrees with No Secondary Morbidity**

Technique	Duration
There is no "correct" order for the following work. You can pick and choose techniques that are appropriate for your client's needs for any given session.	All durations are to the client's tolerance and should last at least as long as it takes to feel the tissue soften and respond.
Begin and end each 60-minute session with long, slow relaxation techniques. Include effleurage, petrissage, compression, and stroking anywhere on the body at the client's request.	5 minutes to begin and 5 minutes to end the session
Apply a hot pack to hypertonic tissue, and a cold pack to spasming tissue. Be keenly aware of the tissue and client's response to the application of both heat and cold.	5–10 minutes for each
Myofascial stretching techniques. Include use of your two flat hands pushing in opposite directions, deep compression or skin rolling. Start superficially and work deep to the client's tolerance. • This work, unlike most of the following protocol, can be performed over the entire back in order to prepare it for deeper, localized work.	
Effleurage, petrissage, compression, digital kneading, muscle stripping, and jostling. Start superficially, advance to medium depth, and then work as deeply as the client will allow. Work slowly, rhythmically as you focus on *one specific area of the affected back.* • When working the splenius capitis muscles, work firmly along the occipital ridge and into the transverse process of the cervical spine. • When working the levator scapulae, work deeply into the occipital ridge and along the medial and superior borders of the scapula. Move the scapula as much as possible. • In your attempts to move the scapula, be sure to perform detailed work into the medial, superior, *and lateral* borders (you will have to work into the axilla). • When working the rhomboids, note which side is convex and which side is concave. Be sure not to stretch overstretched muscles. Digitally knead into the laminar grooves and then into the lateral border of the scapula. Use the heel of your hand to deeply work these muscles and to flush out waste. • With work on the large trapezius, be aware of all bony borders and use them to your advantage. Flow easily up into the base of the skull at the occipital ridge, move down to the top of the shoulders, glide deeply into the thoracolumbar fascia, and work into the cervical and thoracic laminar grooves. Imagine you are trying to lift this large *superficial* muscle off the back, and try to move it so you can get to the underlying musculature.	

(continued)

Technique	Duration
• On the latissimus dorsi, use compression, stripping, apply your focused forearm, and use petrissage on this large muscle. It must be softened before you can approach the underlying musculature. • Strip the finer, underlying obliques. • Imagine the small, hardworking erector spinae group and try to push them off the spine with compression, digital kneading, and stripping. Determine which side is hypertrophic and which is less developed. • Identify the QLs. Try to grip and move them as you perform detailed cross-fiber work along the bottom of the ribs and the superior crest of the pelvis.	
If you are trained in trigger point work, you will have ample opportunities to use your skills, because there will be multiple regions of long-standing hypertonicity that have created knots. Be careful not to be overly aggressive or focused, because trigger point work, performed without control and for too long, will cause post-session pain.	
The gluteal complex has worked hard to help hold the lower back muscles in response to the abnormal spinal curve. Asking the client's permission, perform deep kneading, compression, jostling, petrissage, muscle stripping, deep effleurage, and, if you are trained, trigger point work on the large gluteal muscles. Work from the sacroiliac (SI) joint, to the posterior/superior iliac spine (PSIS), down to the ischial tuberosities.	
The tensor fasciae latae will be hypertonic secondary to the gluteal hypertonicity. Use the heel of your hand or your forearm to compress, strip, and move this tough, dense tissue.	
Your client will have adjusted to her scoliosis by adapting inefficient breathing patterns. *If you are sure no osteoporosis exists in the ribs, if there is no spinal hardware, and if the client has normal "spring" in her costals,* you can perform resisted breathing exercises to both stimulate and move the diaphragm and increase thoracic efficiency.	
After one or two localized areas have been worked, ask your client to stretch her back out to the greatest ROM she is capable of while taking deep breaths. She may lie supine on the table, while spreading her arms out to either side and then bringing them over and above her head as she deeply inhales and exhales. She can also stand at the side of the table, lean over the table, and, using the table as a resisted breathing device, take several deep breaths.	
If the client is constipated secondary to an inefficiently functioning diaphragm and inactivity, offer to perform colon massage.	

- Stretch your arms out to the sides and over your head to work your chest muscles every day.
- Don't stay in one position for long periods.
- Experiment with hot or cold applications to your back (if you don't have inserted hardware).
- Even on days when you are sore, keep moving. Immobility will worsen your symptoms.

Review

1. Define the normal and abnormal spinal curvatures.
2. List muscles that may be affected by scoliosis.
3. Is scoliosis painful?
4. How is scoliosis typically treated?
5. Which medications are typically used to treat scoliosis?
6. How can you assess for the presence of scoliosis?
7. How aggressive is the massage therapy when treating this condition?
8. Would you work on the entire back at the first massage therapy session? Why or why not?

BIBLIOGRAPHY

Dalton E. Symptomatic Scoliosis. *Massage & Bodywork Magazine*. April/May 2006. Available at: http://www.massagetherapy.com/articles/index.php/article_id/1226/Symptomatic-Scoliosis. Accessed July 30, 2010.

Eck JC. Scoliosis. MedicineNet.com. Available at: http://www.medicinenet.com/scoliosis/article.htm. Accessed July 30, 2010.

Hamm M. Impact of massage therapy in the treatment of linked pathologies: scoliosis, costovertebral dysfunction, and thoracic outlet syndrome. *Journal of Bodywork and Movement Therapies* 2006;10:12–20. Available at: http://www.ScienceDirect.com. Accessed July 30, 2010.

Lensman L. Scoliosis and Structural Integration. *Massage & Bodywork Magazine*. April/May 2003. Available at: http://www.massagetherapy.com/articles/index.php/article_id/583/Scoliosis-and-Structural-Integration. Accessed July 30, 2010.

MayoClinic.com. Scoliosis. Available at: http://www.mayoclinic.com/health/scoliosis/DS00194. Accessed July 30, 2010.

Medline Plus. Scoliosis. Available at: http://www.nlm.nih.gov/medlineplus/scoliosis.html. Accessed July 30, 2010.

Rattray F, Ludwig L. *Clinical Massage Therapy: Understanding, Assessing and Treating over 70 Conditions*, Toronto: Talus Incorporated, 2000.

Spine Institute of New York. Scoliosis. Available at: http://www.spineinstituteny.com/conditions/scoliosis.html. Accessed July 30, 2010.

Werner R. *A Massage Therapist's Guide to Pathology*, 4th ed. Philadelphia: Lippincott Williams & Wilkins, 2009.

37

Sprain and Strain

GENERAL INFORMATION

- Torn or stretched ligament = *sprain*
- Torn or stretched muscle or tendon = *strain*
- Primary causes: stressful or traumatic incident or repetitive low-level motions that lead to structural malfunction
- Contributing or predisposing factors: previous injury, inadequate warming before exercise, joint or muscle comorbidities
- Most commonly affected joints: ankles and knees, then fingers, wrists, toes

Morbidity and Mortality

There are no published data on the frequency of sprains or strains. It is a rare, inactive human who has not experienced even a mild joint injury. Although rarely life threatening by itself, the secondary effects of a sprain or strain on soft tissue or bone, combined with compensatory movements, can significantly hinder complete, or correctly aligned, joint healing. Compensation occurs in the contralateral limb and/or proximal or distal joint. In addition, slings, removable casts, or crutches can create hypertonicity or hypotonicity. With or without aids, the sprain or strain itself creates immediate protective voluntary splinting and/or spasm. If the person returns to activity too quickly, a secondary overuse injury can compromise complete healing.

Adhesions naturally and quickly form in and around an injured joint; they can prolong healing and cause a limited, painful limb. Scar tissue, another natural but limiting response to soft tissue injury, although taking weeks to develop, can result in range-of-motion (ROM) limitations. Both adhesions and scar tissue slow healing and can lead to chronic, long-term pain.

Sprains and strains usually heal completely within days, weeks, or months, depending on severity. Although localized tenderness, regional stiffness, radiating pain, and/or weather-dependent aching may persist over the long term, the injured area generally returns to full functioning and strength.

PATHOPHYSIOLOGY

A quick review of bone and joint anatomy will help clarify sprain or strain pathophysiology. Joint and muscle movement is possible because the (soft, mobile) muscles terminate in tendon, and then attach to a (hard, stationary) bone, giving the sanguinous (blood-filled) muscle something to hold onto and work against. An excellent example of a readily palpable muscle-tendon complex is the distal end of the gastrocnemius, which terminates in the Achilles tendon, which then attaches to the calcaneus (heel bone).

Bones are secured to other bones by ligaments—nonsanguinous ropes that intertwine, connect, and keep joints stable. Palpable examples of ligaments are those

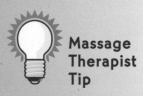

Massage Therapist Tip

When It's Not a Simple Sprain or Strain

Although common, joint injuries can also be serious. Although most simple sprains and strains can be treated at home, be aware that if any of the following symptoms occurs, immediate medical attention is necessary:

- A joint that appears irregular, or one that can bear no weight, may indicate a broken bone or joint dislocation.
- Numbness or tingling associated with the injury may indicate nerve injury.
- A cold or discolored body part may indicate circulation loss and/or damaged blood vessels.
- A fever higher than 100°F accompanied by heat and redness at the injured site may indicate infection.

found on either side of the malleoli and knees. When fascia, muscles, tendons, or ligaments are torn or damaged, bleeding occurs. Visible or invisible swelling and bruising immediately follow interstitially and/or subcutaneously; these signs may not be noticeable for minutes or hours.

Sprain or strain severity is graded, usually in degrees from 1 to 6. A lower degree sprain involves a minor ligament tear or stretch, while a higher degree sprain indicates the breaking of a ligament off the bone and/or a breaking of the bone itself.

Diagnosis is made according to the absence or persistence of swelling, the deformation of the joint, the joint "sound" heard upon injury, the mechanics of the actual incident, the person's medical history (osteoporosis, previous injuries, etc.), and following a thorough examination of the injured joint and surrounding tissue. Immediate X-rays to determine bony involvement may be taken if swelling is not pronounced. X-rays will not indicate soft tissue damage, however, and swelling can adversely affect the accuracy of an X-ray reading; therefore, diagnostic X-rays are often taken a few days post-injury.

OVERALL SIGNS AND SYMPTOMS

Here are the signs and symptoms of a typical low-grade sprain or strain.

- Immediate pain
- Increasing pain after 1–2 days as spasm begins
- Swelling: immediate or within hours
- Spasm
- Popping sound (sprains only)
- Bruising: immediate or within hours or days
- Deformity
- Loss of function of affected joint
- Decreased function of affected limb

SIGNS AND SYMPTOMS MASSAGE THERAPY CAN ADDRESS

Massage therapists are not first-line responders for traumatic injuries. It is not within a massage therapist's scope of practice to perform the compression component of the typical, appropriate rest, ice, compression, elevation (RICE) treatment. The most effective treatment a massage therapist can offer an immediate traumatic injury that involves swelling is lymphatic drainage techniques. These techniques are not covered in this book. All the following information regarding sprains and strains assumes the massage therapist is attending to subacute pain, swelling, and stiffness and/or chronic pain, stiffness, and scarring secondary to an initial (now past) sprain or strain injury.

TREATMENT OPTIONS

The traditional, conservative, and most effective immediate care for a sprain or strain is RICE. Rest means the affected joint is used little or not at all, and weight bearing is limited. The recommended timeframe for resting an injured limb is 7–10 days for mild injuries, and 3–5 weeks for more severe cases. Ice packs are applied immediately to the affected area for up to 20 minutes at a time or three or four times a day for the first 24–72 hours after injury. Ice reduces pain, swelling, and inflammation. A compression bandage is wrapped around the affected joint, but not so tightly as to compromise circulation. Compression helps reduce painful swelling and provides minimal support. The limb is elevated, preferably above the heart. Elevation uses gravity to help reduce swelling and increase venous return.

RICE usually suffices for treating simple sprains and strains—as long as it is followed by vigilant avoidance of overusing the injured joint or limb. Although the use of a healing joint is imperative for proper healing to occur, premature overuse may lead to reinjury. Internal injured structures need time to heal, even in the absence of obvious symptoms. Physical therapy (PT) rehabilitation often follows a relatively serious sprain or strain to ensure the proper return to strength and aligned healing. Imaging studies are necessary if symptoms persist or worsen, or if surrounding structures will not heal. Surgery is rare and indicated only for significant tendon or ligament tears, or if surrounding bony structures must be rebuilt or stabilized.

Preventive techniques include warming and stretching muscles both before and after exercise, creating a safe work or home environment, not trying new exercise regimens or recreational activities without proper training, wearing appropriate footwear, increasing awareness of physical surroundings, and taping or bracing a weak or previously injured joint before athletic activity.

Common Medications

- Nonsteroidal anti-inflammatory drugs (NSAIDs), such as ibuprofen (Motrin, Advil)
- Nonopioid pain reliever fever reducers, such as acetaminophen (Tylenol, Feverall, Anacin, Panadol)

MASSAGE THERAPIST ASSESSMENT

Remembering that the massage therapist is not a first-line health care responder and that new or recent, still swollen joints will not be addressed with massage therapy; the therapist can consider the following assessment points before treatment. She can ask the questions while palpating the injured area to determine ROM restrictions, the presence of scarring and/or adhesions, tenderness, redness, heat, or swelling.

- Did a pre-existing medical condition predispose the client to injury? Conditions might include osteoporosis, frailty, arthritis, previous injury to the same or nearby joint, or compensating from an earlier injury.
- When did the injury occur?
- Did the person hear a popping sound at the time of injury?
- How is the client compensating for the injured limb? Which other structures are affected or painful?
- Which treatment(s) was performed at the time of and immediately after the injury?
- Is the client seeing a physician or PT?
- Is the client taking pain medications? Narcotics? Blood thinners?
- Is the client using any physical aids, such as crutches, splints, or canes?
- What exactly are the current symptoms, and how localized are they? Do they radiate?
- How limited is the ROM compared to previous use and the contralateral side?
- Which movements aggravate symptoms?
- Which activities of daily living (ADLs) are directly affected by the injury?

THERAPEUTIC GOALS

Reasonable goals resulting from the judicious use of common massage therapy techniques include reduced pain and spasm, increased ROM, decreased hypertonicity, reduced spasm, pain of compensating structures, and fewer adhesions and scar tissue.

MASSAGE SESSION FREQUENCY

- Ideally: 60-minute sessions twice a week, until full use and ROM are regained
- Minimally: 60-minute sessions once a week, until full use and ROM are regained

Thinking It Through

What are the effects of limping, the body's compensatory response to an ankle injury? How is the body compensating? Why would a massage therapist be concerned not only with an original site of injury, but also with all compensating structures? How could a distal ankle injury compromise a contralateral shoulder? Could this injury create a headache? Using the example of a right ankle sprain, the therapist thinks through the mechanics of compensation. This exercise will help clarify the treatment approach.

- If the right ankle is swollen, spasming, painful, and unable to bear weight, which proximal joint will contract and experience overuse to help keep weight off the ankle?
- How will the workload of the contralateral ankle be affected?
- What is the effect on the ipsilateral and contralateral hips?
- If the hips are affected, what is the effect on the lower back?
- If the lower back is now spasming as a result of overwork, how will the shoulders most likely react?
- If the trapezius is involved, where does it attach, and how can this lead to a headache?

- Maintenance: 60-minute sessions once a month
- Mildly effective: 60-minute sessions in response to episodic radiating pain; each session must be followed by vigilant self-care exercises

MASSAGE PROTOCOL

As mentioned earlier, massage therapists do not treat a fresh strain or sprain. However, if the injury remains untreated or unmoved, debilitating scar tissue and adhesions will lead to long-term chronic pain. Your job in treating sprains or strains is to use your palpation, listening, and diplomacy skills to discern whether your client has sufficiently healed to allow you to work. You must also convince him to let you perform the sometimes aggressive techniques that will be most effective, and persuade him to return to you with sufficient frequency. Remember that you will also need to break up the adhesions and scars that have already formed. You can assure your client that the skills you have to offer will decrease long-term chronic pain secondary to the compensatory effects of the initial injury.

Your protocol will not merely address the injured site but will also include *every layer of tissue, from the most superficial fascia working all the way to the bone.* The careful, persistent, and thorough use of warming techniques, compression, friction, cross-fiber friction, longitudinal muscle stripping, and diplomatic-but-challenging ROM techniques are the staples of effective joint injury work. In order for complete healing to occur, blood must be brought to the area (even to nonsanguinous ligaments), waste must be flushed toward the heart, and the joints and muscles must be returned to their full functional capacity.

Hot packs can be applied to the injured site and left to warm while you begin work on compensating structures. If you are tempted to apply ice because of swelling, heat, or pain, this is a sign that you are working on the injury too early and that you should stop treatment until these symptoms have subsided.

Compression is always an effective introductory technique and can be applied progressively from light to bone-deep.

Use of your fingertips, thumbs, elbows, and/or forearms can provide extremely effective friction techniques. Attention to the amount or lack of lubricant will significantly affect the efficacy of this work. Although you want to be careful and not bruise the client, you *must* create localized redness, which will indicate effective friction is being performed.

Muscle stripping presupposes your anatomic knowledge of origins and insertions. Be careful not to "cross over" long muscles, causing the uncomfortable and sometimes painful "thump" experienced by the client. (Noncareful forearm effleurage to the long heads of the quadriceps will often result in this painful "thump"; learn to work slightly medial or lateral to the rectus femoris and you'll avoid this uncomfortable technique.) Friction techniques should always be followed by centripetal flushing techniques and ROM.

Pain-free, relaxed, passive, but challenging joint play and ROM techniques will help break up adhesions and scar tissue and avoid long-term joint limitations and chronic pain. These techniques should be performed slightly past the client's comfort zone, but this is definitely not a "no pain, no gain" technique.

Getting Started

Have hot packs, pillows, and bolsters ready for the application of heat and comfortable positioning. Remove throw rugs or obstacles, and rearrange the room for safety if the client is using a cane, walker, or wheelchair. Review the specific injured joint anatomy so you can be sure you address every inch of the muscle, as well as the insertions and origins, and attaching/surrounding tendons and ligaments. Ask yourself repeatedly: Which structures will be compensating for this injury? Keenly observe your client as he comes through your door.

Step-by-Step Protocol for	Severely Strained Right Ankle 3 Weeks Post-Injury	
Technique	**Duration**	
Apply a hot pack to the affected ankle. Perform thorough, deep compression to the entire ipsilateral and contralateral limb.	5 minutes	
Remove the hot pack. Perform compression on the right ankle. Palpate with your fingertips to determine areas of tenderness, scarring, and adhesions. Get client feedback while you work, performing gentle ROM to determine restrictions. Use the ROM performed at this point in the protocol to compare to the ROM performed at the end of the protocol.	3 minutes	
Digital kneading, effleurage, petrissage, ROM, cross-fiber friction, muscle stripping *to the unaffected, proximal, ipsilateral (right) joints before approaching the affected ankle.* • Knee and all immediately surrounding muscles • Hip and all surrounding muscles, including the iliotibial (IT) band	5 minutes	
Place your hands on the injured ankle and simply hold for a few seconds. Then slowly and carefully perform *passive right ankle* ROM, moving it to end-feel as you plantar flex and dorsiflex and move it in a 360-degree circle. Carefully watch the client's reactions and do not cause pain. Ask the client to perform *active* ROM and again watch his response.	2 minutes	
Digital muscle stripping, deep centripetal effleurage performed slowly and rhythmically. • A few inches *above* the affected ankle working on the distal section of the tibialis anterior and gastrocnemius/Achilles tendon complex • Work both anteriorly and posteriorly	3 minutes	
Now begin work on the injured ankle itself. Perform digital muscle stripping, digital and palmar kneading, cross-fiber friction, deep muscle stripping combined with frequent deep centripetal effleurage and frequent, gentle ROM performed carefully and rhythmically. • Into every crevice of both malleoli • Following the tibia and fibula up, proximally, several inches above the malleoli • Into, around, and underneath every tarsal and metatarsal bone; include the plantar surface of the foot • Into, around, and underneath every toe	15 minutes	
Grasp the toes in your fingers and hyperflex and hyperextend them. Repeat ROM of the ankle, now moving slightly beyond end-feel, if necessary, to the point of slight discomfort. Notice if this ROM differs from the original ROM performed during warm-up.	2 minutes	
Leave the affected area. Effleurage, petrissage, knead, vigorously and not necessarily rhythmically. • Ipsilateral gastrocnemius and rectus femoris muscles	2 minutes	

Contraindications and Cautions

• Do not work on a sprain or strain too early in the injury process. Premature massage therapy could release much needed protective voluntary muscle splinting, disturb a hematoma, and/or cause more inflammation.

• ROM techniques that are too aggressive can further injure a joint.

• Determine whether the client is taking narcotics for pain and if he can describe accurate reactions to pressure and discomfort.

• If your client is taking a blood thinner, this contraindicates the use of cross-fiber or deep friction techniques.

• Heat should not be applied if any redness or swelling still exists in the joint or surrounding tissue.

• Heat, redness, pain, swelling, and/or a fever can indicate infection, so avoid massage.

• Be aware of surgically reduced ligaments and of the presence of pins, rods, or other stabilizing hardware in the affected or surrounding joints.

(continued)

Technique	Duration
Reapply the hot pack to the affected ankle. Ask the client which areas of his body are stiff or in pain secondary to compensation. Work these areas for most of the remainder of the session.	20 minutes
Remove the hot pack. Perform passive ROM to the affected ankle. Follow with deep, slightly vigorous centripetal effleurage. Ask the client to perform active ROM to the affected ankle. Compare the difference from the initial ROM exercise.	3 minutes

HOMEWORK

If your client is severely affected by a sprain or strain injury, his self-care instructions from a PT or a physical medicine physician will preclude any of your own. If the injury is minor and/or you are working as a team member with the PT, you are completely within your scope of practice to suggest the following homework assignments:

- Apply heat before stretches, before exercise, or whenever you're feeling stiff. Make sure it's moist heat in the form of a hot water bottle or microwaveable gel pack. A heating pad or rice pack does little but provide palliative comfort.
- Perform your stretching exercises to the point of mild discomfort but not to the point of pain.
- Use your affected joint as much as possible; unless you see swelling or are in pain, do not pamper it. Be aware of compensating movements that will cause long-term pain.
- Do not refer to your affected joint or limb as your "bad" side; the body "takes offense" at being referred to as such, and this negative mind-body connection hampers healing.
- At any resting opportunity, deeply massage the affected joint.
- See a PT for lengthening shortened muscles and strengthening weakened muscles.

Review

1. Define a sprain and a strain and make a clear distinction between them.
2. List massage contraindications for treating a client who has a sprain or strain.
3. Why are X-rays performed immediately post-injury not always an accurate indicator of injury?
4. Name one distinctive sign or symptom that distinguishes a sprain from a strain.
5. Why is applying compression outside the massage therapist's scope of practice?

BIBLIOGRAPHY

Benjamin B. Injuries of the Knee: Essential Principles and Their Applications. *Massage & Bodywork Magazine*. Available at: http://www.massageandbodywork.com/Articles/OctNov2003/essentialprinciples.html. Accessed July 30, 2010.
Benjamin B. Principles of Orthopedic Massage and Their Application to Ankle Sprains. Available at: http://www.massageandbodywork.com/Articles/FebMar2004/ankles.html. Accessed July 30, 2010.
Cluett J. Sprains and Strains. Available at: http://orthopedics.about.com/cs/sprainsstrains/a/asprain. Accessed July 30, 2010.

MayoClinic.com. Sprains and Strains. Available at: http://www.mayoclinic.com/health/sprains-and-strains/DS00343. Accessed July 30, 2010.

MayoClinic.com. Sprain: First Aid. Available at: http://www.mayoclinic.com/health/first-aid-sprain/FA00016. Accessed July 30, 2010.

Rattray F, Ludwig L. *Clinical Massage Therapy: Understanding, Assessing and Treating over 70 Conditions*, Toronto: Talus Incorporated, 2000.

Vorvick L. Sprains. Available at: http://www.nlm.nih.gov/medlineplus/ency/article/000041.htm. Accessed July 30, 2010.

Wedro BC. Sprains and Strains. Available at: http://www.webmd.com/a-to-z-guides/sprains-and-strains. Accessed July 30, 2010.

38

Stress

Definition: Physiologic reactions to real or imagined, normal or extreme, physical, medical, emotional, or psychological events.

GENERAL INFORMATION

- Causes: anxiety, uncertainty, or fear from real or imagined threats; acute one-time events; sustained low-level irritations; medical, emotional, or psychological upset or trauma; illness
- Onset: before, during, after, or long after any of the earlier mentioned causes
- Short-term or lifelong duration
- Experienced in some form by all individuals

Morbidity and Mortality

Stress is considered a major health problem in the U.S. About 33% of Americans report living with extreme stress, and 48% state that their stress has significantly increased for the last 5 years. Although most Americans believe that they are handling stress well, 77% report experiencing physical symptoms, and 73% experience psychological stress-related symptoms. The health conditions and comorbidities associated with stress can affect every aspect of a person's life, including his or her physical, emotional, psychological, interpersonal, and spiritual well-being. Prolonged, unrelenting stress is medically and psychiatrically linked to anxiety and depression.

Medically, persistent severe and/or low-level stress can do the following:

- Cause skin rashes, hives, various skin outbreaks, and hair loss
- Exacerbate chronic obstructive pulmonary disease (COPD), asthma, and other breathing difficulties
- Decrease fertility and erections; cause painful menses and difficulty during pregnancy
- Worsen gastrointestinal problems, such as gastroesophageal reflux disease (GERD), peptic ulcers, irritable bowel syndrome (IBS), ulcerative colitis
- Cause muscular tension in the neck, back, and shoulders
- Exacerbate or cause headaches
- Worsen arthritis
- Lead to insomnia
- Elevate blood pressure, cause an abnormal heartbeat, increase blood clots and hardening of the arteries, increase the propensity for heart attack and heart failure
- Compromise the efficacy of the immune system, thereby increasing the incidence and severity of chronic diseases

Psychologically and emotionally, severe and/or low-level stress can do the following:

- Develop into an inability to deal with large and small problems
- Lead to frustration, increased intolerance, and loss of temper
- Increase fatigue
- Destroy the ability to focus
- Lead to anxiety and depression

PATHOPHYSIOLOGY

The human body functions within the framework of its reaction to stressors. The simple act of breathing depends on the brain's continual need for oxygen; the normal stress set up by that need triggers the automatic and predictable next breath. Every physiologic function the body performs, from digestion to pupil restriction, exemplifies its response to normal stressors.

When imbalance or trauma occurs, such as excess alcohol consumption or a bleeding injury, the body's heightened response to stressors is again predictable and efficient. A temporary, sympathetic state—the "fight-or-flight" response—results in a rush of hormones and chemicals that are necessary to balance or heal. This extreme state lasts only until the physiologic trauma subsides and homeostasis (physiologic equilibrium) is restored. The sympathetic state is neutralized and replaced by a "business-as-usual" parasympathetic ("rest and digest") calm.

The sympathetic state, although a normal reaction to crisis—real or imagined—is not intended to be sustained. The chemical and hormonal flush that rushes through the body to dilate pupils, increase breathing, flood the muscles with blood, slow digestion, and cause mental hypervigilance is as dramatic in the short term as it is caustic (literally) over the long term. The sympathetic state removes the individual from the path of the oncoming car; and once safety is assured, the body, usually within 45 minutes, rids itself of these caustic chemicals and returns to a quiet state of efficient functioning.

Stress becomes a killing disease when the brain is repeatedly tricked into "believing" there is a reason to continue to flood the body with caustic chemicals. Healing, on any level, from the cellular to the psychological, cannot occur if the body is in a sympathetic state. No system—from immune to gastrointestinal—can function normally and/or heal unless the body is in the parasympathetic mode.

OVERALL SIGNS AND SYMPTOMS

- Headache
- Irritability, anxiety, restlessness, crying, anger
- Inability to focus, forgetfulness
- Insomnia
- Rapid speech; persistent, inappropriate laughing
- Social withdrawal
- Increased smoking
- Inappropriate emotional responses
- Drug or alcohol abuse
- Reduced or increased appetite
- Increased heartbeat and/or breathing rate
- Sweating
- Nausea, diarrhea, upset stomach
- Hypochondria
- Multiple joint aches and pains
- Nightmares
- Personality change

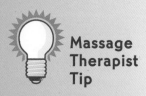

Massage Therapist Tip

Associating Stress with Most Client Conditions

In a society that tends toward self-reliance and glorifies those who "pull themselves up by their bootstraps," it can be an act of courage to acknowledge that life may be overwhelming at times. It is safe to assume, even in the most seemingly perky clients, that major underlying stressors coexist with their primary complaints. Although it is beyond our scope to explore psychological trauma, it certainly is within our regimen of compassionate care to assume that any number of stressors can temporarily defeat most adults, and that these challenges can wear many faces. The challenges of parenting, joining the Armed Forces, losing one's job, an abusive spouse, a dying pet, moving a household, or a wedding can unravel the strongest human. It's best to assume your clients are undergoing great and possibly back-breaking stressors, whether spoken or unspoken. Even the most therapeutic session (as opposed to a strictly relaxing one) should contain a strong element of leaving the body in a parasympathetic state.

SIGNS AND SYMPTOMS MASSAGE THERAPY CAN ADDRESS

Since the body, mind, and emotions cannot heal when the body is in a sympathetic state, and since most massage therapy techniques help put the body into a parasympathetic state, the therapist can decrease many of the earlier mentioned symptoms by performing any calm-inducing techniques with compassion and healing intention.

TREATMENT OPTIONS

Addressing stress is not a clear-cut, direct path from diagnosis to cure. Stress is inherent in our everyday life, whether or not we have health problems. Although stress accompanies every condition from a paper cut to cancer, it is often treated as the "stepchild" of any medical or psychological condition. Some astute health care professionals will identify stress as a comorbidity and will include it in the treatment plan for the primary medical condition. For example, an antidepressant is often prescribed for cancer patients undergoing chemotherapy, and anti-anxiety medications are often prescribed for patients following a car accident or other types of physical trauma.

The pervasive, secondary, life-threatening effects of stress accumulate when the *perceived (untreated) stress* continues well after the trauma of the initial event has been resolved. At that point, treatment options include age- or trauma-related support groups, psychotherapy or psychiatry, medications, mind–body techniques, guided imagery, massage therapy, hypnotherapy, and exercise.

Common Medications

Because stress is so often linked to anxiety and depression, the most commonly prescribed medications for anxiety include those that are proven effective for depression.

- Tricyclic antidepressants, such as amitriptyline hydrochloride (Apo-Ami Triptyline, Endep)
- Selective serotonin reuptake inhibitors (SSRIs), such as escitalopram oxalate (Lexapro)
- Immune regulators, antirheumatics, such as anakinra (Kineret)
- Antihistamines, sedatives, antispasmodics, such as hydroxyzine embonate (Atarax)
- Antidepressants, such as venlafaxine hydrochloride (Effexor)
- Benzodiazepine anxiolytics, sedative hypnotics, such as lorazepam (Ativan)

MASSAGE THERAPIST ASSESSMENT

Because stress is so pervasive, most clients will come to a massage therapist with a self-diagnosis, either as a manifestation of muscular tension or as an accompaniment to some other chronic condition. Because therapists are trained to visually "take the client's emotional pulse," most will be able to determine the presence or absence of stress based on easily discernible signs and symptoms, such as headache and tight shoulders. The treatment can then move ahead to address stress as either the primary condition or a strong, secondary comorbidity.

THERAPEUTIC GOALS

Whether stress is presented as the primary or secondary condition, the treatment goal is to return the body to a parasympathetic state, thereby facilitating physical and/or emotional healing.

MASSAGE SESSION FREQUENCY

Frequency is dictated by either the comorbidity being treated or the muscular effects of the stress itself.

- Ideally: 60-minute sessions once a week

MASSAGE PROTOCOL

Two simple, calming techniques are used by many massage therapists working in high-stress environments, including hospitals, hospices, and nursing homes. These techniques are very effective in treating the stress experienced by agitated psychiatric, pediatric, cancer, intensive care unit (ICU), or cardiac care unit (CCU) patients; or those suffering with intractable pain. The techniques are also effective for addressing unrelenting or day-to-day stress observed in clients in private massage practices.

The following two protocols can be provided alone or in combination with other relaxing Swedish techniques. The duration of the session depends on whether you are treating stress as the primary or secondary condition.

Other massage therapy techniques, such as slow compression and effleurage, stroking, rocking, and energy work, can also be incorporated into the protocols. If you are also addressing muscular hypertonicity of the head, neck, shoulders, and back, the most common massage techniques of heat application, effleurage, wringing, compression, and petrissage are extremely beneficial.

Slow-Stroke Back (or Front) Massage

This protocol assumes the client is positioned prone, but in many cases (as in a hospital or nursing home environment), the patient may be able to lie supine only.

- Stand at the side of the hospital bed or massage table, facing the client's head. Lay your *non-lubricated* hands (either directly on the client's skin or over the clothes) at the base of the client's neck (see Figure 22-1). Using only the weight of your hands (no lighter, because this will be stimulating to the body; and no deeper, because your intent is not to massage muscle) and maintaining full hand (not fingertip) contact, slowly slide your hands down the client's back to her sacrum. It should take you about 1 minute to travel the length of her spine.
- When your hands reach the sacrum, slowly "brush off" your hands to either side of the body.
- Return to the base of the neck immediately and repeat. *This work is unidirectional— running down the spine only.*

Hold and Stroke

This technique can be performed with the client lying in any comfortable position.

- Facing the massage table, standing at about the location of the client's waist, gently place one of your hands on your client's shoulder and the other on her hand. Simply rest *for a full minute.* Focus, and determine your intent. Breathe slowly and evenly. Do nothing. Do not speak.
- Once you are focused, begin stroking *down* the arm with the *non-lubricated* hand that was holding your client's shoulder. Use the weight of your full, open hand; do not use your fingertips. Move slowly. This work is performed to the depth at which you would normally apply lubricant and goes no deeper than superficial fascia.
- Repeat three times on one arm.
- Move silently to the contralateral upper extremity and repeat.
- Use slow-stroke back (or front) techniques to the trunk of the body.

Thinking It Through

Stress is ubiquitous and often shrugged off as a normal part of life; it is not taken as the serious condition it can become. The massage therapist should think through the pervasiveness of common stressors and the danger of ignoring the body's responses.

- Often the most common response to a person's emotional problem is, "No problem, I'm okay," when in fact this is not the case. What effect could this outward state versus inward struggle have on the body?
- It is easy to belittle others for "worrying too much about small things" without finding out the cause of such worry. What are some helpful skills for being a more considerate listener?
- It is common for individuals to experience unrelenting stress, with attendant multiple physical ailments, and still believe they are not at risk for life-threatening disease. How can these people be reached and convinced to address the underlying stressors?
- People who seem hypochondriacal, or who complain of multiple, frequently traveling points of bodily pain, may be experiencing deep stressors. What are some suggestions that might help these people make the connection between their stressors and their body's reactions?

- Moving to the lower extremities, place one hand near the head of the femur and the other as far down the leg as you can comfortably reach. Again, center yourself and focus in silence.
- Repeat the slow stroking down the leg.
- Silently move to the other lower extremity and repeat.
- Finish with about 5 minutes of slow-stroke back (or front) massage.

Getting Started

As simple as these techniques are, they can cause back spasms in a massage therapist who is not used to performing slow, focused work. Be careful to bend your knees, work from your core, breathe deeply, and shift your weight rather than stretch from your shoulders as you perform these highly effective but surprisingly demanding massage therapy techniques.

Warm packs are often very soothing and can be applied anywhere on the client's body. A heated table pad is also comforting. If the client is comfortable with complete silence, consider forgoing the use of music.

HOMEWORK

Think about your own reactions to the stressors in your life, and be reasonable and nonjudgmental as you make the following suggestions for your client's self-care:

- Try to become more aware of your body when you are stressed. Do you raise and tighten your shoulders? Do you hold your breath? When you find yourself tensing up, "shake it out" and try to relax.
- When you're in a private place, either at home or at work, and you have 5 minutes to yourself, practice tensing and relaxing every major muscle group in your body. Start at your feet. Tense your feet as tightly as you can, inhale deeply, then exhale, and release the muscles. Next, tighten your calves as tightly as you can, take a deep breath, and release. Work all the way up your body, tensing and releasing your thighs, abdomen, chest, arms, face, and head muscles. As you exhale during each muscle set, imagine all tension draining out of your body through the bottom of your feet or the top of your head.
- Close your eyes. Imagine your most perfect vacation spot. See the green grass, feel the cool breeze off the ocean on your face. Feel the sand in your toes. Relax your shoulders. Feel your face gently relaxing and smiling. Remember what your body feels like when you are this relaxed, and then open your eyes.
- Find music or nature sound recordings that soothe you. Buy a CD, play it at work through your computer, or go for a walk and listen to it through a headset. Lie on the floor at home, put in your ear buds and listen to your special, relaxing music or sounds. Feel how your body feels when you are completely relaxed, and try to replicate this sensation throughout your day.
- Gently think about all the physical ailments that are produced by the existence of sustained stress. Remember: You can compromise your health and shorten your life if you keep yourself stressed all the time. Try to remove as much stress from your life as you can.
- Pray, meditate, sing, dance, and laugh.

Review

1. Name some of the body's normal physiologic stress responses.
2. What is the difference between the sympathetic and parasympathetic state?
3. Which state is the body's natural healing mode?
4. Is stress really a serious medical condition?
5. List some characteristic symptoms of stress.
6. Describe some bodily symptoms that result from unrelenting stress.

BIBLIOGRAPHY

American Academy of Dermatology. Stress and Skin: How the Mind Matters to Your Skin. Available at: http://www.aad.org/media/background/factsheets/fact_stressandskin.html. Accessed August 8, 2010.

American Psychological Association. Stress Survey: Stress a Major Health Problem in the U.S., Warns APA. October 24, 2007. Available at: http://www.apa.org/news/press/releases/2007/10/stress.aspx. Accessed August 8, 2010.

MayoClinic.com. Stress Symptoms: Effects on Your Body, Feelings and Behavior. Available at: http://www.mayoclinic.com/health/stress-symptoms/SR00008_D. Accessed August 8, 2010.

Rattray F, Ludwig L. *Clinical Massage Therapy: Understanding, Assessing and Treating over 70 Conditions*, Toronto: Talus Incorporated, 2000.

WebMD. Stress. Updated October 12, 2009. Available at: http://www.webmd.com/balance/stress-management/stress-management-topic-overview. Accessed August 8, 2010.

WebMD. Stress Management—Effects of Stress. Available at: http://www.webmd.com/balance/stress-management/stress-management-of-stress. Accessed August 8, 2010.

39

Also known as:

Brain Attack, Cerebrovascular Accident (CVA)

Stroke

Definition: An acute impairment of normal blood flow to a specific area of the brain that lasts longer than 24 hours.

GENERAL INFORMATION

- Causes: atherostenosis (narrowing of major arteries to the brain); a deep brain arterial occlusion (blockage), or an embolus (clot) originating from the heart, from poor cardiac output or a broken aneurysm
- Primary cause: clots, 88% of all strokes
- Increased incidence secondary to blood-clotting disorders, hypertension, heartbeat irregularities, cardiac disease, diabetes, hyperlipidemia (excess lipids in the blood), chronic bronchitis, periodontal disease, changes in age-related brain blood flow, and peripheral vascular disease
- Lifestyle risk factors: inactivity, alcohol consumption, excess stress

Morbidity and Mortality

Every 45 seconds, one U.S. citizen has a stroke, and more than 700,000 people suffer a stroke every year. About 4 million Americans live with the effects of stroke; two-thirds will require rehabilitation. Stroke is the third leading cause of death after heart disease and cancer, and it is the number one cause of disability in adults. Among stroke survivors, 10% recover almost completely, while 25% experience minor impairments; 40% have impairments requiring special care, and 10% need permanent care in a long-term facility. About 15% die soon after having a stroke. Of those experiencing a first stroke, 14% will experience a second stroke within 1 year.

Stroke causes five types of disabilities that result in life-altering comorbidities: paralysis, sensory disturbance, language difficulty, cognitive and memory difficulties, and emotional disturbances. Tendonitis, bursitis, adhesive capsulitis, and rotator cuff tears are common post-stroke complaints. Stroke patients often live with feelings of fear, anxiety, frustration, depression, and grief.

PATHOPHYSIOLOGY

The body's muscles cannot function without direct input from the brain and spinal cord. In addition, mental activity, coordination, imagination, memory, logical thinking, and speech, as well as breathing, heartbeat, and all senses, depend on a fully functioning brain. As with any organ, blood inflow and outflow must be maintained at precise pressures in order for the brain to send thousands of minute commands every second. When either too much blood or not enough blood disrupts the brain's delicate homeostasis, dramatic and serious symptoms immediately occur. The result is a stroke. The longer this blood loss or excess flooding lasts in the brain, the more serious and extensive the damage to the brain and, thus, the rest of the body.

There are two main categories of stroke:

- *Brain hemorrhage:* Blood seeps into the spaces around, or within, the brain, causing pressure and damage to cerebral tissue; a less frequent type of stroke.
- *Ischemic stroke:* Inadequate blood supply causes damage to cerebral tissue; the most common type of stroke.

A mini-stroke, or *transient ischemic attack* (TIA), occurs when the brain's blood supply is briefly interrupted (for less than 24 hours). Microemboli (tiny clots) or microvascular spasms cause a transient reduction in blood flow. The aftereffects of a typical TIA are either subtle, short-lived, or nonexistent. When symptoms are absent, the TIA might not even be noticed, but undetected TIAs can show up on brain scans later. A TIA is often a precursor to a full-blown stroke, occurring months or years after the initial "silent stroke."

Typically, permanent or temporary deficits in speech, memory, movement, and cognition result from damage to the area of the brain that normally regulates these functions. Damage to one side of the brain causes a contralateral response in the body. For example, a right-sided stroke causes functional deficits in the body's left-sided musculature. A stroke frequently results in flaccid paralysis (lack of nerve impulse transmission, so muscles cannot move); spastic paralysis (excess nerve signal transmission, so muscles spasm involuntarily and frequently); or paresthesias (numbness, tingling, changes in sensation). Affected musculature leads to further long-term difficulties, such as shortened tendons, ossified joints, forearm and leg contractures, and pressure sores or open skin ulcers from prolonged immobility. All these complications are accompanied by pain, compromised range of motion (ROM), loss of function, depression, and ironically, an increased risk of further clot formation. The extent of the damage of any stroke is directly related to two equally important factors: the affected brain region, and the timing of both the emergency treatment and post-stroke convalescent therapy.

OVERALL SIGNS AND SYMPTOMS

- Sudden onset of numbness in one arm, one leg, or the face
- Sudden slurred speech
- Sudden impaired vision in one or both eyes
- Sudden inability to repeat a simple phrase
- Sudden drooping of one side of the face or a noticeably uneven smile
- Sudden severe headache of unknown cause

SIGNS AND SYMPTOMS MASSAGE THERAPY CAN ADDRESS

- Massage therapists do not address immediate stroke symptoms, but once the patient is stabilized, massage therapy is appropriate and effective.
- Given the new medical understanding of neuroplasticity, the brain's ability to reroute signals in order to regain function after trauma, massage therapy's contribution to the stroke patient can be essential.
- The effects of massage therapy during rehabilitation are discussed in the Therapeutic Goals section.

TREATMENT OPTIONS

The prompt administration of anticoagulants for blood clot reduction is the best medical treatment. Quick intervention is crucial for minimizing the effects of long-term damage to the brain and body. Rehabilitation begins while the patient is still in the hospital. The success of a treatment plan is determined by the swiftness and skill with

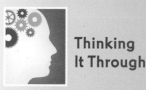

Thinking It Through

More than muscle is affected following a stroke. Joints particularly take a beating, as the weight of the affected muscles pull and the compensating joints work double time. The therapist can consider the ways in which the joints might be affected.

- The weight of the affected arm's pull on the shoulder will affect both ipsilateral and contralateral back and chest muscles as the shoulder girdle rolls anteriorly, pulling the trapezius forward and shortening the pectoralis complex.
- The drag of the affected leg places tremendous pull on the ipsilateral ankle, knee, and hip, while the contralateral hip becomes hypertrophied in the attempt to help swing the leg forward during every difficult step.
- Lower extremity challenges always necessarily directly affect the sacroiliac joints' structure and function.

which it is initiated, the involvement of caregivers, and the patient's determination to overcome obstacles.

Rehabilitation teaches patients how to perform daily tasks with either temporary or permanent muscle loss. Even while in hospital, patients are urged to perform both passive and active ROM exercises and to begin using the stroke-affected limbs. Speech, occupational, recreational, and physical therapy focus on frequent, focused, repetitive exercises. Complementary therapies include acupuncture to relieve pain, increase blood flow, and restore energy. Yoga helps the patient regain balance, muscular control, and strength.

Eighty percent of strokes are preventable by the use of medication and/or lifestyle changes. Medications and a controlled diet can help lower and stabilize blood pressure. The risk of recurrence can be minimized by controlling weight and by avoiding alcohol and cigarette smoking.

Common Medications

The most typical strokes, those caused by a clot blocking blood flow to the brain, are ideally immediately treated with tissue plasminogen activator (tPA), a powerful fast-acting medication that dissolves blood clots. The drawback to this drug's efficacy is that it must be given within 3 hours of the brain attack, thus, the importance of getting the possible stroke patient to the hospital immediately so the evaluation can be performed and then, if appropriate, tPA can be administered.

Drug therapy with blood thinners is the most common post-stroke treatment.

MASSAGE THERAPIST ASSESSMENT

Before working with a stroke patient, the therapist should consult the patient's physician and/or rehabilitation team. Although massage therapy is extremely beneficial to the patient's overall rehabilitation program, it is helpful to know his complete stroke history, the medications he is taking, and any potential risks before assessing, in preparation for planning the sometimes rigorous and often repetitive massage therapy protocols.

Here are some questions to ask the physician, the lead rehabilitation therapist, the patient, and/or the patient's caregiver:

- When did the stroke occur?
- Which medication is the patient taking?
- What is the medical treatment, and what is the rehabilitation program thus far?
- Is the patient taking narcotics or muscle relaxants?
- If contractures exist, for how long? What previous therapy was performed, and what progress was achieved?
- If PT is being performed, what results have been achieved? How can the massage therapist enhance the PT's efforts?
- What is the best way to effectively communicate with this patient?
- Does the patient have seizures or emotional outbursts?
- Does the patient have pain? How does he demonstrate the severity?
- If skin breakdown is a problem, what are the positioning challenges?
- What are his greatest challenges in terms of daily activities?
- What was his general lifestyle before the stroke?

Once the therapist has received a medical clearance to proceed and understands the present therapy and medication regimen, an extensive and thorough palpation examination will search for disuse atrophy, compensating hypertonicity, contractures, low-level barely palpable spasms, and spastic flexors and/or extensors. A thorough written treatment plan should include repetitive techniques and should fit appropriately into the medical care practitioner's goals. Assessment might include any of the following. The therapist should take detailed notes before and after each session.

These notes can be used to prove progression and digression, and they can provide a solid basis for encouragement.

- Postural and balance assessment of sitting, standing, walking, rising out of a chair, getting on/off the massage table, and so forth
- Observation of fine motor skills, such as buttoning and unbuttoning, putting on makeup, writing (These skills can be pantomimed.)
- Observation of gross motor skills, such as putting on clothes, washing hair, catching a ball
- Determining the fist grasping strength
- Palpation of muscles on both the affected and the unaffected side
- Palpation and passive ROM exercises of muscles of both the affected and the unaffected side
- Evaluation of communication facility
- Discovery of edema and any areas of skin breakdown

THERAPEUTIC GOALS

The multiple treatment goals are tied directly to the primary physician's objectives for the patient, and will depend on the point in the rehabilitation process at which the massage therapist enters. The therapeutic goals are to provide a safe, calm, comfortable, and encouraging treatment environment; decrease stress; induce the parasympathetic state; reduce edema; reduce or limit contractures; decrease or eliminate pain; increase muscle use and strength; minimize muscle atrophy and spasticity; decrease muscle hypotonicity and hypertonicity; and stop the pain-spasm-pain cycle.

MASSAGE SESSION FREQUENCY

A stroke patient may not find his way to the benefits of massage until well after the disruption from the initial event has settled down. However, significant rehabilitation is possibly weeks, months, or even years after the stroke occurred, as long as the massage therapist's expertise is applied in frequent sessions, and the patient makes a commitment to improve, including performing homework exercises.

Massage session frequency is determined by the patient's rehabilitation stage and the arena in which the therapist is working. A therapist in a hospital setting could begin treating a stroke patient as soon as 48 hours after the incident, at which point, daily sessions would last only a few minutes. Those in private practice or in a rehabilitation clinic will find it most effective to see the patient at least weekly. However, even in this setting, session duration is often linked to the patient's tolerance and lifestyle, the area of the body being addressed, the limitations of the surroundings, and the conflicting therapeutic appointments. The therapist must learn a way to diplomatically insist that massage is a crucial part of the patient's overall rehabilitation program.

MASSAGE PROTOCOL

"A massage therapist's work is never done" could be the slogan for therapy offered to stroke patients. Except for the small percentage of patients who completely recover, the patient's body is a tapestry for ongoing, lifelong massage therapy. The following list outlines the initial reasons you and your patient may well have a long therapeutic relationship:

- Facial muscles may be hypertonic, hypotonic, spastic, or flaccid. The muscles of expression and eating (essential for self-esteem, socialization, and survival) need daily therapy.

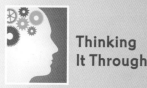
Thinking It Through

The therapist might assume, since the stroke patient might have paralysis, that he cannot "feel" pain. Nothing could be farther from the truth. Stroke patients suffer with a variety of chronic pain syndromes. The therapist can think through the various ways pain can manifest in a body that has experienced a stroke.

- Uncontrolled and spastic muscular movement results in constant flexing and extending of major muscles. Because the muscle is rarely in a fully resting phase, a pain-spasm-pain cycle is continuous.
- A paralyzed limb places an unusual, unrelenting pull at the proximal joint, which can cause radiating pain both proximally and distally.
- The unaffected limb is forced to perform twice the work as it takes over for the weakened side. This compensation leads to hypertonicity, trigger points, and radiating pain.
- The possible disfigurement, the loss of self-control, the need for constant help, and the loss of income and a job obviously lead to anxiety and depression. Not all pain manifests physically.

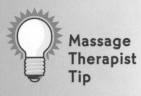

- Flexors are stronger than extensors. Arms, forearms, thighs, and legs, which manifest the muscular difficulties described earlier, are usually severely imbalanced and easily fatigued as the battle rages between compensation and function.
- Joints are either pulled beyond or shortened into abnormal angles. Passive and active ROM exercises must be performed daily, if not hourly, in order to relieve and revive joints.
- Constipation is a common side effect of inactivity and of narcotic and muscle relaxant use. Colon massage is a helpful component of every session.

The massage therapy performed on a stroke patient is different from other types of work you might have performed. It is extremely detailed, specific, repetitive, and slow. You need to observe everything about every muscle you work on and to note the difference from the last session. Your work must place the patient in a profound parasympathetic state while you simultaneously encourage him to do his best and not give up. Techniques vary from session to session, depending on what you hope to accomplish, what he will allow, and what is the level of his pain tolerance that day.

The subsequent step-by-step protocol focuses on a stroke-affected upper extremity. The techniques remain the same for any portion of the body you may need to address. You can use cross-fiber friction on contracted limbs, for example, but modified according to the patient's mood and pain tolerance level. If you do not know where to start, or need a technique to simply get to know the patient, or if he is particularly agitated, you can always perform the slow-stroke back (or front) massage to help quiet your patient and reduce his pain and anxiety (see Chapter 38).

Getting Started

Confirm in the phone interview with your patient or his caregiver how you will need to adjust your massage therapy setting and communication style. Can he speak? Is he using a cane or walker? Will he need multiple pillows for appropriate positioning? Does he experience seizures? Often a significant other, or family member, will want to be in the room to explain the extent of the condition, help with positioning the client, offer feedback about your work, and certainly to listen to homework assignments.

Adequate, comfortable pillowing in the supine position, with a large pillow under his head and knees, may be the best way to accommodate his stiffness and the work you have to perform, without placing further pressure on a limb with limited blood flow. Remember that all your techniques must be slow, rhythmic, predictable, steady, and repetitive. Do nothing to surprise or stimulate the muscle and risk setting off a spasm. The protocol lasts a full 60 minutes and only covers the upper extremity. It is not possible to address an entire body affected by a stroke in one session.

HOMEWORK

Self-care is an ongoing trial for stroke patients, because almost *everything they do takes effort*. Giving your patient a set of boring, repetitive (although necessary) self-care exercises will almost ensure noncompliance. The following homework assignments are not only very helpful, but they are also intended to add humor to his daily regimen. Suggest only those exercises appropriate for his particular challenges.

Facial Paralysis

Explain the homework exercise to your patient as follows, while demonstrating every move with your own face:

- Remember when you learned the vowels A E I O U in school? Over-enunciate each one very slowly while stretching every single muscle in your face and holding the position for several seconds at a time. (*At this point, demonstrate, so he can see how humorous the exercise can be. Exaggerate each move.*)

Step-by-Step Protocol for | Stroke, Upper Extremity

All techniques can be adapted for use on the large muscles and joints of the lower extremity and the hips, as well as the smaller involved muscles and joints of the face, hands, and feet.

Technique	Duration
Apply a warm pack to the affected shoulder and/or elbow.	
Ask your client to take three large breaths. Slow, even, and deep. While he is breathing, place your hands on his chest to make initial contact and establish trust.	1 minute
Compressions, slow, medium pressure, very rhythmic, using your full, open hand • Foot, lower leg, knee, thigh, hip • Abdomen, chest • Ipsilateral hand, forearm, arm, shoulder • Across the top of the shoulders • Down to the contralateral arm, forearm, hand • Down to the contralateral hip, thigh, knee, lower leg, foot • Hold both feet for one moment	2 minutes
Remove the warm pack. Effleurage, petrissage, effleurage, compression, medium pressure, evenly rhythmic but briskly • *Unaffected* shoulder, arm, forearm, hand	2 minutes
Grasp the affected arm gently. • Examine every inch of the tissue. • Palpate every joint, shoulders, elbow, wrist, and every finger joint. • Move every joint to its comfortable end-feel to determine ROM.	3 minutes
Effleurage, deeply to the patient's tolerance, slow, rhythmic • Every inch of the affected arm from shoulder to fingertips	2 minutes
Effleurage, petrissage, digital kneading, effleurage, medium pressure, slow, rhythmic • Every inch of the affected arm from shoulder to fingertips	5 minutes
Digital kneading combined with compressions, medium pressure, very detailed, probing every bony prominence and every palpable joint surface, a little briskly, very rhythmic • Affected side shoulder girdle • Down the arm, into and around the humerus, around the elbow joint, into and around the ulna and humerus • Around and into the wrist bones, into and around each finger joint, into the palm and back of the hand, into the metacarpals	10 minutes

(continued)

Contraindications and Cautions

- The patient may have lost the ability to feel touch, pain, or temperature. Be sure to check it regularly during the session, using the agreed-upon communication style.

- Avoid work on the sternocleidomastoid (SCM) muscle and the anterior neck unless the patient is completely stable and unless you have a physician's clearance.

- If the patient is stabilized and not taking anticoagulants, work on the lateral and posterior neck with light pressure only, one side at a time. Do not stretch the neck.

- If a limb (or even a toe) feels cooler than normal, looks more swollen than normal, or appears brown, the patient should see a physician immediately.

- If a region of broken skin, such as between the toes, under the heel or coccyx, or under the elbows, has a particularly strong smell, the patient should see a physician immediately.

Technique	Duration
Cross-fiber friction, used judiciously. Using your thumb, find the underlying bony prominence, friction back and forth, until you feel the tissue release or see the skin significantly redden. Pay close attention to the patient's reaction; stop if he expresses any discomfort. Follow with ample cephalic effleurage. Cross-fiber friction should be performed after all tissue is well-warmed and prepared; slightly briskly, very rhythmically. • Limited to use at areas of extreme hypertonicity and contracture. Not to be used on the entire limb.	10 minutes
ROM exercises to the affected side. Move joints to end-feel, stop, and then move slightly beyond end-feel. ROM is the last technique after all other techniques have warmed and moved the tissue. Perform *both passive and active* exercises slowly, methodically, rhythmically, with the limb well-supported, and the patient relaxed. Note even the smallest improvements.	10 minutes
Because the unaffected side will be compensating and thus hypertonic, try to allow for at least a few minutes during each session to address the contralateral, compromised limb. The same techniques used on the affected side can be used to address the extreme hypertonicity of the unaffected side, but you may be able to work more briskly and deeply, depending on his tolerance and ability to report discomfort.	10 minutes
Finish the session with firm, steady, long effleurage strokes. • From hand to forearm to arm to shoulder • Across the shoulders • From arm to forearm to hand	5 minutes

- Open your eyes and mouth wide for the "AAAAAAAA."
- Grimace to the point of (feigned) horror and show all your teeth for the "EEEEEEE."
- Open your mouth and eyes wide for the "IIIIIIII."
- Furrow your brow, pull the muscles tight over your cheekbones, and open your eyes wide for the "OOOOOOOO."
- Purse your lips, thrust your jaw forward, and look devilish for the "UUUUUUU."

If you perform the exercises correctly, your facial muscles will feel as if they've had a workout.

Limited Range of Motion at the Shoulder

- Put on your favorite music that has a definite beat. Use music you enjoy that makes you want to move. Perform all of the following exercises *to the beat*.
- Rotate your *unaffected* shoulder both forward and backward, making large circles.
- Move your *unaffected* arm in a wide arc both forward and backward, making large circles.
- Rotate your *affected* shoulder both forward and backward. Making circles as large as you can. After every completed circle, snap your fingers with your *unaffected hand*. The sequence: Large circle (with the beat) with your

affected shoulder, snap your fingers once (with the beat) with your unaffected hand. You may feel clumsy at first, but in time, you'll be moving like a choreographer.

Limited Range of Motion at the Knee and Ankle

- Put on your favorite music that has a definite beat.
- Sit so you are stable and can freely swing your lower leg, from your knee down.
- To the beat, swing your *unaffected* lower leg forward and backward, five times.
- To the beat, swing your *affected* lower leg forward and backward, five times. Each time your toe comes forward, make a fist with your unaffected hand and rap your unaffected knee (to the beat). The sequence: Affected leg swings forward and backward (to the beat), rap fist to knee with unaffected hand. Repeat five times. Don't give up. You will feel awkward at first, but the music will keep you moving. You'll be able to measure progress much more easily as you see how you move from feeling clumsy to moving to the music.

Poor Balance or Limited Hip Movement

(Make sure he is reasonably stable, but needs to improve his balance, or ask his PT or physician if he is ready for this exercise before you assign it.)

- Purchase a big exercise ball appropriate for your height. Inflate it, but not completely; keep it slightly soft.
- Place it next to the sofa, a big easy chair, or to something soft and stable that you can hold onto. (It's not a good idea to put it next to a table with sharp edges.)
- Put on music that has a beat.
- If you think you need a little stabilizing, ask a partner to sit or stand in front of you and place her hands on your knees or hold your hands. Start bouncing to the beat. Begin with little bounces to get your bearings. At first, this will be a very unusual sensation, but in time you'll realize you can bounce and not fall over. As you feel more confident, make the bounces a little bigger. Stay with the beat.
- The first time you bounce, you might last only a few seconds or minutes. That's okay. As easy as this bouncing looks, you are engaging all of your thigh, leg, back, and hip muscles to stay upright and bounce. It's a great exercise and will help you regain balance and become stronger.
- Work up to being able to bounce for a whole song.

Deep-Breathing Technique

Breathing deeply is important for your general health, to avoid respiratory complications, and to help you relax. Whenever you have a moment, or before falling asleep, perform the following breathing exercise:

- Inhale as deeply as you can.
- Hold your breath to the slow count of three.
- Forcibly exhale until you feel as if you can't exhale any more breath. Hold your breath for a second.
- You'll immediately feel as if you must inhale. Do so, and rest for a moment.
- Repeat a few times.
- It's sometimes easier and more fun to purchase a bag of helium balloons and see how far you can blow them up.

Review

1. Describe the pathophysiology of a stroke.
2. Which area of the brain is affected if a stroke patient cannot use his left arm?
3. Explain why is it essential to get a possible stroke patient to the hospital immediately.
4. Name some comorbidities of a stroke.
5. At which point in the disease process can a massage therapist provide helpful therapy?
6. What are some contraindications in the care of a stroke patient?
7. Name the other health care team members who might be involved in a stroke patient's care.

BIBLIOGRAPHY

Fehrs L. Stroke Rehabilitation: 3 Complementary Therapies. Institute for Integrative Healthcare Studies. Available at: http://www.integrative-healthcare.org/mt/archives/2008/05/3_complementary.html. Accessed August 5, 2010.

Iwatsuki H, Ikuta Y, Shinoda K. Deep friction massage on the masticatory muscles in stroke patients increases biting force. *Journal of Physical Therapy Science* 2001;13:17–20.

MedlinePlus. Stroke: An Overview of Reference Sites. Available at: http://www.nlm.nih.gov/medlineplus/stroke.html. Accessed August 5, 2010.

Miesler DW. Stroke Rehab, Part 1: An Overview. *Massage & Bodywork Magazine*. April/May 2000. Available at: http://www.massagetherapy.com/articles/index.php/article_id/297/Stroke-Rehab-Part-1A. Accessed August 5, 2010.

Miesler DW. Stroke Rehab, Part 2. *Massage & Bodywork Magazine*. August/September 2000. Available at: http://www.massagetherapy.com/articles/index.php/article_id/298/Stroke-Rehab-Part-2. Accessed August 5, 2010.

National Institute of Neurological Disorders and Stroke. Post-Stroke Rehabilitation. Available at: http://www.stroke.nih.gov/materials/rehabilitation.htm. Accessed August 5, 2010.

National Institute of Neurological Disorders and Stroke. Stroke Rehabilitation Information. Available at: http://www.ninds.nih.gov/disorders/stroke/stroke_rehabilitation.htm. Accessed August 5, 2010.

Rattray F, Ludwig L. *Clinical Massage Therapy: Understanding, Assessing and Treating over 70 Conditions*, Toronto: Talus Incorporated, 2000.

Rodriguez D. Alternative Therapies for Stroke Treatment. Available at: http://www.everydayhealth.com/stroke/stroke-treatment.aspx. Accessed August 5, 2010.

Werner R. *A Massage Therapist's Guide to Pathology*, 4th ed. Philadelphia: Lippincott Williams & Wilkins, 2009.

40

Temporomandibular Joint Dysfunction

Definition: A group of conditions that cause jaw dysfunction and pain.

GENERAL INFORMATION

- Cause: often unknown
- Common causes, some not well proven: joint adhesions and scarring, intrajoint dysfunctions, hypertonic muscles, trigger points, postural distortions, abnormal teeth alignment, stress, mineral and vitamin deficiencies, osteoarthritis, direct facial trauma, mouth overstretching, habitual head or neck forward jut
- Contributing factors include bruxism (teeth grinding), teeth clenching, aging
- Duration self-limiting, most often weeks to months; rarely long term or debilitating
- Prevalence: more common in women, usually at age 20–40

Morbidity and Mortality

It is estimated that about 10 million Americans are affected by TMJD. Although 75% of adults have signs and symptoms, only 5% actually need treatment. Trigger points in the upper body caused by referred pain, hypertonicity in surrounding muscles caused by TMJ pain, and secondary conditions such as migraine and tension headaches, earaches, and toothaches often accompany this condition.

The prognosis is very good; most cases are treated conservatively and successfully. For many, untreated symptoms are short-lived and do not return.

PATHOPHYSIOLOGY

The TMJs are complicated, synovial, highly innervated, and modified hinge articulations of the mandibular condyles into the fossa of the temporal plates (Figure 40-1). The joint's function is easily palpated by pressing a finger in front of the ear while opening and closing the mouth. A fibrocartilage disc seated between the two bones prevents bone-on-bone contact. In its healthy state, the TMJs are bathed by slippery synovial fluid, which facilitates the chewing, talking, singing, yawning, and laughing movements demanded of such small, compact joints.

The muscles involved in jaw protrusion, retraction, contraction, compression, and side-to-side gliding are shown in Figures 40-2, 40-3, and 40-4. The masseter closes the jaw, the temporalis helps close the jaw and pull the mandible into retraction, and the pterygoids facilitate protrusion and side-to-side deviation. The suprahyoid and infrahyoid muscles form a sleeve that supports the jaw. The digastrics, which open and retract the jaw, form much of the floor of the mouth.

A TMJD diagnosis is difficult to confirm due to the preponderance of conflicting opinions in the medical literature. For example, bruxism is a contributing factor versus there is no proof that teeth grinding causes TMJD; pain is always present versus

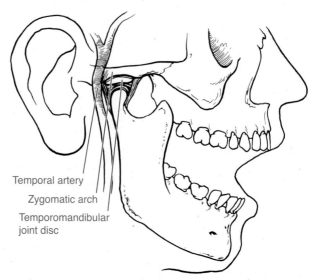

FIGURE 40-1 **The temporomandibular joint. From
Koopman WJ, Moreland LW. *Arthritis and Allied Conditions:
A Textbook of Rheumatology*, 15th ed. Philadelphia:
Lippincott Williams & Wilkins, 2005.**

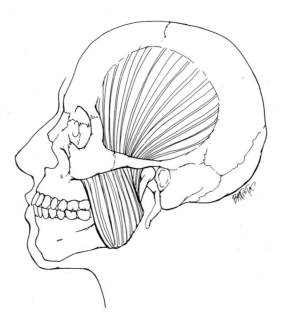

FIGURE 40-2 **The masseter
and temporalis muscles. From
Hendrickson T. *Massage for
Orthopedic Conditions*. Philadelphia:
Lippincott Williams & Wilkins, 2003.**

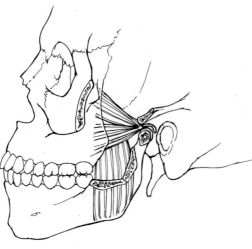

FIGURE 40-3 **The medial and
lateral pterygoids muscles.
From Hendrickson T. *Massage
for Orthopedic Conditions*.
Philadelphia: Lippincott Williams &
Wilkins, 2003.**

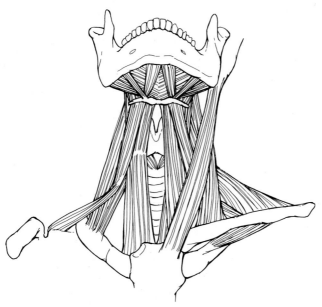

FIGURE 40-4 **The suprahyoid, infrahyoid, and digastric muscles. From Hendrickson T.** *Massage for Orthopedic Conditions.* **Philadelphia: Lippincott Williams & Wilkins, 2003.**

pain is not necessarily a symptom. Given these variances, combined with an absence of a firm medical diagnostic standard, it is not surprising that many cases are not diagnosed, incorrectly diagnosed, or self-diagnosed. Symptoms are often mistaken for migraines, sinus infection, neuralgias, or toothache.

Diagnostic efforts may include a thorough history of jaw clenching, gum chewing, and eating habits, as well as questions about stress management. Palpation will indicate bony or muscular abnormalities. A medical history will indicate past or present arthritis, extensive dental work, and/or facial trauma. Finally, X-rays, CT scans, or MRIs may be done to determine bony and soft tissue damage and displacement.

OVERALL SIGNS AND SYMPTOMS

TMJD generally occurs bilaterally, but it occasionally affects only one side. The following symptoms can occur either bilaterally or unilaterally.

- Asymmetrical jaw movement
- Uncomfortable bite
- Reduced range of motion in the jaw
- Occasional jaw locking
- Popping or clicking sound in the jaw
- Constant, sporadic, or use-related pain; can be sharp, intolerable
- Dull, aching facial pain, sometimes radiating to the neck and shoulders
- Slight facial swelling on the affected side
- Headaches, vertigo, hearing problems, earaches

SIGNS AND SYMPTOMS MASSAGE THERAPY CAN ADDRESS

- TMJD causes the pain-spasm-pain cycle and can also lead to trigger points; many massage therapy techniques effectively reduce localized hypertonicity.
- The condition is often secondary to profound stress, and easing a client into a parasympathetic state is one goal of most therapy sessions.
- Massage therapy techniques focusing on the face, head, neck, and shoulders, combined with relaxing modalities, can relieve muscle pain and anxiety.

TREATMENT OPTIONS

TMJD is usually treated conservatively; rarely is it necessary to resort to aggressive or irreversible measures. Moderate holistic approaches are usually preferred, especially since, inexplicably, symptoms can persist for a short, intense period; disappear; and then return later.

Treatment goals include relieving pain and improving efficient jaw movement. Since there is rarely one right way to treat this condition, several health care specialists may be involved simultaneously. These may include a dentist, a psychotherapist, a physical therapist (PT), a chiropractor, a massage therapist, an orthodontist, or an oral surgeon.

Initial, conservative treatment usually includes resting the jaw by eating soft foods, avoiding gum chewing and big joint movements (such as open-mouthed laughing or biting into a large sandwich), applying warm and/or cold compresses to the joint, and performing gentle mandibular exercises.

A mouth guard is one mildly invasive treatment. Used for decades to address teeth grinding, night clenching, and TMJ disorders, the effectiveness of this oral appliance remains questionable. Its use is intended to be short term; it does not "cure" the condition but instead protects the teeth from destruction. The person's bite could be altered by the long-term use of a mouth guard.

An aggressive treatment is a corticosteroid injection into the joint. Treatments of last resort include dental equilibrations, oral surgery, teeth extraction, facial surgery, and bridgework.

Prevention of occasional jaw pain involves avoiding gum chewing and biting hard objects, eliminating hard or sticky food, and supporting the lower jaw when yawning or laughing.

Common Medications

Muscle relaxants and/or antidepressants may be prescribed if the jaw pain is intolerable or if the emotional stress is uncontrolled. In rare cases, corticosteroid injections directly into the joint are beneficial. Over-the-counter (OTC) pain medication is typically used.

- Nonsteroidal anti-inflammatory drugs (NSAIDs), such as ibuprofen (Motrin, Advil) and naproxen (Aleve, Anaprox, Naprelan, Naprosyn)
- Nonopioid pain reliever fever reducers, such as acetaminophen (Tylenol, Feverall, Anacin, Panadol)

MASSAGE THERAPIST ASSESSMENT

Ideally, the massage therapist works as a member of a health care team. In reality, however, a person will usually come to a massage therapist after having self-diagnosed and has no intention of seeing a physician or dentist. In this situation, the therapist can intelligently assess to determine treatment.

Upon digital palpation, the normal masseter and other jaw muscles should feel as relaxed and almost as pliable as the gastrocnemius, for example. They should be easily mobile at the muscle belly (which is comparatively small), and superior and distal attachments should be palpable. (All facial muscle palpation and assessment should be performed bilaterally, for comparison.) The therapist is looking for hypertonicity and/or unilateral differences.

The client's mouth should easily open from 1.5 to 2.0 inches with no effort or pain. A practical measurement is to ask her to stack three fingers and place them in her mouth vertically (Figure 40-5). A limited or painful opening may indicate TMJ difficulties. The following actions should be performed easily and with no pain: gliding the jaw from side to side, protruding and retracting the jaw, chewing, yawning, and laughing. As the therapist observes the client, he is looking for indications of wincing from pain or lateral deviations.

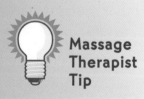

Massage Therapist Tip

Avoiding Intraoral Work

Although the treatment of TMJD can be profoundly aided by massage both inside and outside the mouth, most massage therapy schools do not teach intraoral techniques. Moreover, most states regulate against massage therapists entering any body orifices. Given these restrictions, the assessment and treatment outlined in this chapter focus on work that does *not* enter the oral cavity.

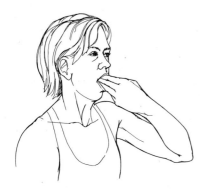

FIGURE 40-5 Determining a normal jaw opening: Ask the client to place three fingers, stacked vertically, into the opening of the mouth. From Hendrickson T. *Massage for Orthopedic Conditions*. Philadelphia: Lippincott Williams & Wilkins, 2003.

The therapist can inquire about past injuries, whiplash, trauma to the face, surgeries, lengthy dental procedures, and (while staying within scope of practice) past emotional traumas that might have caused bruxism. Further inquires about how the pain is managed will help the therapist determine a treatment plan.

THERAPEUTIC GOALS

Since there is a good chance that, left untreated, TMJD will resolve in time, the massage therapist can help hasten the recovery by reducing the pain-spasm-pain cycle before permanent joint damage is done to bone or cartilage. He can also relieve hypertonicity in surrounding muscles; address secondary or contributing factors (e.g., back pain from kyphosis); facilitate smooth, pain-free movement and function of both TMJs; and decrease irritable innervation.

MASSAGE SESSION FREQUENCY

- 60-minute sessions twice a week when the pain is severe
- 60-minute sessions once a week until recovery is complete
- 60-minute sessions once a month for maintenance

MASSAGE PROTOCOL

You will notice in the following protocol that extensive time is spent first relaxing the client, then softening superficial localized tissue, well before detailed or deep therapeutic work begins. The reason is multifaceted. The face is personal, rife with emotional agendas, and cannot be invaded as directly as the gastrocnemius, for example. A client who habitually clenches and grinds her teeth, when startled or distrusting, will clench and grind harder. Effective therapy to this region must be relatively deep, and trust must be gained and superficial tissue must be softened before "to the bone" deep work can be accomplished.

Getting Started

For easy access to relevant anatomic structures, position the client supine while working on the TMJ. Assure the client that, although you are focusing on her jaw, it is essential that she disrobe so you can easily get to the muscles that may contribute to her condition. The prolonged prone position, with the face compressed in the face cradle, may not be comfortable for the client's jaw. Side-lying is always a good alternative (with the neck supported and with a pillow between the knees) and is often the position in which many people sleep. Have hot towels or cold packs ready. Be sure to begin and end the session with relaxation techniques performed away from the face, neck, and jaw.

During the entire protocol, the client should be able to easily breathe, swallow, and speak. At no time should your pressure or hand positions compromise these functions.

Thinking It Through

It is not possible to separate TMJ problems from hypertonicities and imbalances in the rest of the body. Thinking through the following will clarify the importance of avoiding "spot work" when treating this condition and will prompt the therapist to investigate distal, seemingly unrelated, variances contributing to TMJD.

- Is there a leg-length variance? This common condition would lead to lateral pelvic tilt that affects spinal alignment, which in turn leads to head/neck misalignment, thus directly affecting the TMJ.
- Does the client have either scoliosis or kyphosis? Spinal curvatures ultimately cause imbalances at the cranial-spinal junction, therefore forcing the TMJ to adjust.
- Does the client carry her head forward or jut her jaw forward several hours a day, while sitting at a computer, for example? This position creates mandibular imbalance, which places direct abnormal pressure on the TMJ.
- Does the client have a sunken chest? This condition is common among radical mastectomy survivors, long-time smokers or asthmatics, or those with long-term kyphosis. A sunken chest pulls on the pectoralis complex, thus pulling the mandible forward.

Contraindications and Cautions:

- While treating the anterior neck muscles, do not compress the carotid artery.

- While treating the sternocleidomastoid (SCM), do not simultaneously work both sides.

- When palpating for the mastoid process and working on the occipital ridge to release the digastrics, be careful not to compress the styloid process.

- Ask permission before placing your hands anywhere near the face, jaw, or anterior neck.

Step-by-Step Protocol for Temporomandibular Joint Dysfunction

Technique	Duration
With the client positioned comfortably supine, perform relaxation techniques anywhere on the body (other than the jaw and face) that the client requests. (Scalp, feet, hands, and abdomen are some options.) If the client allows, place a warm compress on one or both sides of the jaw. She can help hold it in place.	5 minutes
Ask the client to perform full range-of-motion (ROM) movements at her jaw. Note imbalance and ask about pain or restrictions. Compression, effleurage, petrissage, digital kneading, effleurage, pressure to tolerance, slow, long, evenly rhythmic strokes • Occipital ridge • Superior trapezius • Posterior cervical spine musculature • Superior pectoralis major (pushing down with your fingers under the clavicle) • Pectoralis minor • Superior deltoids	8 minutes
With permission, place your soft hands and fingers on the anterior and lateral neck. Staying superficial and without compromising underlying structures, imagine your hands are glued to the *skin only* (you are also moving fascia at this point) and glide your hands around this region, moving in all directions, gently tugging the skin to its farthest comfortable extension, then allowing it to return and relax.	2 minutes
With slightly more pressure and more focused work, repeat the previous technique while applying sufficient pressure on the anterior and lateral neck so that you can palpate underlying *muscles*. Again, your hands and fingers are soft and open.	2 minutes
With permission, place your soft hands on either side of the client's face. Rest a moment. Repeat the previous technique by slowly and carefully moving the skin (fascia) of the entire face first and then progressing to palpating underlying muscles. Use broad, slow, noninvasive strokes but tug the tissue—the epidermis, dermis, underlying fascia, and superficial muscles—so that they begin the softening process and become accustomed to your touch. Now the real work begins.	3 minutes
Compression, skin rolling, plucking, pressure to tolerance, evenly rhythmic • From the chin to the TMJ, following the line of the mandible and along the zygomatic arch	3 minutes

(continued)

Technique	Duration
Digital kneading, in a gentle to-and-fro motion, at origin and insertion first, then move to the muscle belly, pressure to tolerance, evenly rhythmic, working one side of the face/jaw at a time. • SCM • Masseter • Temporalis • Medial and lateral pterygoids • Suprahyoids and infrahyoids • Digastrics	10 minutes (for both sides)
Rest for a moment, stroke the face, and then place your open, soft, still hands and fingers on the face and jaw.	A couple of breaths
Repeat your digital kneading techniques as listed previously, but move to a pressure that creates *slight* discomfort in its depth and stretch. Pain is not necessary for effective treatment. *Remember to stay on the bony prominences when working origins and insertions, and use caution when working on the muscle belly; stay well away from the most delicate and easily compromised structures, such as lymph nodes and major arteries and veins.*	10 minutes (for both sides)
Effleurage, medium pressure, with a soft, open hand, slow, evenly rhythmic • Occipital ridge • Superior trapezius • Deltoids • Pectoralis major • Anterior, posterior, lateral neck	2 minutes
Muscle stripping, used with great caution, focusing on the tiny muscles alone and not compromising underlying structures, working slowly, watching the client's reaction, interspersing frequent stroking and effleurage • SCM • Masseter • Temporalis • Medial and lateral pterygoids • Suprahyoids and infrahyoids • Digastrics	10 minutes (for both sides)
Ask the client to perform full ROM movements at her jaw. Note imbalance and ask about pain or restrictions. Note differences from the beginning of the session.	
Medium pressure, compression, effleurage; long, smooth, stroking techniques to the entire worked surface of the face, neck, and shoulders	2 minutes
Perform relaxing techniques anywhere else on the body other than the face, head, and neck.	3 minutes

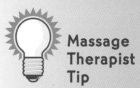

Massage Therapist Tip

Using Caution in the Anterior Neck

There is good reason for all massage therapy schools to teach that the anterior neck is an "endangerment zone." The small, compact area is dense with easily damaged tissue. Lymph nodes are nestled under the mandible. Major arteries and veins are easily palpable, and incorrect or rigorous compression can compromise circulation to and from the brain. The small fragile styloid process can be moved with pressure that is too aggressive. All of this does not contraindicate your work; instead, it forces you to stay completely focused on the positions of your fingers and hands. With a keen awareness of the anatomy that you touch and the pressure you use, you'll be able to work safely in this delicate region.

HOMEWORK

Working in your favor is the fact that TMJD will often spontaneously resolve. You can help move this recovery forward more quickly by making some homework assignments. As always, it is best to work with a PT or a physician, but in the (most probable) absence of either, you can safely suggest the following self-care exercises.

- Think "swan neck." Think of your neck as long, relaxed, and easily moved. When you feel yourself clenching or grinding, quickly open your mouth, take a big breath, and elongate your neck.
- Become aware of when you clench or grind. Gently place your fingers to your jaw, stroke it slowly, and try to relax.
- Try placing your tongue lightly at the roof of your mouth, which makes it impossible to clench your teeth.
- *Gently* stretch the muscles of your face and neck. Stretch your facial muscles by reciting the vowels AEIOU throughout your day.
- Here is the normal, relaxed posture for your head and neck; practice it throughout the day: shoulders down and relaxed, jaw free of tension, lips closed, teeth slightly apart, tongue gently touching the roof of your mouth behind the teeth.
- Breathe through your nose, not your mouth.

Review

1. List some of the names that refer to this condition.
2. Which bones meet to create the TMJ?
3. Name the muscles that are involved in normal jaw functions.
4. What are some cautions in working on clients who have TMJD?
5. How is TMJD usually treated?

BIBLIOGRAPHY

Barriere P, Zink S, Riehm S, et al. Massage of the lateral pterygoids muscle in acute TMJ dysfunction syndrome. PubMed 2009. Available at: http://www.ncbi.nlm.nih.gov/pubmed/19162287. Accessed August 5, 2010.

Cross N. Snap, Crackle and Pop, Part I. *Massage Today*. May 2001;1(05). Available at: http://www.massagetoday.com/mpacms/mt/article.php?id=10249. Accessed August 5, 2010.

Luchau T. The Temporomandibular Joint, Part 2. *Massage and Bodywork*. September/October 2009;121–126.

McKesson Health Solutions. UIHealthcare.com 2002–2003. TMJ (Temporomandibular Joint Syndrome). Available at: http://www.uihealthcare.com/topics/generalhealth/ghea3523.html. Accessed August 5, 2010.

National Institute of Dental and Craniofacial Research. TMJ Disorders. June 18, 2009. Available at: http://www.nidcr.nih.gov/OralHealth/Topics/TMJ/TMJDisorders.htm. Accessed August 5, 2010.

O'Rourke P, Hamm M. Jaws: how massage can help clients dealing with temporomandibular dysfunction. *Massage Therapy Journal* Winter 2008;65–74.

Rattray F, Ludwig L. *Clinical Massage Therapy: Understanding, Assessing and Treating over 70 Conditions*, Toronto: Talus Incorporated, 2000.

Shiel W. Temporomandibular Joint (TMJ) Syndrome. WebMD 2009. Available at: http://www.emedicinehealth.com/temporomandibular_joint_tmj_syndrome/article_em.htm. Accessed August 5, 2010.

Upledger J. TMJ: Primary Problem, or Tip of the Iceberg? *Massage Today*. August 2002;02(08). Available at: http://www.massagetoday.com/mpacms/mt/article.php?id=10531. Accessed August 5, 2010.

Werner R. *A Massage Therapist's Guide to Pathology*, 4th ed. Philadelphia: Lippincott Williams & Wilkins, 2009.

Zieve D, Juhn G, Eltz D. TMJ Disorders. MedlinePlus. March 27, 2009. Available at: http://vsearch.nlm.nih.gov/vivisimo/cgi-bin/query-meta?v%3Aproject=medlineplus&query=tmj+disorders&x=12&y=10. Accessed August 5, 2010.

41

Tendinosis

Definition: Injury and damage to a tendon.

GENERAL INFORMATION

- Primary cause: joint overuse due to athletic, recreational, or occupational activities
- Secondary causes: sudden joint injury, aging
- Commonly affected joints: elbow, wrist/forearm, shoulder, knee, heel/ankle
- Risk factors: frequent overhead motions, using vibratory tools or forceful exertion, working in awkward positions, repetitive movements, obesity
- Prevalent in middle age
- Often associated with systemic diseases, such as rheumatoid arthritis and diabetes

PATHOPHYSIOLOGY

Tendons are thick, fibrous bands located at the muscle's distal and proximal ends. All muscle/joint movement is possible because of this fulcrum-and-lever, highly effective biomechanical arrangement. Collagen and elastin within the tendinous tissue provide strength and elasticity, respectively. Inflammation of, or damage to, the tendon can occur anywhere along its path, but it usually happens at the juncture between tendon and bone. Rarely, in severe cases, the muscle can rupture off the bone. Temporarily or permanently weakened surrounding muscles often accompany tendinosis because of disuse atrophy at the painful site and overuse hypertonicity at the contralateral joint.

Diagnosis is medically confirmed by a variety of muscle resistance examinations. The patient generally reports a history of a specific, repeated activity leading to joint pain, tenderness, and self-imposed restrictions. X-rays, CT scans, or MRIs are rarely ordered and then only to rule out more complicated, possibly contributing, conditions. Self-diagnosis is the norm, however, as sufferers use the same previously mentioned criteria (usually combined with Internet research and colleagues' or friends' war stories) to confirm their condition.

OVERALL SIGNS AND SYMPTOMS

- Warmth to the touch
- Mild redness
- Mild swelling
- Decreased range of motion (ROM) secondary to pain
- Pain and tenderness upon palpation along the tendon path, often near the joint; at night and at rest; worse with activity

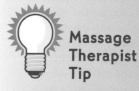

Massage Therapist Tip

An "Itis" without Inflammation

Although the term *tendonitis* is commonly used both inside and outside the medical profession, *tendinosis* and *tendinopathy* are more appropriate names because they encompasses the overall cellular (not necessarily inflammatory) and functional damage that results from a tendon injury. All four classic signs of inflammation—redness, swelling, heat, and pain—do not accompany many tendon injuries. It has now become questionable whether inflammation is a serious component of these injuries at all. You might think of a tendinopathy as a cellular and fibrous disorganization of the normally functioning muscle and tendon fibers. You will have the most success with clients if you work to repair damaged collagen and flush out joint waste instead of attempting to decrease a possibly nonexistent inflammation.

SIGNS AND SYMPTOMS MASSAGE THERAPY CAN ADDRESS

- The massage therapist approaches this condition primarily as a disorganization of cellular tendon components (and sometimes as a mild inflammatory process) and secondarily with respect for the client's pain, discomfort, and diminished ROM.
- Therapeutic techniques can address localized cellular nourishment and cleansing, as well as healing painful joints and atrophied, underused, or overused muscles.

TREATMENT OPTIONS

Thinking It Through

The importance of rest in healing overuse injuries is well documented. Also well established is the damage to the body caused by prolonged immobility. The massage therapist who addresses overuse injuries must often delicately balance these two physiologic realities while treating and when assigning homework. Here are some questions that might arise:

- Is the injury work-related or recreation-related? How will this affect the client's ability to truly rest?
- Does the client understand that rest is important until the joint begins to heal, but then movement, albeit not full-throttle use, is essential?
- If the client is using a brace or splint, how long is he wearing it, and is it making the joint weaker or dependent? What is the effect on surrounding and contralateral joints?
- Is he inclined to "muscle his way through" the pain and keep using the joint while ignoring the therapeutic necessity of rest?
- Is he inclined to overrest until there is absolutely no pain? Does he understand the importance of mild use and stretching?

Initial treatment focuses on relieving pain and reducing any inflammation. Subsequent treatment includes strengthening and stretching the joint-tendon-muscle unit to ensure the return to full function. Rest, or ceasing offending activities, is essential. Rest, however, is not synonymous with complete immobilization. Severely restricting all normal limb use leads to joint weakness, thereby impeding healing and causing secondary difficulties. Ice application is helpful for acute, throbbing pain when the tendon appears inflamed. Warm packs are appropriate when the inflammation or acute pain has subsided, and for dull, achy pain. Self-care without medical attention, combined with rest, simple home remedies, and over-the-counter (OTC) pain and anti-inflammatory medications, can resolve most cases of tendinosis.

If simple personal restraint is not possible or convenient, a physician may suggest a splint or removable brace, a cane, or crutches for short-term use. If pain persists and normal activities are compromised for more than a few days, a sports medicine physician or rheumatologist should be consulted. In severe cases, when the tendon ruptures off the bone, surgical repair is necessary.

Preventive techniques include avoiding or altering the performance of a repeated activity, stretching before and especially after activity, and striving for ergonomically correct body mechanics. If mild symptoms recur, vigilant ice application and self-imposed rest can completely prevent exacerbation.

Common Medications

Corticosteroid injections around the affected joint can reduce inflammation and pain. Repeated injections, which can lead to a weakened and possibly ruptured tendon, are not recommended.

- Nonsteroidal anti-inflammatory drugs (NSAIDs), such as naproxen (Aleve, Anaprox, Naprelan, Naprosyn)
- Nonopioid pain reliever and fever reducers, such as acetaminophen (Tylenol, Feverall, Anacin, Panadol)

MASSAGE THERAPIST ASSESSMENT

Because tendinosis is often self-diagnosed, the massage therapist has an opportunity to use keen assessment skills. If the client complains of a painful joint associated with specific overuse (e.g., hammering, playing tennis, continual wrist twisting on the job); has relative, but not complete, relief upon rest; and reports a chronic pattern of occurrence, the therapist is probably dealing with a tendinopathy. Gentle palpation and passive and active ROM movements will further confirm the assessment. It is advisable to look at other structures related to the shoulder to determine if there is accompanying pain in the triceps, flexors, or extensors. Trigger points harbored in surrounding muscles can contribute to elbow joint pain.

If, however, the client presents with a painful joint that has resulted from no obvious overuse, or if the joint is reddened, warm to the touch, swollen, and/or the client suffers from an autoimmune disorder or diabetes, the therapist should refer him to a physician before treating.

THERAPEUTIC GOALS

It is reasonable for the massage therapist to help relieve pain and inflammation (if inflammation is present), help the reorganization and rebuilding of healthy collagen, flush the joint of cellular irritants, improve ROM, and decrease anxiety, which often accompanies overuse injuries.

MASSAGE SESSION FREQUENCY

Unless the therapist is trained in lymphatic drainage techniques, the injured limb should not be addressed during the acute, very painful stage. Once the acute pain has quieted, the client can be seen regularly.

- 60-minute sessions once a week, until most symptoms subside
- 60-minute sessions every other week, for 2 weeks, after all symptoms subside
- 60-minute monthly maintenance sessions

MASSAGE PROTOCOL

The following protocol addresses forearm flexor tendinosis manifesting at the wrist. You can use these same techniques on any similarly affected joint. You do not treat this condition as if it is an inflammation. The cross-fiber and frictioning techniques are not intended to create a temporary region of localized inflammation as much as they are used to help reorganize collagen fibers. This reorganization is facilitated by increasing the presence of fresh arterial blood, which is full of essential reparatory nutrients, to the region and by flushing waste from the joint. As with any injury, working on the painful site for a full 60 minutes would be inappropriate and painful. Half of the protocol addresses the injury, while the other half addresses contralateral, compensatory hypertonicity.

Getting Started

Positioning for the client's comfort level is essential. Have plenty of pillows ready. Treatment will include whole-body relaxation techniques, so more than partial disrobing is necessary. Ice packs and warm packs can be helpful. (Even though you are not treating this as an inflammation, ice packs can quiet the pain.)

The protocol will require you to cause temporary, localized discomfort. Diplomacy and tact are necessary to persuade the client to bear the sometimes uncomfortable—but never painful—techniques. It is important to be patient and keenly aware of the effects of your pressure and methods. As always, "no pain, no gain" is *not* the massage therapist's mantra.

HOMEWORK

Self-care is the norm when treating tendinopathies. The vigilance and consistency with which the client performs the following exercises can significantly speed healing.

- Immobilization is essential only in the early stages of your injury. Once the acute pain subsides, gentle use and movement are important.
- Apply ice packs any time you are in pain—10 minutes on, and then take the ice off once every hour.
- Apply hot or warm packs when the pain is dull and achy.
- Experiment with OTC "hot/cold" creams and gels; some can be beneficial.
- When you are not in acute pain, grip the belly of your affected muscle and squeeze it like a sponge. Move it around as much as possible. Stroke the muscle deeply from one joint to another, working in the direction of your heart.

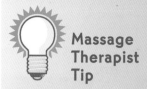

Massage Therapist Tip

Telling Him He Can't Play Tennis

You will face many challenges when attempting to treat a tendinopathy, because the offending activity is either essential for the client's livelihood or necessary for his enjoyment. He'll be most anxious to return to full activity; however, the client's adamant desire to be fully functional can seriously thwart your therapeutic efforts. A single hour of even stellar massage therapy will have little effect if the client immediately returns to the same unmodified behavior. You will need to use all of your diplomatic skills to convince him that he must be patient and temporarily halt the offending activity, while assuring him that if he follows your advice, and possibly the advice of his physician, he will play tennis again, pain free.

Contraindications and Cautions

- Warm packs are not appropriate when the joint shows any signs of inflammation.
- Causing pain (moving beyond the necessary feeling of discomfort) is not therapeutic or respectful of the injury.
- If the injury does not respond well and relatively quickly to rest and immobility (within days to a couple of weeks), urge the client to see a physician.
- Deep friction techniques are contraindicated if the client is taking anti-inflammatory medications.

Step-by-Step Protocol for Tendinosis of the Wrist

Technique	Duration
Greet the client's body with overall warming compression. Offer relaxation techniques to one specific area to begin the session.	5 minutes
Compression, light-then-medium pressure, evenly rhythmic • Shoulder, arm, forearm, palm	3 minutes
Effleurage, light-then-medium pressure, evenly rhythmic, work cephalically • Shoulder, arm, forearm, palm	2 minutes
Compression and effleurage, deep pressure, evenly rhythmic • Forearm and palm	2 minutes
Digital stripping (using your thumb is most helpful), start with light pressure and then move in as deeply as the client can tolerate. Work slowly, in between, in, and around all tendons and muscles; perform thorough and detailed work. This area is dense with long, stringy muscles. • Palm • Distal forearm • Mid-forearm • Proximal forearm	8 minutes
Effleurage, medium pressure, briskly • Palm, forearm, arm	1 minute
Cross-fiber friction, as if strumming guitar strings; start with light pressure, then move in as deeply as the client can tolerate. • Palm • Distal forearm • Mid-forearm • Proximal forearm	5 minutes
Find the point at which the client reports the most pain. It could be no larger than a quarter or as large as a few inches. Gently stroke the region for a few seconds, and then compress it slightly more deeply. Then effleurage it even more deeply. Now do cross-fiber friction as deeply as the client can tolerate. At the point where he is uncomfortable, stop and compress the area with your thumb, hold it still, and then slowly release the compression. Ask the client to continue to breathe; ask him about his favorite hobby or sports team to distract him. This may not be comfortable, but it is very beneficial. Stroke the region when you are done. Then perform slow, careful, passive ROM at the wrist, holding the stretch a little at the end-feel.	3 minutes
Effleurage, petrissage, effleurage, stroking, medium pressure, slow, evenly rhythmic • Arm • Forearm • Palm	1 minute

(continued)

Technique	Duration
Treat compensating, hypertonic muscles at the shoulder joint or contralateral forearm.	25 minutes
Finish the session by performing more overall relaxing techniques.	5 minutes

Try to grasp the tendon between your thumb and index finger where it attaches to the bone. Wiggle it back and forth slowly.
- Soak the joint and limb in a warm Epsom salts bath.
- As soon as the acute pain subsides, stretch the muscle by performing slow ROM exercises. Hold the stretch in every direction for a few seconds.
- Be sure not to overrest the joint or overuse splints or protective devices.
- Rearrange your workspace for better ergonomics and body mechanics.
- Once you are pain-free and have returned to full function, be keenly aware of *any* hint of recurrence. Immediately ease up on activities, apply ice, do self-massage, and use any variety of OTC anti-inflammatory topical products.

Review

1. What is tendinosis?
2. List some of the other names for the condition.
3. Is it classically an inflammatory process?
4. Describe the normal treatment for tendinosis.
5. What are some beneficial self-care techniques?

BIBLIOGRAPHY

Almekinders LC. Tendonitis and other chronic tendinopathies. *Journal of the American Academy of Orthopedic Surgery* 1998;6:157–164. Available at: http://orthopedics.about.com/cs/sportsmedicine/a/tendonitis. Accessed August 8, 2010.

Benjamin B. Weakness and Tendon Injuries. *Massage Today*. November 2003;3(11). Available at: http://www.massagetoday.com/mpacms/mt/article.php?id=10815. Accessed August 8, 2010.

Brosseau L, Casimiro L, Milne S, et al. Deep transverse friction massage for treating tendinitis. *Cochrane Database Syst Rev.* 2002:CD003528. Available at http://www.ncbi.nlm.nih.gov/pubmed/11869672. Accessed August 8, 2010.

Ehrlich SD, Albert JD, Cacchio A. Tendinitis. University of Maryland Medical Center website, June 11, 2008. Available at: http://www.umm.edu/altmed/articles/tendinitis-000163.htm. Accessed August 8, 2010.

Ingraham P. Friction Massage Therapy for Tendonitis. SaveYourself.ca. Available at: http://saveyourself.ca/articles/frictions.php. Accessed August 8, 2010.

Levesque MC. (Reviewer). What Is Tendinitis? WebMD. September 21, 2009. Available at: http://www.webmd.com/osteoarthritis/guide/arthritis-tendinitis. Accessed August 8, 2010.

Lowe W. When Is It Tendinitis? *Massage Today*. July 2001;1(07). Available at: http://www.massagetoday.com/mpacms/mt/article.php?id=10287. Accessed August 8, 2010.

Steele M, Norvell JG. Tendonitis. EMedicine. March 31, 2008. Available at: http://www.emedicine.medscape.com/article/809692-overview. Accessed August 8, 2010.

Vorvick L. Tendinitis. MedlinePlus. August 11, 2008. Available at: http://www.nlm.nih.gov/medlineplus/ency/article/001229.htm. Accessed August 8, 2010.

Werner R. *A Massage Therapist's Guide to Pathology*, 4th ed. Philadelphia: Lippincott Williams & Wilkins, 2009.

Zeballos A. Tendinitis. EMedicineHealth. 2009. Available at: http://www.emedicinehealth.com/tendinitis/article_em.htm. Accessed August 8, 2010.

42

Thoracic Outlet Syndrome

Definition: Upper extremity pain and/or compromised function resulting from compression, irritation, or injury to the neurovascular structures of the anterior neck.

GENERAL INFORMATION

- Controversial cause, diagnosis, and treatment
- Classified as neurogenic, venous, or arterial based on the structures affected
- Neurogenic TOS causes: neck injury, whiplash, fall, repetitive movement
- Venous TOS causes: subclavian vein obstruction secondary to congenital anatomic anomalies or arm overuse, as in pitching, swimming, weight lifting, or working with the arms above the head; also poor posture, pregnancy, or obesity
- Arterial TOS causes: subclavian artery (axillary artery) stenosis or aneurysm secondary to a cervical rib congenital anomaly
- Mimicked by trigger points in the primary neck muscles
- Onset usually between ages 20 and 50
- Prevalence: three times more common in women

Morbidity and Mortality

Reported statistical occurrence varies widely. Some medical professionals question whether the syndrome exists at all. TOS symptoms are often shared with or mistaken for, or are comorbid with, spinal cord injuries or neoplasms, diabetes, hypothyroidism, superficial thrombophlebitis, carpal tunnel syndrome, multiple sclerosis, rotator cuff injuries, ulnar nerve compression at the elbow, fibromyalgia, brachial plexitis, and vasculitis.

The prognosis for all forms of TOS is good. Neurogenic TOS rarely progresses but does take longer to resolve. Venous and arterial TOS usually resolve relatively quick with appropriate treatment. If left untreated, however, permanent nerve damage and, in rare cases, loss of limb use can occur.

PATHOPHYSIOLOGY

The thoracic outlet spaces are located anterolateral, bilaterally between the clavicle and T-1, the first rib. The structures involved in TOS are shown in Figure 42-1. The brachial plexus, which is a bundle of the C-5, C-6, C-7, C-8, and T-1 spinal nerve roots, exits the spinal cord at the base of the skull. The plexus then traverses down the neck in a usually predictable pattern from underneath the clavicle and first rib then out toward the axilla, where it branches to continue down the anterior, medial, lateral, and posterior arm. It is a sensory *and* motor nerve network consisting of five major nerves: the median, radial, ulnar, musculocutaneous, and axillary. The brachial plexus controls shoulder, arm, and hand muscle sensations and movements. Sensations travel *to* the brain, and motor signals are issued *from* the brain through this nerve bundle. Thus, a person can both feel the heat of a coffee mug and grasp the mug to bring it to the mouth.

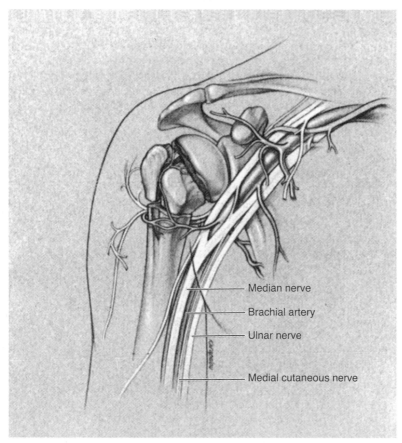

FIGURE 42-1 **Anatomic structures involved in, and affected by, TOS. The plexus traverses down the neck from underneath the clavicle and first rib, then out toward the axilla. From Koval KJ, Zuckerman, JD. *Atlas of Orthopaedic Surgery: A Multimedia Reference*. Philadelphia: Lippincott Williams & Wilkins, 2004.**

All forms of TOS are entrapment syndromes of either the brachial plexus or the veins and arteries that feed the shoulder, arm, and hand. The nerves and vessels may be trapped between the anterior and middle scalenes, between the clavicle and T-1, and/or between the pectoralis minor and rib cage. As in any other part of the body, nerve compression or compromise results in pain along the nerve pathway and/or loss of function of the limb. The severity of the pain and the degree of functional loss correlate to the extent of injury to the nerve.

Neurogenic symptoms, from compression of the brachial plexus, occur in 95% of TOS cases. Nerve roots at C-8 and T-1 are usually involved, causing pain and paresthesias (numbness and tingling) along the ulnar nerve pathway. Nerve root involvement at C-5, C-6, and C-7 occurs almost as often, with neurogenic symptoms radiating to the neck, ear, upper chest, upper back, and outer arm along the radial nerve pathway.

Venous or arterial TOS occurs when veins or arteries that travel under the clavicle are compressed. The subclavian artery (axillary artery) sends oxygenated blood to, and the subclavian vein drains deoxygenated blood from, the upper extremity. Compression of these delicate structures leads to compromised blood flow, which manifests as color changes, such as blanching (paleness) and cyanosis (bluish color), as well as an uncomfortable cooling of the upper extremity. Neurogenic TOS is far more prevalent than the two vascular forms.

Diagnosis is difficult and sometimes controvesial. Symptoms can be subjective and chronic and related to other medical conditions. Sensory symptoms are difficult to measure. Physical examination findings are often completely normal. As a result, a typical diagnosis may be nerve compression syndrome rather than TOS. However,

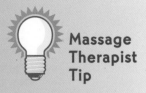

Massage Therapist Tip

Being Aware of Possible Thrombus

When blood vessels are compressed, blood does not flow freely, and pooled blood is an ideal environment for the formation of a blood clot or thrombus. Thrombi are life threatening, especially in the neck because of the proximity to the brain and lungs. As you palpate your client's cervical and upper arm regions before the treatment, be aware of the classic signs of localized thrombi: swelling, heat, pain, and warmth. You'll notice that these are identical symptoms to venous or arterial TOS; however, don't take a chance and proceed with any techniques that might move the thrombus. If you notice any of these symptoms, discontinue your treatment and refer the client to a physician.

attempts are sometimes made to pin down an exact diagnosis by performing specific tests. Provocative tests (techniques that duplicate or exacerbate the patient's complaints), although commonly used, are considered unreliable. Although the elevated arm stress test (EAST) is also considered inconclusive, it is the one that is used most often for screening for TOS. Neck X-rays may indicate skeletal abnormalities. Chest X-rays can indicate clavicular deformities, pulmonary disease, or tumors. Arteriographies and venographies can show evidence of blood flow abnormalities. Nerve conduction evaluations are the best indicators of neurogenic TOS.

OVERALL SIGNS AND SYMPTOMS

The phrase, *constellation of symptoms,* is often used when describing TOS symptomology due to the varying and widespread nature of the complaints. Symptoms can be unilateral or bilateral.

Neurogenic TOS symptoms:

- Pain, usually along the middle upper arm, forearm, fourth and fifth fingers
- Paresthesias, usually involving all fingers, especially the fourth and fifth fingers and the forearm
- Arm and/or hand weakness
- Arm and/or hand cold intolerance
- Neck pain, usually at the trapezius or the chest below the clavicle
- Headache in the occipital region

Venous and arterial TOS symptoms are very similar. Affected arm cyanosis is specific to venous TOS. The absence of a pulse in the affected arm is specific to arterial TOS.

Venous and arterial TOS symptoms:

- Arm swelling
- Hand and/or finger paresthesias
- Arm and/or hand pain, pallor, or paresthesias

SIGNS AND SYMPTOMS MASSAGE THERAPY CAN ADDRESS

- The massage therapist can address the pain, paresthesias, and compensating hypertonicity and trigger points that accompany this condition.
- *Note:* The origin of TOS is located in what most massage schools describe as an endangerment zone, so discovering signs and symptoms should be approached with caution.

TREATMENT OPTIONS

Treatment usually involves conservative measures of physical therapy (PT) combined with pain relief medications. Rarely is surgery necessary. Patients are counseled to avoid prolonged periods of overhead arm positioning, such as sleeping supine with arms extended up and behind the head, or sleeping prone with arms above the head.

Common Medications

Patients whose symptoms prompt an emergency room visit may be suffering from painful venous or arterial TOS and will be given intravenous (IV) anticoagulants (heparin) immediately. This situation, however, is rare. Muscle relaxants may be prescribed temporarily. More commonly, the following medications are used to address TOS.

- Nonsteroidal anti-inflammatory drugs (NSAIDs), such as ibuprofen (Motrin, Advil)
- Nonopioid pain reliever and fever reducers, such as acetaminophen (Tylenol, FeverAll, Anacin, Panadol)
- Tricyclic antidepressants, such as doxepin hydrochloride (Sinequan)
- Anticoagulants, such as warfarin sodium (Coumadin)

MASSAGE THERAPIST ASSESSMENT

Assessing for the presence of TOS is well outside the scope of practice for most massage therapists. Given the complexity of the condition, the fact that it often mimics other systemic diseases, and that even the simple test of pulse taking is not taught in most massage therapy schools, it is wiser for the massage therapist to wait until after the client has been diagnosed by a medical professional. After this assurance, a detailed verbal assessment of symptoms, combined with range-of-motion (ROM) exercises and palpation for temperature changes and localized pain, can give the therapist sufficient information to initiate treatment. If there is any doubt about the origin of the client's pain, however, or if swelling and heat are present, it is best to refer the client immediately to a physician.

THERAPEUTIC GOALS

Even with the complexity of this condition, it is reasonable to expect that the massage therapist can aid in decreasing pain, relaxing hypertonic muscles, reducing sympathetic nervous system activity, increasing circulation to compromised structures, and teaching the client more efficient postural, breathing, and compensating habits.

MASSAGE SESSION FREQUENCY

- Ideally: 60- to 90-minute sessions, twice a week, when the client is first diagnosed and pain and discomfort are at their worst.
- 60- to 90-minute sessions once a week, when the pain decreases. Continue this frequency until all symptoms are relieved.
- 60-minute sessions every other week for 3 months.
- 60-minute monthly maintenance as part of the client's self-care regimen.
- Infrequent work will not produce the desired results.

MASSAGE PROTOCOL

The best approach to treating TOS is directly related to its etiology. The specific structures—anterior scalenes, pectoralis minor, and costoclavicular region—correlate to the manifesting symptoms. Compensating and postural muscles must also be addressed. In an ideal world and with the client getting medical and/or PT treatment, you will know the exact origin of the TOS. The diagnosis might be "TOS of neurogenic origin" or "TOS of vascular origin," for example. Remembering that all forms of TOS are entrapment syndromes of either the brachial plexus or the arteries and veins that feed and drain the shoulder, arm, and hand, you would check your anatomy books to review that the nerves and vessels may be trapped between the anterior and middle scalenes, between the clavicle and T-1, and between the pectoralis minor and rib cage. You would then have a clear map for proceeding.

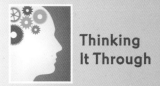

Thinking It Through

Muscular bracing is a common side effect of TOS. The condition begins insidiously and progresses to the point of sometimes severe compromise of the neck, upper back, and upper extremity. As a result, the person braces for pain and compensates by using alternative muscles for a period of months or years. By the time the massage therapist gets involved, the entire upper body may well be compromised. The therapist can consider why the following muscles may respond as a result of bracing and self-limiting movements from TOS pain.

- Sternocleidomastoid (SCM)
- Trapezius
- Latissimus dorsi
- Scalenes
- Cervical and thoracic erector complex
- Pectoralis major and minor
- Deltoids
- Occipitofrontalis
- Temporalis
- Masseter

In the real world, however, it is more likely that your client will present with a vague set of upper extremity symptoms after having visited several physicians and experiencing little relief. While being appropriate in your comments about the medical profession, you can make it clear that—unless the TOS has a pathologic origin (tumor or thrombus)—it is a *structural problem* ideally treated by intelligent massage therapy and that you will most probably be able to provide relief. The generalized approach of treating the entire shoulder girdle, neck region, and upper back in the following protocol is based on the real-world scenario. It assumes entrapment of either the brachial plexus or the subclavian vein or artery from postural or overused etiology.

Getting Started

Positioning will be a challenge. Side-lying, which could be the perfect position to approach cervical, clavicular, and upper shoulder problems, may be out of the question because of client discomfort. The prone position may be ruled out for the same reason. Working with the client comfortably pillowed in the supine position may be your only option and that is the position assumed in the following protocol. Of course, the client leads the way.

Do not apply hot or cold packs to any swollen structures in the neck, shoulder, or upper extremity when treating this condition. If you are not sure that there is no thrombus, hot packs can exacerbate TOS.

Use caution during stretching techniques so you do not reproduce or exacerbate this condition. For example, if she tells you that laying her arm over her head causes numbness and tingling, do not perform either passive or active ROM exercises approaching that position.

It is worth repeating that this work is performed in what is most commonly called an endangerment zone, for good reason. The neck is congested with vascular and nervous structures that, if compressed for too long, can compromise brain function. Be sure to focus, keep a clear head, remember your anatomy, and proceed gently.

There is a lot to be done in this protocol, so it departs from the normal 60-minute session and moves to a more appropriate 90-minute session.

HOMEWORK

Whether or not you are working with a PT or a physician, you can safely recommend gentle homework assignments to ensure your client's ongoing shoulder mobilization and improved posture.

- The doorway stretch: Do this once a day. (See Figures 5-4, 5-5, 5-6, and 6-1.)
- Stand up straight. Make slow, big circles with your arms, one arm at a time. Circle several times backward then circle several times forward. If you experience pain or tingling, stop.
- Maintain good posture. Don't slouch. If you find yourself slouching when you are sitting or standing, take a big breath and purposefully roll your shoulders backward several times. Pretend that you are hanging your shoulders on a very straight hanger that is positioned behind you, and allow them to gently stay there.
- Teach yourself exercises for whole-body relaxation.
- Lay on the floor in a position reminiscent of making "snow angels" when you were a kid. Make "carpet angels" by reproducing that slow, even, full ROM movement of both arms and legs. Do not cause pain. When you're done, rest with your arms fully outstretched from your shoulders and breathe deeply.
- Take frequent breaks from any activities that make your symptoms worse.

Step-by-Step Protocol for **Neurogenic Thoracic Outlet Syndrome of the Right Upper Extremity**

Technique	Duration
With the client supine and you sitting at her head, gently lay your hands on the anterior neck. Rest a moment.	1 minute
Soften the fascia by slowly and gently, but firmly, stretching the tissue in all directions. Thoroughly work the following regions: • Anterior, lateral, posterior neck • Above and below the clavicle • As far down the anterior chest as modesty allows • Over the superior trapezius • Over the deltoid	5 minutes
Plucking, briskly, firmly, with keen awareness of staying on the superficial tissue, not involving the muscles yet. (*Avoid any throbbing vessel; it is probably the carotid artery.*) • Anterior, lateral, posterior neck • Above and below the clavicle • As far down the anterior chest as modesty allows • Over the superior trapezius region • Over the deltoid region	5 minutes
Passive ROM, slowly, gently, moving to end-feel. Ask the client to take a full breath, and move slightly beyond comfortable end-feel. Be sure not to cause any pain. • The head and neck: side to side, then ear to shoulder. (*Avoid hyperflexion and hyperextension at the neck.*) • The affected shoulder. After performing normal ROM, carefully pull the shoulder down toward the client's feet. Grasp the arm at the biceps and forearm, not at the joints, to perform this passive stretch. • The elbow, wrist, and all fingers.	7 minutes
Compression, effleurage, petrissage, effleurage, trying to reach all origins and insertions; medium pressure, slowly rhythmic • Superior trapezius where it attaches to the occipital ridge • Superior trapezius at the shoulders • Scalene complex • SCM • Pectoralis major and minor • Deltoid complex • Biceps and triceps (spend the least amount of time here)	10 minutes
By now, you have identified areas of hypertonicity and/or trigger points. (See Chapter 43 for trigger points.) Return to the areas of extreme hypertonicity. Digitally knead, effleurage, petrissage, and muscle strip these regions with care. Use medium pressure in the neck region, medium-to-deep pressure elsewhere. Use caution not to compromise underlying vessels. Work slowly and evenly rhythmic.	15 minutes

Contraindications and Cautions:

• Be aware of possible comorbidities. Proceed only after considering contraindications for all existing medical conditions.

• Heat or cold should not be applied to the neck, chest, arm, or hand regions without physician's permission.

• Even in the presence of trigger points and extreme hypertonicity, aggressive techniques such as stripping or too aggressive ROM, are contraindicated.

(continued)

Technique	Duration
Stand at the client's affected side. Ask her to slide to the edge of the table. Lay her arm over the edge of the table, down toward the floor. (If this exacerbates symptoms, skip this step.) Place the heel of your hand at the position of the pectoralis minor, near the coracoid process. Slowly but firmly press directly down into the client's pectoralis minor until you feel the coracoid process. Press for a few seconds and release. Repeat once again. Then return the client to the normal position on the table.	5 minutes
Digital kneading, effleurage, petrissage, deep to the client's tolerance, evenly rhythmic • Along the occipital ridge • Into the superior trapezius and out onto the deltoids	5 minutes
Effleurage and stroke the entire area you have been working to soothe any irritated structures (and the client).	5 minutes
Repeat the initial, introductory techniques of softening the fascia and plucking. Perform them much more deeply and with more vigor this time. Aim to produce superficial redness from your plucking. Work to muscle depth when moving the fascia. Finish by stroking the area you worked again to soothe.	7 minutes
Repeat the *passive* ROM exercises, same as the previous step, especially the shoulder pull. Ask the client to perform *active* ROM to determine any increased ROM and pain relief.	5 minutes
Return to the most hypertonic and compromised structures. Compression, muscle stripping, petrissage, effleurage, deep to the client's tolerance, a little more swiftly.	15 minutes
Effleurage the entire area to soothe. Work more firmly than your normal effleurage but work very slowly.	5 minutes

Review

1. Why is TOS so difficult to diagnose?
2. Describe other conditions that mimic the symptoms of TOS.
3. Explain why heat would be inappropriate to apply to a swollen cervical region where a thrombus is suspected.
4. Name 10 muscles that might be affected by TOS.
5. Explain the difference in symptoms based on TOS of neurogenic origin as opposed to TOS of vascular origin.

BIBLIOGRAPHY

BenEliyahu D. Posttraumatic Cervico-Axillary Syndrome (Thoracic Outlet Syndrome). *Dynamic Chiropractic*. May 1998;16(12). Available at: http://www.chiroweb.com/mpacms/dc/article.php?id=37242. Accessed August 8, 2010.

Chang AK, Bohan JS. Thoracic Outlet Syndrome. Emedicine Medscape. Available at: http://emedicine.medscape.com/article/760477-overview. Accessed August 8, 2010.

Dalton E. Thoracic Outlet Syndrome. April–May 2007 Newsletter. Available at: http://erikdalton.com/newsletter/07April_May_Newsletter.htm. Accessed August 8, 2010.

MayoClinic. Thoracic Outlet Syndrome. November 8, 2008. Available at: http://www
    .mayoclinic.com/health/thoracic-outlet-syndrome/DS00800. Accessed August 8, 2010.
Muscolino JE. Freedom from Thoracic Outlet Syndrome. *AMTA Massage Journal* Winter 2006.
    Available at: http://www.amtamassage.org/journal/winter06_2journal/
    winter06_2_art3-2.html. Accessed August 8, 2010.
National Pain Foundation. Thoracic Outlet Syndrome, 2009. Available at: http://
    www.nationalpainfoundation.org/articles/577/what-is-it. Accessed August 8, 2010.
Rattray F, Ludwig L. *Clinical Massage Therapy: Understanding, Assessing and Treating over 70
    Conditions*, Toronto: Talus Incorporated, 2000.
Shiel WC Jr. Thoracic Outlet Syndrome. February 20, 2008. MedicineNet. Available at:
    http://www.medicinenet.com/thoracic_outlet_syndrome/article.htm. Accessed
    August 8, 2010.

43

Trigger Points

Definition: A localized area of muscle hypertonicity that radiates in a predictable pain pattern.

GENERAL INFORMATION

- Cyclical causes: insufficient cellular energy (adenosine triphosphate [ATP]) to a specific muscle area secondary to localized ischemia (restricted blood flow), from prolonged muscle contraction, leading to further insufficient ATP
- Contributing factors: poor posture; repetitive motion; muscle compensation from injury, accident, or prolonged inactivity; nutritional deficiency; chronic infection; sleep deprivation; depression
- Usually occurs in skeletal muscles, especially the trapezius, rhomboids, sternocleidomastoid (SCM), masseter; can occur in organs and bones
- Common in most adults, either latent or active, at some point in life; rare in children
- Often associated with chronic headaches, tendonitis, bursitis, arthritis, and stress
- Often incorrectly referred to as "knots"; the more correct term is "nodule"

PATHOPHYSIOLOGY

In order to function, every cell needs oxygen delivered via the bloodstream. In addition to pain, the body's response to insufficient blood supply can be dramatic. The person might faint or convulse; the affected body part might turn blue, decay, and fall off.

The causes of insufficient blood supply are numerous, but in the case of trigger points, the cause is subtle and cellular. Nodules are created as follows: (1) a small fragment of the muscle contracts; (2) this fragment pulls on another, progressively tightening, band of muscle; (3) blood flow to the constricted region is reduced because of the tightness; (4) oxygen debt occurs; (5) local ischemia follows; (6) this cycle of poorly vascularized cellular muscle structures causes an involuntary painful contraction; (7) the lack of oxygen, combined with the sustained contraction, causes pain signals to flood the region; (8) pain is experienced in the focal and more frequently in the referred pain zone that characterizes the muscle harboring a TrP.

Localized pain that radiates away from a central muscle nodule is known as *referred pain*, and it is a characteristic component of trigger points. The patterns of radiating pain are reproducible, predictable, and unique to the muscle affected. For example, an active trigger point in the SCM can be expected to refer pain to the face, ear, jaw, head, and around the eye (Figure 43-1). As is often the case with pain, the body compensates in a holding pattern in an effort to gain relief. This compensation creates *satellite trigger points*, secondary nodules resulting from radiating pain.

Persistently restricted or weakened muscles may develop *latent trigger points* that do not refer pain and are not painful unless palpated. Latent TrPs can be seen as *active*

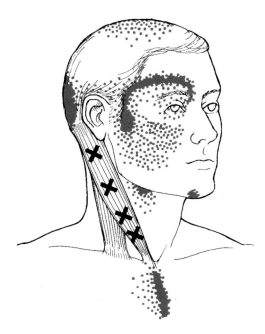

FIGURE 43-1 **The referred pain pattern of SCM trigger points. MediClip image. Philadelphia: Lippincott Williams & Wilkins, 2003.**

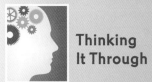

Thinking It Through

Why not use force or attempt to "dig out" trigger points? That has been the mistaken but accepted approach for years and, sometimes, it works. So what if the client experiences temporary pain if he ultimately gets relief? Plus, isn't it common knowledge that massage therapy to tight muscles *should* hurt in order to be effective? Thinking through the pathophysiology of a trigger point will further illuminate why brute force is not only unnecessary, potentially harmful, and disrespectful to the body, but also scientifically unsound. The therapist can follow the subsequent logic to come to a different understanding of TrP treatment.

- If trigger points, physiologically speaking, originate from cellular regions of ischemia . . .
- And ischemia means restricted blood flow . . .
- Why would an elbow, a tool, or a knuckle applied deeply and for a prolonged period *that has the purposeful effect of restricting blood flow* be considered appropriate treatment for this condition?
- Why, instead, not use slow, medium-depth, almost pumping techniques to try to *flood the region with blood*, thereby decreasing ischemia and delivering much-needed nutrients?

trigger points waiting to happen. If ischemia persists and if the cellular flood of pain signals accumulate sufficiently in a latent trigger point, it can turn into an actively painful, radiating trigger point very quickly. Active TrPs cause exquisite local and radiating pain, even when the muscle is at rest.

OVERALL SIGNS AND SYMPTOMS

- Hypertonicity palpable as a taut band
- A palpable nodule usually in the muscle belly
- Often a palpable twitch when the nodule is stimulated by a "snapping palpation"
- Dramatic response from the client (wincing, pulling away), called a jump sign, upon direct TrP palpation
- Visible holding pattern of compensating structures
- Shooting pain radiating from the focal point, which may or may not seem directly related
- Dull, aching, throbbing, and burning pain at the focal point
- Pain at rest or with activity, often worse with activity

SIGNS AND SYMPTOMS MASSAGE THERAPY CAN ADDRESS

- Relieving hypertonicity is a centerpiece for most massage therapy and is regularly addressed with many traditional techniques.
- Compensatory hypertonicity and pain, as well as the accumulation of cellular debris and metabolic waste, are also treated with basic massage skills.

TREATMENT OPTIONS

Most people do not seek medical attention for muscle tightness alone. Temporary muscular discomfort is usually self-treated with over-the-counter (OTC) creams or patches that claim to provide relief. Those in pain may also take OTC anti-inflammatory

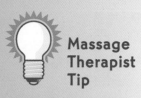

Massage Therapist Tip

When the Client Says, "Go Ahead, Beat Me Up"

A nagging myth surrounding the relief of muscle nodules is held by many, usually male, clients. The thinking is as follows: "I'm in pain, so I'm going to the strongest massage therapist I can find. She will really hurt me with her therapy. This is good and I know I'll be sore the next day, but that means I got my money's worth and it's supposed to hurt in order for it to work." It takes tact and persistence to reverse this attitude. Try this: Honor the client's request by saying you understand this is how he has been treated in the past, and perhaps it worked for him. Let him know there's another way to think about trigger point treatment that's much more effective. Tell him his body is like an onion, and you're going to "peel" (work on) one layer at a time until you get down to the most affected region. So, rather than "take a knife" to this onion, you'll carefully peel each layer away until you get to the core. Once you identify the source of his pain, you'll work on it, deeply and thoroughly, but not to the point of pain he is used to (or may want). Aggressive, deep work further injures the tissue and is counterproductive. Let him know this is a different—but more effective and less painful—way of working out his TrPs. This explanation will quiet most clients who insist on pain for perceived gain. Unfortunately, you may lose those who demand brute force massage therapy. Ultimately, your hands—and your professional reputation—will be better off if they seek treatment elsewhere.

medications, apply hot or cold packs, and (erroneously) rest the affected area. If pain becomes intolerable, a sports medicine physician or physical therapist may treat with noninvasive, conservative techniques.

Common Medications

Medications are not usually prescribed. In extreme cases of multiple, intolerable trigger points, as in people with cerebral palsy, partial paralysis, Lou Gehrig's disease, and conditions that involve unrelenting hypertonicity, muscle relaxants may be prescribed.

MASSAGE THERAPIST ASSESSMENT

Asking questions about the client's general state of health and activity will give the therapist a sound baseline to start her assessment. A client's report of a recent accident that has produced compensating patterns, or prolonged inactivity, a desk job, or complaints about pain that "won't go away, burns and shoots from here to here," will help clarify the appropriate treatment.

A word of caution about the assessment: The quality of the pain should be described as dull, aching, nagging, steady, throbbing, and sometimes burning. The specific terms used for describing neurologic pain (shooting, tingling, numbness, and burning) are similar and may muddy the therapist's assessment. Knowing, or having a picture reference that indicates, typical trigger point referral patterns will help differentiate between TrP and neurological pain.

Asking about the duration of the pain and how the client has been self-treating will further help determine a treatment plan.

THERAPEUTIC GOALS

Decreasing pain and hypertonicity in the immediate and referred regions, increasing circulation to the affected muscles, increasing range of motion (ROM), restoring normal muscle resting length, and reducing secondary stress and tension—all of these are reasonable therapeutic goals for treating trigger points.

Palpation restores ROM to the tissues, and compression acts to move the myofascia. A properly trained therapist would move the muscle through ROM. Because improper technique will often stimulate TrPs and not deactivate them, the therapist's goal is to use techniques that precisely avoid a flare-up.

MASSAGE SESSION FREQUENCY

Trigger points can both develop and resolve quickly. However, they often reside in the muscle belly for weeks or months and thus need frequent, consistent treatment and self-care. Most people begin to notice relief in about 4–6 visits. If no resolution occurs, then therapy may not be effective and a perpetuating factor or another pathology may be present. At this point, a client should be referred to another health care practitioner for evaluation.

The following frequency suggestions assume that the client's symptoms are decreasing with massage therapy treatment and that he is doing his homework assignments.

- 60-minute sessions twice a week until resolution, for severe cases
- 60-minute sessions once a week, for normally painful cases
- 60-minute sessions once a month, for maintenance and prevention, after resolution

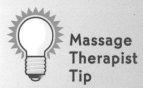

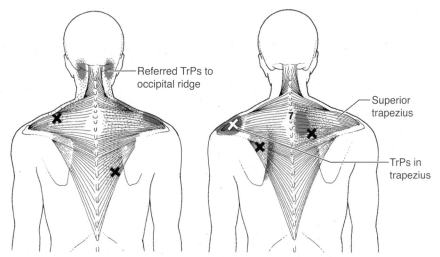

Referred TrPs to
occipital ridge

Superior
trapezius

TrPs in
trapezius

FIGURE 43-2 **Superior trapezius trigger points refer pain along the entire body of this large muscle as well as at the occipital ridge on either side of the muscle attachment. MediClip image. Philadelphia: Lippincott Williams & Wilkins, 2003.**

MASSAGE PROTOCOL

Trigger point pressure release is the application of slowly increasing, nonpainful pressure over a trigger point until a barrier of tissue resistance is encountered. Contact is then maintained until the tissue barrier releases, and pressure is increased to reach a new barrier to eliminate the trigger point tension and tenderness. Rather than "digging" into the tight muscle, thereby causing a painful response to which the body will react, constrict, and shut down, you will be respectfully, slowly, and carefully approaching the taut band of muscle and the surrounding area in order to flood the region with fresh blood. This will help release the constriction, remove the ischemia, flush waste products, alleviate pain, and increase function and ROM. The methods are simple.

Before and after ROM is used to demonstrate initial restrictions and then subsequent, post-treatment improvement. Heat, effleurage, petrissage, and intermittent deep stroking and kneading are used to bring blood into the restricted area, and remove metabolites from it. The medium-pressure fingertip pumping used at the center of the nodule replaces the sustained-pressure, elbow-to-the-bone techniques. No instruments are necessary.

Stubborn or long-standing trigger points will require several sessions for resolution. Homework is essential to keep the region flushed with blood and to prevent reconstriction of the muscle fibers. The following protocol focuses on trigger point treatment of the superior trapezius (Figure 43-2), as this is one of the most common complaints you will encounter.

Getting Started

Have hot packs ready. Be patient.

You'll notice that there are no durations indicated for the techniques in this protocol. With any soft tissue work, you must be keenly aware of the tissue's condition before moving mechanically onto the next step. In the case of trigger point work, you will want to train yourself to remain very aware of the depth to which you are working, the tissue's response, the presence of any spasms or tissue flinching, the width of the taut muscle band, the presence of "Rice Krispies," and whether or not the TrP is softening. It would be impossible to impose time restrictions on this process. Do not overwork the tissue in which the trigger points are embedded. Try, instead, to approximately spread your time evenly between all the steps, spending the most time directly on the trigger points themselves.

Contraindications and Cautions

- Clients taking daily aspirin or anticoagulants are at risk for serious bruising resulting from any form of prolonged deep work.

- Be keenly aware of the medical history of those clients whose trigger points do not resolve after several sessions. Seemingly persistent localized muscle pain can be an indicator of cancer recurrence or other systemic diseases.

- Although you may be well-intentioned, overzealous work at a focused point of pain can cause extremely uncomfortable soreness or even pain for the client the next day. Monitor the depth and vigor with which you perform this work.

Step-by-Step Protocol for **Trigger Point in the Right Superior Trapezius**

Technique	Duration*
Position the client in a right side-lying position. Start by treating the left side. Tuck a moist hot pack into the space between the table and the client's affected right shoulder. Leave it in place as you treat the left shoulder. Keep the hot pack away from the lateral neck region.	
Stroking, effleurage, skin-rolling, petrissage, kneading, forearm effleurage, forearm compressions, light-then-medium pressure, slowly, evenly rhythmic • Along the occipital ridge • Into the entire trapezius muscle. Include the attachments at the shoulder, along the scapula, into the cervical and thoracic spine regions. Attempt to "grip" the muscle frequently, and move it as much as you can. • Reach over, respectfully, and work the superior pectoralis major. • Finish by using your forearm and stretching/pulling the shoulder away from the neck, down toward the feet. Note: There may be a satellite TrP or radiating point of pain in the left trapezius, but that is not your focus right now. You are softening related structures in order to work into the primary trigger point on the right.	
Remove the hot pack. Roll the client to his other side. Warm this entire area by repeating the same steps you performed on the unaffected side before you begin the actual trigger point work. Stroking, effleurage, skin-rolling, petrissage, kneading, forearm effleurage, forearm compression, light-then-medium pressure, slowly, evenly rhythmic. • Along the occipital ridge • Into the entire trapezius muscle. Include the attachments at the shoulder, along the scapula, into the cervical and thoracic spine regions. Attempt to "grip" the muscle frequently and move it as much as you can. • Reach over, respectfully, and work the superior pectoralis major. • Finish by using your forearm and stretching/pulling the shoulder away from the neck, down toward the feet.	
Using gentle palpation and digital kneading, ask the client to help identify the *exact* location of the offending trigger point. You will feel a palpable nodule under your fingers, and/or a feeling of "Rice Krispies" in the tissue immediately surrounding the nodule. Sometimes, I draw a circle around the nodule with a nonpermanent marker in order to save time and to be able to return to the exact spot again as the protocol demands.	
With your full open hand, grasp as much tissue *around the trigger point and including the trigger point region. The TrP should be situated almost near the palm of your hand.* Hold this position, just grasping the superior trapezius in a medium-pressure grasp for a few seconds. Wiggle the tissue around a bit. Feel as if you are actually lifting the trapezius off the bone but not yanking it. Return the tissue to its normal position, stroke it for a few seconds, and repeat.	

(continued)

Technique	Duration*
With open, flat hands, deeply effleurage and knead the area surrounding the trigger point, *moving your hands in the direction of the trigger point*. Imagine you are forcing blood directly into the most painful and affected area. This action is similar to that of kneading bread, rhythmically, with both hands working toward the center of the trigger point.	
Stand back and ask the client to move his arm in a full ROM arc. Ask him to move his arm and shoulder in every plane, a full 360 degrees, bending his elbow, pulling his shoulder back, bringing it forward. (This is as much for distraction as for assessment). Ask him to report pain and restriction.	
Return to the trigger point. With gentle fingers, palpate the trigger point. Ask the client to identify the exact path of referred pain. Now, the real work begins. With the client's shoulder in a relaxed position, with firm fingers or soft knuckles, apply a pumping-like pressure to the center of the trigger point and all along the path of the referred pain. Your compressions are at the rate of about one per second. These compressions should not cause pain, although they might cause mild discomfort. This is detailed, focused work. Stay centered.	
Sweep the entire area with broad effleurage strokes. Ask the client how he's doing. Allow him to stretch if he needs to.	
Now, ask the client to stretch his shoulder into the position that duplicates his worst pain. This may be a position in which he stretches his head to the side and forces the shoulder down. Ask him to move the shoulder *just an inch or two to relieve the worst pain*. This is the position he will hold for your next step.	
Repeat the previous poking-compression steps along the path of the trigger point and radiating pain while the client holds this stretched position. You will perform this step in a little less time than the previous step because it is difficult for the client to hold this position for long.	
Allow the client to rest, and broadly effleurage the area.	
Palpate for the trigger point and taut band of surrounding muscles. Effleurage, petrissage, kneading, plucking, hacking, medium-to-deep (nonpainful) pressure at a brisk pace. • Along the occipital ridge • Into the entire trapezius muscle. Include the attachments at the shoulder, along the scapula, into the cervical and thoracic spine regions. • Reach over, respectfully, and work the superior pectoralis major.	
Position the client prone. Using any techniques, working briskly, and with medium-to-deep pressure, massage the entire back from the sacrum to the occipital ridge.	
Position the client supine. Ask him to stretch—full extension—both arms over his head and bring them down to his sides. Repeat this several times. The movement is reminiscent of "making snow angels" except the legs are not engaged.	

Contraindications and Cautions: (cont.)

- Although a trigger point does not manifest all the symptoms of a thrombus (blood clot), to the layperson or the inexperienced massage therapist, the two can be confused. If *any* swelling, redness, or heat is present along with the exquisite radiating pain of the typical trigger point, you should halt all work (that means anywhere on the body) and refer the client to a physician. It's possible to inadvertently move a thrombus into an embolus by attempting to work on a presumed nodule.

- If the trigger point is injury-related and accompanied by local inflammation, the application of heat to the region is contraindicated.

- If the trigger point is secondary to an overstretch injury, passive and active stretching exercises are contraindicated.

- The application of ice to a "burning" trigger point may worsen symptoms.

(continued)

Technique	Duration*
Position the client seated on the side of the table with you standing behind him. Maintain appropriate draping and provide a footstool for back support. Effleurage and petrissage, medium pressure, working briskly. • Bilateral superior trapezius • Bilateral superior deltoids • Occipital ridge	
Finish by performing strong, open-handed, full effleurage to the entire neck, back, and arms. Ask the client to repeat full ROM of both shoulders and report pain and restriction.	
Assign ample homework including stretches, stress management, and the application of hot packs.	

*Durations are not given for trigger point work because the pace and duration depends on how the tissues respond to the work. For further explanation, see Getting Started section.

HOMEWORK

The stress of daily life can be as responsible for muscle nodules as the more medically precise cause of localized ischemia. This painful and radiating problem will consistently recur unless the client realizes that he must manage both his stress level and his muscles. Diplomatically, let your client know that homework is not optional; it's mandatory.

- As soon as you become aware of your muscles tightening, stop what you're doing. Move. Stretch. Slowly roll your head. Place your right hand on your head, almost over to the top of your left ear, and gently press your head down to the right shoulder. Repeat on the other side. Raise your shoulders to your ears and hold them for a few seconds. Force your shoulders down as far as they'll go, hold for a few seconds. Slowly roll your shoulders forward, one at a time, in large circles. Roll them backward, one at a time.
- The doorway stretch—do this once a day. See Figures 5-4, 5-5, 5-6, and 6-1.
- Take a huge inhale as you raise your arms up over your head. Exhale as you bring your arms back to your sides. Let your body fall forward, and try to touch the floor.
- Find effective relaxation techniques. Perform these every day.
- Daily, until your next massage therapy session, apply moist hot packs to the trigger point region. Replace them before they become cool.

Review

1. What is the physiologic cause of trigger points?
2. Name the most common locations for TrP formation.
3. Describe the difference between referred pain and satellite trigger points.
4. Why is sustained pressure no longer considered an effective TrP treatment?
5. Explain why cold application would not be an effective therapy for a "burning" TrP.

BIBLIOGRAPHY

Chaitow L, DeLany J. Trigger Points: A Different Version of the Truth. *Massage Today*. February 2006;6(02). Available at: http://www.massagetoday.com/mpacms/mt/article.php?id=13364. Accessed August 8, 2010.

Finando D, Finando S. *Trigger Point Therapy for Myofascial Pain: The Practice of Informed Touch*, Rochester, VT: Healing Arts Press, 2005.

Hong CZ. Pathophysiology of myofascial trigger point. *Journal of the Formosan Medical Association* 1996 Feb;95(2):93–104. Available at: http://www.ncbi.nlm.nih.gov/pubmed/9064014. Accessed August 8, 2010.

Rattray F, Ludwig L. *Clinical Massage Therapy: Understanding, Assessing and Treating over 70 Conditions*, Toronto: Talus Incorporated, 2000.

Simons DG. Cardiology and myofascial trigger points. *Texas Heart Institute Journal* 2003;30(1):3–7. Available at: http://www.ncbi.nlm.nih.gov/pmc/articles/PMC152827/. Accessed August 8, 2010.

Simons DG, Hong CZ, Simons LS. Endplate potentials are common to midfiber myofascial trigger points. *American Journal of Physical Medicine & Rehabilitation* 2002 Mar;81(3):212–222. Available at: http://www.ncbi.nlm.nih.gov/pubmed/11989519. Accessed August 8, 2010.

Simons DG, Travell JG, Simons LS. *Travell & Simons' Myofascial Pain and Dysfunction: The Trigger Point Manual 2nd ed.*, Philadelphia: Lippincott Williams & Wilkins, 1999.

Srbely J, Dickey JP. Stimulation of myofascial trigger points causes systematic physiological effects. *The Journal of the Canadian Chiropractic Association* June 2005;49(2):75. Available at: http://www.ncbi.nlm.nih.gov/pmc/articles/PMC1840017/. Accessed August 8, 2010.

Starlanyl D. Overlooking Myofascial Trigger Points: The Key to Your Pain? December 9, 2004. Available at: http://thyroid.about.com/od/fibromyalgiacfscfids/a/devinstarlanyl_3.htm. Accessed August 8, 2010.

Werner R. *A Massage Therapist's Guide to Pathology*, 4th ed. Philadelphia: Lippincott Williams & Wilkins, 2009.

Whiplash

Definition: A hyperextension soft tissue injury of
the neck.

GENERAL INFORMATION

- Caused by a sudden acceleration and/or deceleration of the head and neck
- Most common cause: front-to-back, back-to-front, or side-to-side motor vehicle collision
- Other causes: sports injury, a blow to the head, a fall, a violent shaking of the body
- Onset: 24–48 hours following the triggering incident
- Duration: About 6 weeks
- Describes multiple injuries to numerous neck tissues

Morbidity and Mortality

Although "whiplash" is not a clinically correct term, its use persists when describing the multiple problems following a neck injury. While 95% of whiplash injuries involve superficial damage to muscle and tendons only, treatment confusion exists because so many neck, shoulder, and back structures can be affected long after the initial injury. For example, compensatory trigger points can lead to muscular dysfunction and pain that can linger for months or years.

Whiplash is rarely life threatening. The short-term prognosis is usually good, and most people recover within several weeks. About 40% of patients may experience symptoms after 3 months; 18% may still suffer after 2 years. Prolonged periods of partial disability are not unusual. There are no reliable statistics about long-term prognosis. However, a previous whiplash injury can double the risk of developing severe symptoms from a second whiplash incident.

PATHOPHYSIOLOGY

The neck is one of the most vulnerable regions of the body. It is densely packed with arteries, veins, lymphatic vessels, muscles, tendons, and ligaments, most of which intricately work to keep the brain alive, the body moving, and the immune system responsive. When the neck is injured, the following structures can be affected:

- Diaphragm
- Intercostal muscles
- Entire erector system
- Chewing and jaw muscles
- Scalenes
- All rectus and capitis structures
- Trapezius
- Levator scapulae

- Cervical and thoracic vertebrae, as well as surrounding muscles, tendons, ligaments, fascia, and blood vessels
- Cervical and thoracic nerve roots, as well as the vagus and phrenic nerves

Conditions resulting from injury to these delicate and essential structures range in severity from temporary vertigo to permanent paralysis. Although most whiplash injuries affecting soft tissue (muscles, tendons, ligaments) are transient, the lingering chronic pain and emotional stress reflect the profound fear surrounding injury to this area.

Diagnosis is made by a physician who inspects the patient's head and neck for visible signs of trauma. X-rays determine cervical spine fracture. CT scans may be ordered if extensive soft tissue injury is suspected.

OVERALL SIGNS AND SYMPTOMS

Pain usually begins within 24–48 hours after the incident. It is not unusual, however, for the following symptoms to occur days, weeks, or months later. The sooner after the incident symptoms manifest, the more serious the injury.

- Neck ache and/or tenderness
- Neck and shoulder spasms
- Shoulder pain
- Low-back pain
- Headache
- Tinnitus (ringing in the ears)
- Limited neck range of motion (ROM)
- Neck swelling
- Arm or hand paresthesias (if neurologic structures are affected)

SIGNS AND SYMPTOMS MASSAGE THERAPY CAN ADDRESS

- Scar tissue from sprained or strained muscles can be addressed with massage techniques.
- Massage can relieve the generalized stiffness of the neck and compensating structures.
- The stress that accompanies any accident or injury can be reduced with soothing massage therapy techniques.
- Fascial stretches can soften constricted fascia.

TREATMENT OPTIONS

The first medical step in whiplash treatment is to determine if any life-threatening or possibly permanent paralytic neck damage has occurred. Once the patient is evaluated and stabilized, conservative treatment can begin. Neck immobilization, usually by the fitting of a neck brace, has been the traditional whiplash treatment. New thinking includes the understanding that artificial and lengthy immobilization of already injured (immobilized) tissue can promote further damage and prolong rehabilitation. Health care practitioners now suggest early and gentle neck movement, limited physical activity, and rest following an accident or neck injury. If a neck brace is prescribed, it should be worn intermittently and for short periods. Prolonged rest, although initially beneficial, is not the key to recovery.

Patients are often sent home from the ER with instructions to apply ice (to reduce inflammation) and take over-the-counter (OTC) pain relievers. Massage, neck rest, bed rest, ROM exercises starting 72 hours after injury, and avoiding excessive neck strain for 1–2 weeks are the normal home treatments. Patients are encouraged

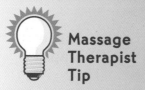

Massage Therapist Tip

No Massage Immediately After Whiplash

As massage therapists, we sometimes can do real harm, and prematurely treating whiplash is a prime example. We are not first-line responders. As desperate as a client might be ("It was just a fender bender; I don't want to go to the ER or to my doctor, and my neck is killing me") and as determined as you are to relieve pain, *you must not touch or treat a whiplash victim for at least 3 days after the accident.* You can do real, permanent, damage to the neck or brain if you prematurely relax muscles that are guarding the injured neck. This muscle splinting is the body's way of compensating and protecting the injured area. A client must seek professional medical treatment for a neck injury. Once the voluntary splinting has relaxed and she has been cleared for massage therapy, you can proceed but not before.

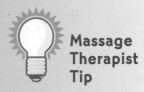

Massage Therapist Tip

Wearing a Neck Brace

If a client is wearing a neck brace, ask whether it was prescribed by a physician. Sometimes a whiplash victim will borrow a neck brace from a friend who had an accident in the past, for instance. Inform your client that prolonged immobility from wearing a neck brace can cause more problems and further injury. She should wear a neck brace only if it was prescribed by a physician and only for the suggested duration. Remember, *you cannot remove or affix a neck brace before or after treatment*. This is outside your scope of practice.

Thinking It Through

Secondary gain is a term used in chronic pain management. It refers to the perceived advantages a patient may get by "holding on to her pain" well after the physiologic symptoms should have passed. Think through why your understanding of secondary gain might be a component in your treatment of certain clients.

- An unhappily married client was the passenger in a car her husband was driving when a collision occurred. What might be her secondary gain if she continues to complain about this perceived husband-induced accident?

---

to revisit their physician or the ER if they experience dizziness, fatigue, irritability, or continued shoulder or arm pain.

Prevention includes wearing a seat belt, using proper headgear when doing high-impact sports, and not shaking a child in a way that could injure the neck.

Common Medications

- Nonsteroidal anti-inflammatory drugs (NSAIDs), such as ibuprofen (Motrin, Advil) and naproxen (Aleve, Anaprox, Naprelan, Naprosyn)

MASSAGE THERAPIST ASSESSMENT

It is important for the massage therapist to take a detailed history before treating a client with whiplash. The answers to the following questions will help determine safe treatment.

- When did the accident occur?
- What pain have you experienced since?
- When did the pain begin?
- Where is the pain?
- Are you experiencing any dizziness or vertigo?
- Are you experiencing spasms? Where?
- Are you experiencing any numbness and tingling down your arm?
- Did you hit your head?
- Have you seen a physician or gone to the ER?
- Are you taking painkillers or muscle relaxants now?

If the acute pain and spasms have quieted, if the incident occurred at least 3 days ago, and if the client is taking neither narcotics nor muscle relaxants, the therapist can proceed with assessment and then treatment.

The neck and shoulder structures should be palpated for hypertonicity and trigger points. Gentle neck ROM should be performed. If the therapist is qualified, palpation of every spinous process, from the cervical to the lumbar spine, will determine tenderness or rotation, as well as hypertonicity in the surrounding muscles.

THERAPEUTIC GOALS

Relieving hypertonicity and trigger points in the neck and surrounding tissue, improving neck ROM, relieving secondary back pain, providing a listening ear for possible secondary gain issues, and relieving stress are reasonable treatment goals for the massage therapist.

MASSAGE SESSION FREQUENCY

- 60-minute sessions twice a week (beginning no sooner than 3 days after the incident), until all pain and hypertonicity are resolved
- 60-minute sessions once a week for 1 month
- 60-minute maintenance sessions once a month

MASSAGE PROTOCOL

Although it may appear as though I have tried to scare you away from treating whiplash, that's not the case. You can provide highly effective treatment with the simplest of techniques and relieve much of the pain experienced by most whiplash sufferers.

Step-by-Step Protocol for	Cervical Strain 5 Days After a Motor Vehicle Collision	
Technique	**Duration**	
Position for client's comfort and access. Well-supported side-lying may be the best option		
Apply warm packs to the posterior cervical neck. Leave in place while you perform general relaxation techniques *anywhere else in the body other than the neck and shoulders.* Remove the packs.	5 minutes	
Using no lubricant, gently cup the client's neck with your hands and rest for a moment. Using your full, open, soft hands, gradually increase pressure to perform fascial stretching, making slow, large circles. • Work the entire posterior and lateral neck region. • Work up into the occipital ridge and down to C-7/T-1. • Move down to the superior trapezius and out over the deltoids		
Apply lubricant. Palpate the entire area listed previously for taut muscle bands and trigger points. In this case, the deeper muscles supporting the neck as well as the trapezius will be directly affected and will be hypertonic.	2 minutes	
Effleurage, light to medium, slow, evenly rhythmic • Posterior, lateral neck • Trapezius down to T-12 • Out over bilateral deltoids • Pectoralis major	3 minutes	
Effleurage, petrissage, effleurage, medium pressure, slow, evenly rhythmic • Posterior, lateral neck • Trapezius down to T-12 • Bilateral deltoids • Pectoralis major	3 minutes	
Digital, palmar, and fist kneading, light-to-medium pressure, slow, evenly rhythmic. (You can perform gentle trigger point work at this point.) • Posterior, lateral neck • Trapezius down to T-12 • Bilateral deltoids • Pectoralis major	5 minutes	
Stroking, effleurage, slightly more briskly, medium pressure, all of the previously listed tissue	2 minutes	
Digital probing, kneading, mobilization, and stripping, light-to-medium pressure, evenly rhythmic, working one side at a time. (Again, trigger point work is appropriate at this time.) • Bilateral sternocleidomastoid (SCM) from the mastoid process to the insertion on the clavicle	5 minutes	

Thinking It Through (cont.)

- A disgruntled employee was driving a forklift on the job when he was hit by another vehicle from behind. What might be his economic gain if he suffers from perceived continued pain?
- A lonely widow experiences a minor whiplash from a fall. What might her emotional gain be if she continues to need medical attention?

Contraindications and Cautions:

- Do not remove a neck brace (cervical collar) prescribed by a physician in order to perform your therapy. *If the client has been instructed that she can take it off at will, she should remove and replace it herself.*
- *No pain or discomfort should ever be caused by any of your techniques.*
- If there is any chance of a fracture, concussion, displaced disc, or serious injury, do not attempt massage therapy; refer the client to a physician.

(continued)

Contraindications and Cautions: (cont.)

- Avoid working both sides of the neck simultaneously (e.g., the SMC). This can cause discomfort and vertigo.
- Be sure that the normal, protective, and essential cervical muscle splinting has quieted before you perform any massage therapy techniques intended to relax these muscles. *Serious damage can be done to the neck structures if you relax muscles that are trying to hold the head and spine in place.*
- Be keenly aware of the location of the carotid arteries. Do not apply direct pressure to them or to the nearby tissues.
- If palpation of a spinous process indicates rotation or elicits a painful response, do not proceed with the treatment and instead, refer the client to a physician or chiropractor.
- Do not assign or perform neck stretches unless you are working as part of a health care team and have a written or verbal order from a physical therapist (PT) or a physician.

Technique	Duration
Digital probing, kneading, mobilization, and stripping; light-to-medium pressure, evenly rhythmic, working one side of the spine at a time (Trigger point work may be done at this time.) • Deep cervical muscles, tendons, and ligaments • Work up as high under the occipital ridge as you can reach, then down to C-7	5 minutes
Digital probing, kneading, mobilization, and stripping; light-to-medium pressure, evenly rhythmic, working one side at a time • Bilateral scalenes	5 minutes
Effleurage, using broad, slow strokes with your open hand • All previously worked tissue	5 minutes
Dry the skin of all lubricant. Fascial stretching, performed deep to client's tolerance. • All previously worked tissue • Offer a scalp massage	10 minutes
Stroking, performed with an open, soft hand, slow, evenly rhythmic • Anterior, posterior, and lateral neck • Pectoralis major • Trapezius • Deltoids	3 minutes
Finish as you started. Cup the neck in your soft hands and rest for a moment.	2 minutes

Myofascial techniques, probing effleurage, petrissage, and some kneading—performed without aggression—will serve your client well and give you satisfactory tissue response. The following protocol treats a very common form of whiplash: cervical strain secondary to a front-to-back motor vehicle collision 5 days after the accident.

Getting Started

Hot packs can provide comfort and soften the tissue. Stay away from the carotid arteries when placing a hot pack on the neck. Positioning may be a challenge. A recommended position is the client seated on the side of the table, feet firmly planted on a footstool, with pillows supporting each elbow. All work should be firm, not aggressive. Don't use so much pressure that the client must "push against you" to keep her neck aligned. Support her head with your free hand if you find she is not strong enough to hold her head in place during your treatment.

HOMEWORK

Unless you have been trained and are certified as a personal trainer, strengthening exercises—especially work on the neck muscles—is outside your scope of practice. Offering supportive encouragement for continuous but gentle activity will be your goal in assigning homework to this client.

- Wear your neck brace only for the amount of time prescribed by your physician.

- You may need to adjust how you sleep for a few days. Sitting comfortably in a big armchair, with pillows, might provide the needed back and neck support.
- Rest your head, neck, and back, but don't overdo the periods of rest. Gently perform your daily activities without overstretching or causing pain.

Review

1. List the structures that might be involved in a whiplash injury.
2. What are other names for whiplash?
3. Describe voluntary muscle splinting.
4. Why is treating a client whose neck is still spasming and in voluntary splinting a contraindication for massage therapy?
5. As a massage therapist, why are you not allowed to apply or remove a client's neck brace?
6. Explain what is meant by secondary gain.

BIBLIOGRAPHY

Benjamin B. Whiplash. *Massage Today*. October 2007:07. Available at: http://www.massagetoday.com/mpacms/mt/article.php?id=13699. Accessed August 8, 2010.
Bentley H. Whiplash: How to Heal a Pain in the Neck. Available at: http://www.massagetherapy.com/articles/index.php/article_id/1107/whiplash. Accessed August 8, 2010.
Cunha J. Whiplash. EmedicineHealth. Available at: http://www.emedicinehealth.com/whiplash/article_em.htm. Accessed August 8, 2010.
Eck J, Shiel W. Whiplash. Medicinenet. Available at: http://www.medicinenet.com/whiplash/article.htm. Accessed August 8, 2010.
Lowe W. Whiplash. *Massage Magazine*. July/August 2003. Available at: http://www.massagemag.com/Magazine/2003/issue104/assess104.php. Accessed August 8, 2010.
Naqui SZ, Lovell SJ, Lovell ME. Underestimation of severity of previous whiplash injuries. *Annals of the Royal College of Surgeons of England* January 2008;90(1):51–53. Available at: http://www.ncbi.nlm.nih.gov/pmc/articles/PMC2216717. Accessed August 8, 2010.
Rattray F, Ludwig L. *Clinical Massage Therapy: Understanding, Assessing and Treating over 70 Conditions*. Toronto: Talus Incorporated, 2000.

Index

Page numbers followed by *f* indicate figure and page numbers followed by *t* indicate table.

A

ABC range-of-motion exercises, 47
acceleration flexion-extension neck injury. *See* whiplash
acquired immunodeficiency syndrome. *See* HIV, AIDS
active trigger points, 324–325
acute bursitis. *See* bursitis
acute muscle spasms, 192–194
acute pain, 28
adhesion, 260
adhesive capsulitis. *See* frozen shoulder
AEIOU facial exercises, 69, 298–300
American Psychiatric Association, 242
American Society for Surgery of the Hand, 78
ankles
    limited motion range, 301
    ROM exercises, 48*f*
    strain protocol, 285–286
ankylosing spondylosis (AS)
    assessment, 57–58
    client homework, 59–62, 61*f*
    contraindications, 60
    defined, 56
    massage protocol, 58–59, 60–61*t*
    morbidity/mortality, 56
    pathophysiology, 56
    session frequency, 58
    signs, symptoms, 56–57
    therapeutic goals, 58
    treatment options, 57
anterior neck massage, 309
AS. *See* ankylosing spondylosis
assessment, defined, 8
ataxic CP, 85
athetoid CP, 85

B

Batavia, M., 6
battle fatigue. *See* post-traumatic stress disorder
Bell's palsy
    assessment, 65
    client homework, 69
    contraindications, 67
    defined, 63
    facial massage, 65–66, 66*f*
    facial nerve, 63, 64*f*
    massage protocol, 65–66, 67–68*t*
    morbidity/mortality, 63
    pathophysiology, 63
    session frequency, 65
    signs, symptoms, 63–64
    therapeutic goals, 65
    treatment options, 64
blood, moving, 10
brain attack. *See* stroke

bursae, 72*f*
bursitis
    acute knee bursitis protocol, 75*t*
    assessment, 73
    bursae, 72*f*
    chronic knee bursitis protocol, 76*t*
    client homework, 74
    contraindications, 75
    defined, 71
    massage protocol, 74
    pathophysiology, 71
    session frequency, 73
    signs, symptoms, 71–72
    therapeutic goals, 73
    treatment options, 72–74

C

carpal tunnel syndrome (CTS)
    assessment, 80
    avoiding, 81
    client homework, 81–84
    contraindications, 82
    defined, 78
    massage protocol, 81, 82–83*t*
    median nerve, 78, 79*f*
    pathophysiology, 78, 79*f*
    session frequency, 81
    signs, symptoms, 79–80
    therapeutic goals, 80–81
    treatment options, 80
cartilage, 203, 204*f*
cerebral palsy (CP)
    assessment, 86–87
    client homework, 92–93
    contraindications, 89–90
    defined, 85
    massage protocol, 88, 89–92*t*
    medications, 86
    pathophysiology, 85
    real effects of, 86
    resisted breathing exercises, 87, 88*f*
    session frequency, 87
    signs, symptoms, 85–86
    spasm response, 88
    therapeutic goals, 87
    treatment options, 86
cerebrovascular accident. *See* stroke
cervical disc disease. *See* degenerative disc disease
cervical sprain/strain. *See* whiplash
CFIDS. *See* chronic fatigue syndrome
CFS. *See* chronic fatigue syndrome
Charley horse. *See* muscle spasm
chemotherapy-induced peripheral neuropathy (CIPN)
    assessment, 199
    client homework, 200–202

contraindications, 201–202
defined, 196
foot examinations, 200
massage protocol, 199–200, 201–202
morbidity, mortality, 197
pathophysiology, 197
session frequency, 199
signs, symptoms, 197–198
therapeutic goals, 199
treatment options, 198–199
chronic bursitis. *See* bursitis
chronic fatigue syndrome (CFS)
    assessment, 96
    client homework, 97–100
    contraindications, 98
    defined, 94
    importance of listening, 95
    massage protocol, 97, 98–99*t*
    morbidity, mortality, 94
    pathophysiology, 94–95
    session frequency, 97
    signs, symptoms, 95
    therapeutic goals, 96
    treatment options, 95–96
chronic pain, 28
CIPN. *See* chemotherapy-induced peripheral neuropathy
clapping. *See* cupping
client, defined, 4
client homework
    assigning, 6–7, 45
    deep breathing, 51–52
    Epsom salts baths/soaks, 46
    heat/cold application, 46
    proper stretching technique, 172
    purposeful walking, 52
    resources for, 54
    ROM exercises, 46–48, 47–50*f*
    scope of practice, 45–46
    strengthening, 51, 51*f*, 52*f*
clinical massage, 2–9
cold application
    client homework, 46
    effectivity, 114, 170
    icing injuries, 272
    physiologic effects, 19–20
colon sections, 101, 102*f*
compensation, 283
constipation
    assessment, 103–104
    causes, 101
    client homework, 108
    colon sections, 101, 102*f*
    defined, 101
    flatulence, 105
    impaction, 102
    massage protocol, 104–105, 105*f*, 106–107*t*

pathophysiology, 101–102
PD, 212
session frequency, 104
signs, symptoms, 102–103
therapeutic goals, 104
treatment options, 103
contractures, 214, 260
contraindications, 5–6
CP. *See* cerebral palsy
craniomandibular pain syndrome.
    See temporomandibular joint
    dysfunction
cross-fiber friction
    defined, 17, 18*f*
    physiologic effects, 17–19
    for scars, 261*f*
CTS. *See* carpal tunnel syndrome
cupping, 13, 15*f*
CVA. *See* stroke

D
DDD. *See* degenerative disc disease
decreased range of motion, 23
deep breathing, 51–52, 301
deep hip rotators, 219*f*
degenerative disc disease (DDD)
    assessment, 113
    client homework, 116–117
    contraindications, 116
    defined, 110
    dermatomes, 111
    establishing client relationship, 115
    heat, cold application, 114
    massage protocol, 114, 114*f*, 115–116*t*
    morbidity, mortality, 110
    muscle spasms, hypertonicity, 112–113
    pathophysiology, 110–112, 111*f*
    signs, symptoms, 112
    therapeutic goals, 114
    treatment options, 112–113
degenerative joint disease. *See* osteoarthritis
delayed onset muscle soreness (DOMS)
    assessment, 120
    client homework, 122–123
    contraindications, 121
    defined, 118
    massage protocol, 120–122, 121–122*t*
    pathophysiology, 118
    session frequency, 120
    signs, symptoms, 119
    therapeutic goals, 120
    topical product application, 120
    treatment options, 119–120
dermatomes, 111
diabetic peripheral neuropathy (DPN)
    assessment, 199
    client homework, 200–202
    contraindications, 201–202
    defined, 196
    foot examinations, 200
    massage protocol, 199–200, 201–202*t*
    morbidity, mortality, 196–197
    pathophysiology, 197
    session frequency, 199
    signs, symptoms, 197–198
    therapeutic goals, 199
    treatment options, 198

*Diagnostic and Statistical Manual of Mental
    Disorders (DSM)* (American
    Psychiatric Association), 242
digital kneading, 12
dish towel stretches, 48, 48*f*
DOMS. *See* delayed onset muscle
    soreness
doorway stretches, 48–50, 49*f*, 50*f*
DPN. *See* diabetic peripheral neuropathy
dry gangrene, 197
*DSM. See Diagnostic and Statistical Manual
    of Mental Disorders*

E
effleurage
    application, 4–5
    defined, 11, 12*f*
    physiologic effects, 11–12
emotion, 23, 28–29
Epsom salts baths/soaks, 46
erector spinae muscles, 114*f*
exercise regimes, 169–170

F
facial massage, 65–66, 66*f*
facial nerve, 63, 64*f*
facial paralysis, 298–300
fibrocartilaginous spinal disc, 111*f*
fibromyalgia syndrome (FMS)
    assessment, 126–127
    client homework, 128, 130
    contraindications, 129
    defined, 124
    desensitizing skin, 128
    massage protocol, 127–128, 128–129*t*
    pathophysiology, 124–125, 125*f*
    session frequency, 127
    signs, symptoms, 125–126
    therapeutic goals, 127
    tissue abnormalities, 126
    treatment options, 126
fibrosis, 23
fibrotic adhesion, 260
fist kneading, 12
flashbacks, 242, 244
flatulence, 105
FMS. *See* fibromyalgia syndrome
foot examinations, 200
frozen shoulder
    assessment, 133
    client homework, 134–136
    contraindications, 135
    defined, 131
    massage protocol, 134, 135–136
    morbidity, mortality, 131
    pathophysiology, 131–132, 132*f*
    signs, symptoms, 132
    therapeutic goals, 133–135
    treatment options, 133
functional scoliosis, 274

G
gait cycle, 229
gate control theory of pain, 24–27, 26*f*
gluteus muscles, 219*f*, 220*f*
golfer's elbow. *See* tendinosis
guarding, 191–192

H
hacking, 13, 15*f*
headache, migraine
    assessment, 139
    client homework, 141–142
    contraindications, 140
    defined, 137
    massage protocol, 139–141, 140–141*t*
    morbidity, mortality, 137
    pathophysiology, 137–138
    sensations of, 139
    session frequency, 139
    signs, symptoms, 138
    therapeutic goals, 139
    treatment options, 138–139
headache, tension
    assessment, 145
    client homework, 149
    contraindications, 147–148
    defined, 143
    massage protocol, 145–149, 146*f*,
        147–148*t*
    pathophysiology, 143, 144*f*
    session frequency, 145
    signs, symptoms, 143–144
    therapeutic goals, 145
    treatment options, 144
    trigger points, 144
healthy lifestyle modeling, 119
heat application
    client homework, 46
    effectivity, 114
    physiologic effects, 19–20
hip movement, 301
hip socket neuropathy. *See* piriformis
    syndrome
HIV, AIDS
    assessment, 153–154
    client homework, 156
    contraindications, 455
    defined, 150
    massage protocol, 154–156, 155–156*t*
    morbidity, mortality, 150–151
    nonjudgmental treatment, 153
    pathophysiology, 151
    session frequency, 154
    signs, symptoms, 151–153
    therapeutic goals, 153–154
    treatment options, 153
hold and stroke massage, 179, 244,
    291–292
homework. *See* client homework
hoola hoop exercises, 47
human immunodeficiency virus (HIV). *See*
    HIV, AIDS
hunchback. *See* hyperkyphosis
hyperkyphosis
    assessment, 160–161
    client homework, 161–165
    contraindications, 162
    defined, 158
    massage protocol, 161, 162–165*t*
    pathophysiology, 158–159
    session frequency, 161
    signs, symptoms, 159
    therapeutic goals, 161
    treatment options, 160

hypertonicity, 10, 22, 112–113. *See also* muscle spasm
hypertrophic scar, 260

I

ice application. *See* cold application
iliotibial band, 167, 168*f*
iliotibial band syndrome (ITBS)
   assessment, 169–170
   client homework, 170–175, 173*f*, 174*f*
   cold application, 170
   contraindications, 171
   defined, 167
   massage protocol, 170, 171–173*t*
   pathophysiology, 167, 168*f*
   session frequency, 170
   signs, symptoms, 168–169
   treatment goals, 170
   treatment options, 169
impaction, 102
inflammation, 261–262
insomnia
   assessment, 178
   client homework, 180–181
   defined, 176
   massage protocol, 178–180, 179*f*, 180*t*
   morbidity, mortality, 176
   pathophysiology, 176–177
   session frequency, 178
   signs, symptoms, 177
   therapeutic goals, 176
   treatment options, 177–178
intraoral work, 306
ischemia, 22, 24
ITBS. *See* iliotibial band syndrome

J

jaw muscles, 304*f*, 305*f*
jogger's heel. *See* plantar fasciitis
joints, 253*f*, 295
jumper's knee. *See* tendinosis

K

keloid scar, 260
knees
   bursitis protocols, 75*t*, 76*t*
   limited motion range, 301
   OA massage protocol, 208–209*t*
knots. *See* trigger points
knuckle kneading, 12

L

latent trigger points, 324
lumbago. *See* degenerative disc disease

M

malignant MS, 184
massage
   clinical *vs.* relaxation, 2
   effects of, 138
   in nursing homes/hospitals, 178
massage therapy. *See* therapy
median nerve, 78, 79*f*
medical massage, 2
medications
   generic/trade names, class, action, 32
   knowledge of, 31–32

off-label, 198
   prolonged NSAID use, 228
   relevant to therapy, 33–43*t*
Melzack, R., 25
migraines. *See* headache, migraine
MPD syndrome. *See* temporomandibular joint dysfunction
multiple sclerosis (MS)
   assessment, 185
   client homework, 188–189
   contraindications, 187
   defined, 182
   injections, 184–185
   limb stretching, 186
   massage protocol, 186, 187–188*t*
   morbidity, mortality, 182
   pathophysiology, 182–184, 183*f*
   session frequency, 186
   signs, symptoms, 184–185
   therapeutic goals, 185–186
   treatment options, 185
muscle cramp. *See* muscle spasm
muscle knots. *See* trigger points
muscle spasm
   assessment, 191
   client homework, 192–195
   contraindications, 191–194
   defined, 112–113, 190
   massage protocol, 192, 193–194*t*
   pathophysiology, 190
   session frequency, 192
   signs, symptoms, 190–191
   therapeutic goals, 191
   treatment options, 191
muscular activity, pain, 22–29
muscular bracing, 319
myelinated motor nerves, 183*f*
myofascial pain dysfunction (MPD) syndrome. *See* temporomandibular joint dysfunction

N

neck braces, 334
NeuroMassage, 5
neuromuscular scoliosis, 274
neuropathy. *See* chemotherapy-induced peripheral neuropathy (CIPN); diabetic peripheral neuropathy (DPN)
nodules. *See* trigger points
non-acute muscle spasms, 194–195
nonsteroidal anti-inflammatory drug (NSAID), prolonged use of, 228

O

OA. *See* osteoarthritis
objective, 8
Occupational Safety and Health Administration (OSHA), 78
off-label medications, 198
OSHA. *See* Occupational Safety and Health Administration
osteoarthritis (OA)
   assessment, 206
   client homework, 207–209
   contraindications, 208–209
   defined, 203

heat, cold application, 205
   massage protocol, 206–207, 208–209*t*
   morbidity, mortality, 203
   pathophysiology, 203–204, 204*f*
   session frequency, 206
   signs, symptoms, 204–205
   therapeutic goals, 206
   treatment options, 205

P

pain
   animals, 29
   chronic, acute, 28
   compensation, 226
   effective treatment, 27
   gate control theory, 24–27, 26*f*
   muscular activity, physiology, 22–29
   perception, emotions, 28–29
   perception, therapy, 26*f*, 27
   scales of, 27–28, 27*f*, 28*f*
   from stroke, 297
   trigger point treatment, 325–327
pain-spasm-pain cycle
   breaking, 24–25, 25*t*
   defined, 22–24, 23*f*
parasympathetic state, 255
Parkinson's disease (PD)
   assessment, 212–213
   client homework, 216
   constipation, 212
   contractures, 214
   contraindications, 215
   defined, 210
   massage protocol, 213, 214–215*t*
   morbidity, mortality, 200
   pathophysiology, 200
   session frequency, 213
   signs, symptoms, 211
   therapeutic goals, 213
   treatment options, 211–212
patient, defined, 4
PD. *See* Parkinson's disease
peripheral nerves, 79
petrissage, 12–13, 13*f*
pincement, 13, 14*f*
piriformis muscle, 220*f*
piriformis syndrome
   assessment, 221–222
   client homework, 225
   contraindications, 223
   defined, 218
   massage protocol, 222–224, 223–224*t*
   morbidity, mortality, 218
   pathophysiology, 218–221, 219*f*, 219*t*, 220*f*
   session frequency, 222
   signs, symptoms, 221
   structural, functional components, 219*t*
   therapeutic goals, 222
   treatment options, 221
   using discretion, 222
pitcher's shoulder. *See* tendinosis
plan, defined, 8–9
plantar fasciitis
   acute, massage protocol, 229–231, 230–231*t*
   assessment, 228–229

chronic, massage protocol, 229–231, 232–233*t*
client homework, 231–233
contraindications, 230
defined, 226
morbidity, mortality, 226
pain compensation, 226
pathophysiology, 226–227, 227*f*
session frequency, 229
signs, symptoms, 227–228
therapeutic goals, 229
treatment options, 228
policeman's heel. *See* plantar fasciitis
polysomnography, 177
post-polio syndrome (PPS)
    assessment, 236–237
    assistive device use, 236–237
    client homework, 239–240
    contraindications, 238
    defined, 235
    massage protocol, 237–239, 238–239*t*
    morbidity, mortality, 235
    pathophysiology, 235
    reassuring the client, 235
    session frequency, 237
    signs, symptoms, 236
    therapeutic goals, 237
    treatment options, 236
post-traumatic stress disorder (PTSD)
    assessment, 243
    client homework, 246
    contraindications, 245
    defined, 241
    flashbacks, 242, 244
    massage protocol, 244
    morbidity, mortality, 241
    pathophysiology, 241–242
    referring the client, 243
    session frequency, 243
    signs, symptoms, 242–243
    sleep, 242
    therapeutic goals, 243
    treatment options, 243
pounding, 13, 16*f*
PPS. *See* post-polio syndrome
Primary Raynaud's. *See* Raynaud's phenomenon
protocol, defined, 4
pseudo sciatica. *See* piriformis syndrome
psychological pain manifestations, 23
PTSD. *See* post-traumatic stress disorder

R
radiculopathy. *See* sciatica
range of motion (ROM)
    decreased, 23
    passive, active, 20–21
    stretching exercises, 47–50*f*
Raynaud's phenomenon
    assessment, 249
    client homework, 251
    contraindications, 250
    defined, 247
    handshakes, 248
    massage protocol, 250–251, 250*t*
    morbidity, mortality, 247
    pathophysiology, 247–248

sensations of, 249
    session frequency, 249
    signs, symptoms, 248
    therapeutic goals, 249
    treatment options, 248–249
referred pain, 324
referring out, 53
relaxation massage, 2
repetitive stress injury (RSI), 78
resisted breathing exercises, 87, 88*f*
rest, ice, compression, and elevation (RICE), 3
rheumatoid arthritis (RA)
    assessment, 255
    client homework, 257
    contraindications, 256
    defined, 252
    massage protocol, 255–257, 256*t*
    medication side effects, 254
    pathophysiology, 252–253, 253*f*
    session frequency, 255
    signs, symptoms, 253–254
    therapeutic goals, 255
    treatment options, 254–255
RICE. *See* rest, ice, compression, and elevation
Roberts, L., 4–5
rocking, 16–17, 17*f*
ROM. *See* range of motion
RSI. *See* repetitive stress injury

S
satellite trigger points, 324
scars
    assessment, 262
    client homework, 264–265, 265*f*
    contraindications, 263
    cross-fiber friction, 261*f*
    defined, 259
    inflammation, 261–262
    massage protocol, 262–264, 263–264*t*
    pathophysiology, 259–260
    session frequency, 262
    signs, symptoms, 260–261
    therapeutic goals, 262
    timing for work, 262
    treatment options, 261–262
Scheuermann's kyphosis, 158
sciatic nerve, 219*f*, 220*f*
sciatica
    assessment, 269
    client homework, 272
    contraindications, 271
    defined, 266
    encouraging movement, 269
    massage protocol, 270, 271*t*
    morbidity, mortality, 266
    pathophysiology, 266–267, 267*f*, 268*f*
    session frequency, 270
    signs, symptoms, 268
    therapeutic goals, 270
    treatment options, 269
SCM release. *See* sternocleidomastoid release
scoliosis
    assessment, 276
    client homework, 277–280

contraindications, 278
    defined, 273
    long-term effects, 276
    massage protocol, 276–277, 278–279*t*
    morbidity, mortality, 273
    pathophysiology, 273–274
    session frequency, 276
    signs, symptoms, 274–275
    therapeutic goals, 276
    treatment options, 275
scope of practice, 3, 45–46
secondary gain, 334–335
Secondary Raynaud's. *See* Raynaud's phenomenon
self-care instructions. *See* client homework
shell shock. *See* post-traumatic stress disorder
shoulders
    joint anatomy, 132*f*
    limited motion range, 300–301
    ROM exercises, 47*f*
skin desensitizing, 128
skin rolling, 12
sleep, 177
slow-stroke massage, 178–179, 179*f*, 244, 291
SOAP. *See* subjective, objective, assessment, and plan
soldier's heart. *See* post-traumatic stress disorder
spasm, 22–23. *See also* muscle spasm
spastic CP, 85
spinal curvatures, labeling, 273, 274*f*
spinal nerves, 267*f*, 268*f*
splinting, 23, 191–192
sprains, strains
    assessment, 283
    client homework, 286
    compensation, 283
    contraindications, 285
    defined, 281
    increased severity, 282
    massage protocol, 284, 285–286*t*
    morbidity, mortality, 281
    pathophysiology, 281–282
    session frequency, 283–284
    signs, symptoms, 282
    therapeutic goals, 283
    treatment options, 282–283
sternocleidomastoid (SCM) release, 146
strains. *See* sprains, strains
strengthening, 51, 51*f*, 52*f*
stress
    assessment, 290
    client homework, 292
    in combination with other conditions, 290
    contraindications, 292
    defined, 288
    importance of recognizing, 291
    massage protocol, 291–292
    morbidity, mortality, 288–289
    pathophysiology, 289
    session frequency, 291
    signs, symptoms, 289–290
    therapeutic goals, 290
    treatment options, 290

stretching
    client homework, 47–48, 47–50*f*
    proper technique, 172
    types of, 47–50*f*
stroke
    assessment, 296–297
    client communication, 298
    client homework, 298–301
    client pain, 297
    contraindications, 299
    defined, 294
    effect on joints, 295
    massage protocol, 297–298, 299–292*t*
    morbidity, mortality, 294
    pathophysiology, 294–295
    session frequency, 297
    signs, symptoms, 295
    therapeutic goals, 297
    treatment options, 295–296
stroke application, 4–5
stroking, 10–11, 11*f*
subjective, defined, 7–8
subjective, objective, assessment, and plan
        (SOAP), 7–9
swimmer's shoulder. *See* tendinosis

T
tapotement, 13–16
tapping, 13, 14*f*
temporomandibular joint dysfunction
        (TMJD)
    anterior neck massage, 309
    assessment, 306–307, 307*f*
    client homework, 311
    contraindications, 308
    defined, 303
    intraoral work, 306
    massage protocol, 307, 308–309*t*
    morbidity, mortality, 303
    pathophysiology, 303–305, 304*f*, 305*f*
    related issues, 307
    session frequency, 307
    signs, symptoms, 305
    therapeutic goals, 307
    treatment options, 306
tender points, 127
tendinopathy. *See* tendinosis
tendinosis
    assessment, 312
    client homework, 313–315

    contraindications, 314
    defined, 311
    massage protocol, 313, 314–315*t*
    pathophysiology, 311
    rest, immobility, 312–313
    session frequency, 313
    signs, symptoms, 311–312
    therapeutic goals, 313
    treatment options, 312
tendonitis, 311
tennis elbow. *See* tendinosis
tennis heel. *See* plantar fasciitis
tension-type headache (TTH). *See* headache,
        tension
terrible triad, 28–29
therapeutic massage. *See* clinical
        massage
therapists
    healthy lifestyle modeling, 119
    as part of health care team, 133
    referring out, 53
    training requirements, 2–3
therapy
    contraindications, 5–6
    medication knowledge, 31–32
    practice scope, 3
    relevant medications, 33–43*t*
thoracic disc disease. *See* degenerative disc
        disease
thoracic outlet syndrome (TOS)
    assessment, 319
    client homework, 320
    contraindications, 321
    defined, 315
    massage protocol, 319–320,
        321–322*t*
    morbidity, mortality, 315
    muscular bracing, 319
    pathophysiology, 316–318, 317*f*
    session frequency, 319
    signs, symptoms, 318
    therapeutic goals, 319
    thrombi, 318
    treatment options, 318–319
thrombi, 318
TIA. *See* transient ischemic attack
TMJ disorder. *See* temporomandibular
        joint dysfunction
TMJ syndrome. *See* temporomandibular
        joint dysfunction

TMJD. *See* temporomandibular joint
        dysfunction
topical product application, 120
TOS. *See* thoracic outlet syndrome
Touch Research Institute, 4–5
transient ischemic attack (TIA), 295
treatment protocol, 4
trigger points (TrPs)
    assessment, 326
    client homework, 330
    contraindications, 328–329
    defined, 23, 324
    massage protocol, 327, 327*f*, 328–330*t*
    pathophysiology, 324–325, 325
    session frequency, 326
    signs, symptoms, 325
    therapeutic goals, 326
    treatment options, 325–326
    treatment pain, 325–327
    vs. tender points, 127
TrPs. *See* trigger points
TTH. *See* headache, tension

V
voluntary splinting, 23

W
Wall, P., 25
wallet sciatica. *See* piriformis syndrome
Walton, T., 4
wear-and-tear arthritis. *See* osteoarthritis
whiplash
    assessment, 334
    client homework, 336–337
    contraindications, 335–336
    defined, 332
    massage protocol, 334–336, 335–336*t*
    morbidity, mortality, 332
    neck braces, 334
    pathophysiology, 332–333
    session frequency, 334
    signs, symptoms, 333
    therapeutic goals, 334
    treatment options, 333–334
    treatment timing, 333
The Wizard of Oz, 20
Wong-Baker FACES Pain Rating
        Scale, 28*f*
wringing, 12
wrist tendinosis, 314–315*t*